Marc A. Reymond, Wiebke Solass

PIPAC

PIPAC

Pressurized IntraPeritoneal Aerosol Chemotherapy –
Cancer under Pressure

Edited by
Marc A. Reymond, Wiebke Solass

DE GRUYTER

Editors
Marc A. Reymond, M.D., M.B.A.
Professor of Surgery
Ruhr University Bochum
Marien Hospital Herne
Surgical Oncology & Therapy Ctr. Peritoneal Carcinomatosis
Hölkeskampring 40
44625 Herne
marc.reymond@marienhospital-herne.de

Wiebke Solass, M.D.
Ruhr University Bochum
Marien Hospital Herne
Surgical Oncology & Therapy Ctr. Peritoneal Carcinomatosis
Hölkeskampring 40
44625 Herne
wiebke.solass@marienhospital-herne.de

ISBN 978-3-11-034594-0
e-ISBN 978-3-11-036661-7

Library of Congress Cataloging-in-Publication Data
A CIP catalog record for this book has been applied for at the Library of Congress.

Bibliographic information published by the Deutsche Nationalbibliothek
The Deutsche Nationalbibliothek lists this publication in the Deutsche Nationalbibliografie; detailed bibliographic data are available on the Internet at http://dnb.dnb.de.

Cover image: Marion Nelle, Ruhr-Universität Bochum
Typesetting: le-tex publishing services GmbH, Leipzig
Printing and binding: Hubert & Co. GmbH & Co. KG, Göttingen
♾ Printed on acid-free paper
Printed in Germany

www.degruyter.com

The least thing that forms in the world is always the product of a great coincidence.

Le Phénomène humain (1955)
Pierre Teilhard De Chardin

The editors of The Book of PIPAC wish to dedicate this work to the memory of P. A., B. E. and E. M., the first patients treated with PIPAC. Their memory will stay with us forever.

Preface

Peritoneal dissemination is a common route of cancer metastasis. The benefit of administering chemotherapy directly into the peritoneal cavity is supported by preclinical and pharmacokinetic data. In comparison to intravenous (IV) treatment, intraperitoneal (IP) administration results in a several-fold increase in drug concentration within the abdominal cavity. There is now growing evidence from clinical studies showing a survival advantage for IP chemotherapy in various tumor types, including ovarian, gastric and colorectal cancer.

However, while the use of intraperitoneal chemotherapy is slowly gaining acceptance, it is not universal, largely due to the greater toxicity associated with this approach. Moreover, efficacy of intraperitoneal chemotherapy is limited by poor distribution within the abdominal cavity and by poor tissue penetration.

A new way of administering intraperitoneal chemotherapy is the application of cytotoxics in the form of a pressurized aerosol into the abdominal or thoracic cavity. Pressurized IntraPeritoneal Aerosol Chemotherapy (PIPAC) is applied through laparoscopic access using two balloon trocars in an operating room equipped with laminar air flow. In the first step, a normothermic capnoperitoneum is established with a pressure of 12 mm Hg. A cytotoxic solution (about 10% of a normal systemic dose) is nebulized with a micropump into the abdominal cavity, and maintained for 30 minutes. The aerosol is then removed through a closed suction system.

Applying an aerosol in the peritoneal cavity allows a homogeneous distribution of the chemotherapeutic agent within the abdomen. Furthermore, an artificial pressure gradient is generated that overcomes tumoral interstitial fluid pressure, an obstacle in cancer therapy. This is resulting in a higher local drug concentration compared to conventional intraperitoneal or intravenous chemotherapy. At the same time the plasma concentration of the chemotherapeutic agent remains low, so that side effects and organ toxicity are minimal.

In the first clinical studies with limited number of patients in ovarian, gastric and colorectal cancer, as well as peritoneal mesothelioma, PIPAC has obtained encouraging tumor response rates and survival, with a relatively low side effects profile. Larger clinical trials, including prospective randomized trials are currently ongoing to examine if these data can be reproduced and extrapolated to other situations.

From the theoretical point of view, PIPAC is a generic technology with potential applications in various pathologies, with various therapeutic principles, and in different anatomic locations. Prevention and therapy of intraperitoneal cancer dissemination is certainly the most promising indication for PIPAC technology, followed by intrathoracic applications (PITAC), which opens new research avenues in therapy of mesothelioma. Since a therapeutic aerosol can also be distributed within organ cavities, potential applications such as Pressurized IntraVesical Aerosol Chemotherapy (PIVAC) in bladder cancer or intraluminal endoesophageal application in Barret's dysplasia

(PILAC) are under investigation in the animal model. Application of chemosensibilizers such as Dbait (see Chapter 9) might improve efficacy of radiochemotherapy, for example for locally unresectable pancreatic cancer. Finally, administration of cytolytic viruses in form of a pressurized aerosol might improve uptake into tumor tissues, a significant limitation in current protocols of intraperitoneal gene therapy.

Innovation is a difficult process that needs to face serious challenges and difficulties. We have met strong resistance from opinion leaders, from reviewers and from grant agencies, and in some cases this resistance went obviously well beyond critical peer-review and scientific arguments. However, the increasing number of academic centers implementing PIPAC technology and the growing interest into our clinical research program compensates this fierce resistance. Finally, only solid scientific data will provide answers to the open questions, and we are working hard to provide the medical community with these data as soon as possible.

Acknowledgments

The Editors of *The Book of PIPAC* would like to recognize the contributions of an outstanding group of contributors, including B. Bürkle, M. Dutreix, C. Eveno, A. Herbette, R. Kerb, T. Mürdter, M. Pocard, M. Schwab, J. S. Sun and all associated scientists.

They also underline the decisive input of two engineers, A. Hetzel and T. Schwarz, for the development and laboratory validation of the technical devices. We are also grateful to Frank Pölzing, M. D. (vet.), who organized all preclinical experiments.

We wish to thank all of those responsible for the publication of this book, including Till Meiner, Nicole Karbe, Kathleen Prüfer and the team of De Gruyter, for their support throughout this process.

Of note, the editors invited junior faculty members to work closely with the senior editors, including Timur Iusupov, Nathalie Jonscher, Nadia Khalili-Harbi, Marielle Hummels, Benedikt Methling, Georgi Nadiradze, Katharina Nordhausen, Katharina Odendahl and others. They rapidly became an invaluable source of new concepts in patient care, and a limitless source of energy.

We thank the Familiy Klee Foundation for the innovation award 2014 that allowed us to publish this book and to organize the first PIPAC symposium.

Last but not least, we are greatful to T. Freitag, G. Godolias and S. Lauer for their vision and support for developing our clinical PIPAC research program at Marien Hospital Herne, Ruhr University Bochum.

Contents

Preface — **vii**

Acknowledgments — **ix**

M. A. Reymond
1 **Introduction — 1**

M. A. Reymond
2 **Peritoneal carcinomatosis: a neglected disease — 5**
2.1 An unmet medical need — **5**
2.2 Role of the physician in provision of care in advanced peritoneal cancer — **6**
2.3 Palliative care in peritoneal carcinomatosis — **7**

W. Solass and M. A. Reymond
3 **Normal and diseased peritoneum — 11**
3.1 Ontology — **11**
3.2 Anatomy — **11**
3.2.1 Blood supply — **12**
3.2.2 Lymphatics — **13**
3.2.3 Lymphatic stomata — **13**
3.2.4 Milky spots — **14**
3.2.5 Greater omentum — **14**
3.2.6 Peritoneal nerves — **16**
3.3 Physiology of peritoneum — **17**
3.3.1 Peritoneum-plasma barrier — **17**
3.3.2 Intraperitoneal Hydrostatic Pressure — **18**
3.4 Pathophysiology of peritoneal carcinomatosis — **19**
3.4.1 Epithelial-mesenchymal transition — **19**
3.4.2 Interstitial intratumoral fluid pressure — **21**
3.4.3 Ascites — **22**
3.4.4 Hormonal changes — **24**

W. Solass and M. A. Reymond
4 **Diagnosis and staging of peritoneal carcinomatosis — 27**
4.1 Diagnostic workup — **27**
4.2 Imaging studies — **27**
4.2.1 Computer tomography (CT scan) — **28**
4.2.2 Magnetic Resonance Imaging (MRI) — **28**

4.2.3 Ultrasound — 29
4.2.4 FDG-Positron emission tomography (PET) — 29
4.3 Diagnostic laparoscopy — 30
4.3.1 Peritoneal Cancer Index — 30
4.4 Peritoneal or pleural cytology — 32
4.4.1 Gastric cancer — 32
4.4.2 Ovarian cancer — 33
4.4.3 Colorectal cancer — 33

C. Demtröder, U. Giger-Pabst, W. Solass, and M. A. Reymond
5 Therapy of peritoneal carcinomatosis — 35
5.1 Systemic palliative chemotherapy — 35
5.2 Intraperitoneal chemotherapy — 36
5.3 Drug uptake into tumoral tissue — 37
5.3.1 Diffusion — 37
5.3.2 Convection — 39
5.4 Effect of peritonectomy on drug clearance — 40
5.5 Influence of intraperitoneal drug concentration — 41
5.6 Tissue penetration of various drugs — 41
5.6.1 Doxorubicin (see also page 199) — 42
5.6.2 Cisplatinum (see also page 198) — 43
5.6.3 Oxaliplatinum — 43
5.6.4 Taxanes (Paclitaxel, Docetaxel) — 43
5.7 Perioperative intraperitoneal chemotherapy — 44
5.7.1 CHPP — 44
5.7.2 NIPS — 45
5.7.3 EIPL — 46
5.7.4 EPIC — 46
5.8 Intraperitoneal chemotherapy for ascites — 47
5.9 Limitations of intraperitoneal chemotherapy — 47
5.9.1 Poor drug penetration — 47
5.9.2 Poor surface exposition — 48
5.9.3 Local toxicity — 48
5.9.4 Peritoneal sclerosis — 49
5.10 Intraperitoneal immunotherapy — 50
5.10.1 Catumaxomab — 50
5.10.2 Bevacizumab — 51
5.10.3 Immunoradiotherapy — 51
5.11 Intraperitoneal cytolytic virotherapy — 52
5.12 Nanodrugs — 52
5.13 Combined CRS with HIPEC — 53
5.13.1 Cytoreductive surgery (CRS) — 53

5.13.2 Hyperthermic IntraPEritoneal Chemotherapy (HIPEC) — 54
5.13.3 Colorectal cancer — 55
5.13.4 Ovarian Cancer — 56
5.13.5 Gastric Cancer — 56
5.13.6 Learning curve and expertise — 57
5.13.7 Evidence of cost effectiveness — 57
5.13.8 Safety — 58
5.13.9 Indications for CRS and HIPEC — 58

W. Solass and M. A. Reymond
6 Assessing tumor response in peritoneal carcinomatosis — 67
6.1 Natural history of peritoneal carcinomatosis — 67
6.2 RECIST criteria — 67
6.2.1 RECIST criteria in peritoneal carcinomatosis — 68
6.3 Laparoscopy in peritoneal carcinomatosis — 68
6.4 Histology for determining tumor response — 69
6.5 Tumor markers for determining tumor response — 70
6.5.1 Gastric cancer — 70
6.5.2 Ovarian cancer — 70
6.5.3 Colorectal cancer — 71
6.6 Determining clinical benefit rate in peritoneal carcinomatosis — 71

M. A. Reymond, B. Hu, A. Garcia, T. Reck, F. Köckerling, J. Hess, and P. Morel
7 Principle of therapeutic capnoperitoneum — 73
7.1 Material and methods — 74
7.1.1 Design of the prototype — 74
7.2 Results — 75
7.2.1 In vitro trial — 75
7.2.2 In vivo trial — 76
7.3 Discussion — 77
7.3.1 Increasing exposure of the peritoneal surface — 78
7.3.2 Increasing hydrostatic intraabdominal pressure — 78
7.3.3 Applications of therapeutic capnoperitoneum — 79

W. Solass, A. Hetzel, T. Schwarz, G. Nadiradze, E. Sagynaliev, and M. A. Reymond
8 PIPAC Technology — 83
8.1 Aerosol — 83
8.2 Pressure — 86
8.3 Micropump — 86
8.4 High-pressure injector — 87
8.5 Training and documentation — 89
8.6 Limited sales — 89

M. A. Reymond, A. Tannapfel, C. Schneider, H. Scheidbach, S. Köver, A. Jung, T. Reck, H. Lippert, and F. Köckerling
9 Preclinical experiments — 91
9.1 Xenograft intraperitoneal model in the pig — 91
9.1.1 Material and methods — 92
9.1.2 Anesthesia — 92
9.1.3 Operative procedure: sigmoid colectomy — 92
9.1.4 Postoperative care — 93
9.1.5 Cell line — 93
9.1.6 Labeling of HeLa cells — 93
9.1.7 Immunohistochemistry — 94
9.1.8 In vitro study of chromate toxicity — 94
9.1.9 Intraoperative complications — 94
9.1.10 Port site recurrence — 94
9.1.11 Postoperative course — 95
9.1.12 Discussion — 96
9.2 Staining experiments with aerosolized methylene blue in the pig — 98
9.2.1 Introduction — 98
9.2.2 Material and Methods — 99
9.2.3 Results — 100
9.2.4 Discussion — 102
9.3 Ex vivo experiments with Dbait on diseased peritoneum — 106
9.3.1 Material and methods — 107
9.3.2 Study design — 108
9.3.3 Nebulizer — 108
9.3.4 Patient characteristics, cytoreduction, and intraperitoneal hyperthermic chemotherapy — 109
9.3.5 Tumor characteristics — 109
9.3.6 Experimental protocol — 109
9.3.7 Microscopic analysis — 109
9.3.8 Results — 110
9.3.9 Discussion — 112

W. Solass, R. Kerb, T. Mürdter, U. Giger-Pabst, D. Strumberg, C. Tempfer, J. Zieren, M. Schwab, and M. A. Reymond
10 First PIPAC in-human application — 115
10.1 Introduction — 115
10.2 Methods — 115
10.2.1 Patients — 115
10.2.2 Surgical procedures — 116
10.2.3 Safety and Efficacy assessments — 117
10.2.4 Histology and immunohistochemistry — 117

10.2.5 Clinical Pharmacology — **117**
10.3 Results — **117**
10.3.1 Patient 1 — **117**
10.3.2 Patient 2 — **118**
10.3.3 Patient 3 — **119**
10.4 Safety — **121**
10.5 Clinical Pharmacology — **121**
10.6 Discussion — **122**

A. Blanco, U. Giger-Pabst, W. Solass, J. Zieren, and M. A. Reymond
11 Renal and liver toxicities — 127
11.1 Patients and methods — **127**
11.1.1 Study Design — **127**
11.1.2 Ethics — **128**
11.1.3 Patients — **128**
11.1.4 Therapy — **128**
11.1.5 Sampling — **129**
11.2 Statistical Analysis — **129**
11.3 Results — **129**
11.4 Discussion — **131**

C. B. Tempfer, I. Celik, W. Solass, B. Buerkle, U. Giger-Pabst, J. Zieren, D. Strumberg, and M. A. Reymond
12 PIPAC in ovarian cancer — 135
12.1 Off-label use — **135**
12.1.1 Patients and methods — **136**
12.1.2 Results — **137**
12.1.3 Discussion — **140**
12.2 PIPAC-OV1: a Phase-2 trial in the third-line palliative situation — **143**
12.2.1 Objectives — **143**
12.2.2 Study design — **143**
12.2.3 Target subject population — **143**
12.2.4 Investigational product, dosage, and mode of administration — **144**
12.2.5 Duration of treatment — **144**
12.2.6 Endpoints — **144**
12.2.7 Patient reported outcomes (PROs) — **145**
12.2.8 Pharmacokinetics — **145**
12.2.9 Safety — **145**
12.2.10 Statistical methods — **145**
12.2.11 Current stage — **145**
12.3 PIPAC-OV2: a Phase-1 dose-finding study — **145**
12.4 PIPAC-OV3: a prospective Phase-2-3 randomized trial — **146**

G. Nadiradze, W. Solass, J. Zieren, D. Strumberg, M. A. Reymond, and U. Giger-Pabst
13 PIPAC in gastric cancer — 147
13.1 Off-label use — **148**
13.2 Results — **149**
13.3 Discussion — **154**
13.4 PIPAC-GA1: a Phase-2 trial in the third-line palliative situation — **158**
13.4.1 Objectives — **158**
13.4.2 Study design — **159**
13.4.3 Target subject population — **159**
13.4.4 Investigational product, dosage and mode of administration — **159**
13.4.5 Duration of treatment — **159**
13.4.6 Study endpoints — **159**
13.4.7 Current stage — **160**

U. Giger-Pabst, W. Solass, C. Demtröder, D. Strumberg, J. Zieren, and M. A. Reymond
14 PIPAC in colorectal cancer — 161
14.1 Patients and methods — **162**
14.2 Results — **164**
14.3 Discussion — **167**

W. Solass, U. Giger-Pabst, C. Demtröder, D. Strumberg, J. Zieren, and M. A. Reymond
15 PIPAC in mesothelioma — 171
15.1 Patients and methods — **171**
15.2 Results — **172**
15.3 Conclusions — **172**

K. Odendahl, W. Solass, C. Demtröder, U. Giger-Pabst, C. Tempfer, D. Strumberg, A. Münker, and M. A. Reymond
16 Quality of Life after PIPAC — 175

M. A. Reymond
17 PIPAC and HIPEC — 179
17.1 PIPAC as a neoadjuvant therapy before HIPEC — **181**

N. Jonscher, M. Hummels, U. Giger-Pabst, E. Karljalainen, J. Zieren, N. Büchner, M. A. Reymond, and M. Beshay
18 Pressurized IntraThoracic Aerosol Chemotherapy (PITAC) — 183
18.1 Patients — **184**
18.2 Technique — **184**
18.2.1 First in-human use — **184**
18.3 Results — **185**

N. Khalili-Harbi, A. Herbette, W. Solass, U. Giger-Pabst, E. Engin, A. Giese, M. Dutreix, and M. A. Reymond
19 Future applications of therapeutic capnoperitoneum — 187
19.1 Study design — 187
19.2 Regulatory background and animals — 187
19.2.1 Staining — 187
19.2.2 Macroscopy — 187
19.2.3 Microscopic analysis — 188
19.3 Pressurized IntraVesical Aerosol Chemotherapy (PIVAC) — 188
19.4 Pressurized IntraLuminal Aerosol Chemotherapy (PILAC) — 190
19.5 Discussion — 192

W. Solass, U. Giger-Pabst, J. Zieren, and M. A. Reymond
20 Occupational health and safety aspects — 195
20.1 Methods — 195
20.1.1 Ethical, legal and regulatory background — 195
20.1.2 Methodology — 195
20.1.3 Nebulizer — 196
20.1.4 Operating room characteristics — 196
20.1.5 Chemotherapy — 197
20.1.6 Experimental protocol — 197
20.2 Results — 198
20.2.1 Identification of hazardous substances and dose — 198
20.2.2 Identification of possible exposure ways — 200
20.2.3 First PIPAC simulation with NaCl 0.9% solution — 200
20.2.4 Second PIPAC simulation with smoke and an artificial leak — 200
20.2.5 Information and training of the team of volunteers — 200
20.2.6 Performance of the first PIPAC procedures with chemotherapy — 201
20.3 Conclusions — 201
20.4 Second assessement — 204
20.5 Biological monitoring — 204

U. Giger-Pabst and M. A. Reymond
21 PIPAC: Risks and dangers — 207
21.1 Bowel access lesions — 207
21.2 Simultaneous PIPAC and cytoreductive surgery — 207
21.3 Port-site metastases — 208
21.4 Tumor invasion of the laparotomy scar — 209
21.5 Subcutaneous toxic emphysema — 209
21.6 Therapy-resistant ascites — 210
21.7 Small bowel obstruction — 210
21.8 Secondary CRS and HIPEC — 211

M. A. Reymond
22 Outlook — 215
22.1 Radio- and Chemosensibilizers — **216**
22.2 Nanodrugs — **216**
22.3 Multimodal therapy — **216**
22.4 Preventive application in cancer — **217**
22.5 Applications outside cancer therapy — **217**

U. Giger-Pabst and M. A. Reymond
23 How to start a PIPAC program at your own institution? — 219
23.1 Regulatory aspects — **219**
23.1.1 Compassionate use program or off-label use? — **219**
23.1.2 Drug or medical product? — **220**
23.1.3 CE certification — **220**
23.1.4 Reimbursement — **220**
23.2 Technology access — **221**
23.3 Occupational health and safety — **221**
23.4 In-house Information and training — **222**
23.5 Research — **222**

U. Giger-Pabst and M. A. Reymond
24 Training and Standard Operating Procedures — 223
24.1 Training — **223**
24.2 Safety checklist for PIPAC — **223**
24.3 Peritoneal and pleural carcinomatosis index — **225**
24.3.1 Extent of Pleural Carcinomatosis (EPC) score — **225**
24.4 Registry data — **225**

Index — **227**

List of contributors

Cédric Demtröder, M.D.
Ruhr-University Bochum
Dept. of General Surgery
Marien Hospital Herne, Ruhr University Bochum
cedric.demtroeder@marienhospital-herne.de

Urs Giger-Pabst, M.D
Ruhr-University Bochum
Dept. of General Surgery
Marien Hospital Herne, Ruhr University Bochum
urs.pabst@marienhospital-herne.de

Marc A. Reymond, M.D., M.B.A.
Professor of Surgery
Ruhr University Bochum
Marien Hospital Herne
Surgical Oncology & Therapy Ctr. Peritoneal Carcinomatosis
Hölkeskampring 40
44625 Herne
marc.reymond@marienhospital-herne.de

Wiebke Solass, M.D.
Ruhr University Bochum
Marien Hospital Herne
Surgical Oncology & Therapy Ctr. Peritoneal Carcinomatosis
Hölkeskampring 40
44625 Herne
wiebke.solass@marienhospital-herne.de

Dirk Strumberg, M.D.
Professor of Internal Medicine
Ruhr-University Bochum
Dept. of Hemato-Oncology
Marien Hospital Herne, Ruhr University Bochum
dirk.strumberg@marienhospital-herne.de

Clemens Tempfer, M.D., M.B.A.
Professor of Gynaecology
Ruhr-University Bochum
Dept. of Gynaecology and Obstetrics
Marien Hospital Herne, Ruhr University Bochum
clemens.tempfer@marienhospital-herne.de

Jürgen Zieren, M.D.
Professor of Surgery
Ruhr-University Bochum
Dept. of General Surgery
Marien Hospital Herne, Ruhr University Bochum
juergen.zieren@marienhospital-herne.de

M. A. Reymond

1 Introduction

In the last century, medical progress and better life conditions have lengthened human life expectation. A paradoxical consequence of this development is the increasing cancer incidence in the ageing population, so that malignant diseases become more frequent in everyday medical practice.

Upon initial diagnosis of advanced cancer, virtually all patients want to continue to live and to live well. For the patients, longer survival may justify tolerating side effects and high financial costs. In the first phase of palliative therapy, patients are usually treated with combination systemic chemotherapy, which is usually effective. For example, in advanced gastric cancer, modern chemotherapy increases the median survival to 7–10 months. However, systemic chemotherapy has limitations and physicians are aware that response rates are not very high, although they are real and evidence-based. For example, in gastric cancer, first-line chemotherapy regimens including CF (cisplatin plus infusional 5-FU) or ECF (cisplatin plus infusional 5-FU plus epirubicin) achieve response rates of 20–40%. Median time to tumor progression is 4–5 months. Patients with HER-2-positive gastric cancer have an improved prognosis with the monoclonal antibody trastuzumab in addition to chemotherapy with a platinum compound and a fluoropyrimidin.

When the tumor becomes platinum-resistant, the situation becomes more complex. Expected response rates of systemic palliative chemotherapy are inferior to those of first-line chemotherapy, but expected side effects will remain or might even increase. For example, in gastric cancer, second-line combinations are currently being evaluated in various clinical trials, including docetaxel (DCF), oxaliplatin (EOX, FLO), capecitabine (EOX, cisplatin-Xeloda) and irinotecan (ILF). The benefit of chemotherapy seems to be limited to patients with a good performance status, and treatment toxicity and discomfort are substantial, in particular with regimens containing cisplatin and infusional 5-FU [1]

When patients develop peritoneal carcinomatosis, and this is the main topic of this book, systemic chemotherapy has not been shown to have a significant benefit. In gastric cancer, for example, despite short-duration response rates (43%) for visceral metastases with epirubicin-, cisplatin-, and 5-FU-based regimens, the response rate for peritoneal carcinomatosis is less than 14%. Peritoneal carcinomatosis is considered as the terminal stage of the disease, and most oncologists have regarded it as a condition only to be treated with symptomatic care because most patients with carcinomatosis die within six months [2].

In this situation, hope for continued, high-quality life leads many well-informed patients to seek treatment beyond the standard of care. Many patients today obtain information about their disease from the Internet. They have read testimonials of long-term survivors, and even though they might be well informed about survival statistics, they hope to be the exception to the rule. Examples of this phenomenon in peritoneal surface malignancies are the numerous discussion fora on the benefits of angiogenesis inhibitors or of surgical therapies combined or not with HIPEC. In general, this information is received without enough criticism and arouses exaggerated expectations of a cure.

In this situation, enrolment in clinical trials should be offered to the patients, with the possibility of therapeutic benefit. If they are ineligible for appropriate clinical trials, patients should be given information about the off-label use of products that may offer benefit to a person with their specific medical characteristics. In some cases, such patients may be realistic candidates for expanded-access protocols of experimental drugs or procedures [3]. This is the moment when experimental therapy with Pressurized IntraPeritoneal Aerosol Chemotherapy (PIPAC) can be offered to peritoneal carcinomatosis patients.

The current situation has to be contrasted to the one of our grandparents, where therapeutic options were much more limited and information was only available from the physician, so that the incurability of a disease was discussed earlier, and more extensively. Recently, I received following testimonial from the son of a PIPAC patient: *"You can not imagine how important it is to have hope. Not false hope. Real hope. A real alternative. My mother has great courage. She is a phenomenal fighter. What she needed was hope that somewhere someone had a science-based approach that she could believe in"*. However, false hope interferes with acceptance of, and preparation for, the inevitable consequences of disease progression. Unfortunately, the scientific and medical communities are responsible for much of the misguided optimism that patients frequently bring to the treatment room. The numerous press releases of cancer leagues and academic institutions reporting on progress in cancer therapy combined with the marketing campaigns of the major pharmaceutical companies clearly lead the uninformed observer to believe that we have made far more progress against cancer than we actually have [3].

Once it becomes clear that the expectations of extended life will not be realized, many patients modify their expectations and hopes to include values such as life and death with dignity, empowerment in the transition from life to death, and compassion and understanding during the process [3]. The very essence of medicine (at least, in all modern cultures) involves both curing and caring, and the two are of equal importance [4]. Once hope for health and normal life fades, new hope arises for good quality of life in the time remaining. Good quality in the final stages of life includes dignity and the absence of symptoms, in first-line absence of pain [3]. In this situation, physicians should find more time for compassion. They should put emphasis on caring for the patient and to resist the hopeless insistence on cures that has emerged as a by-product of technical progress [5] and mass media communication.

Bibliography

[1] Rivera F, Vega-Villegas ME, López-Brea MF. Chemotherapy of advanced gastric cancer. Cancer Treat Rev. 33, 4 (2007) 315–324.

[2] Sadeghi B, Arvieux C, Glehen O et al. Peritoneal carcinomatosis from non-gynecologic malignancies: results of the EVOCAPE 1 multicentric prospective study. Cancer 88 (2000) 358–363.

[3] Erwil RL. Therapy for Advanced Stage Cancer: What Do Patients Want and Expect? A Patient Advocate's Perspective.The Oncologist 15, suppl 1 (2010) 11–12.

[4] Pellegrino ED, Thomasma DC. Helping and Healing. Religious commitment in Health Care. Washington: Georgetown University Press, Caring and Curing, pp 26–38, 1997.

[5] Welte T. Progress means change – reflections on two articles about pleural disease. Dtsch Arztebl Int; 110, 18 (2013) 311–312.

M. A. Reymond

2 Peritoneal carcinomatosis: a neglected disease

Recently, an international consensus statement on peritoneal carcinomatosis was produced by representatives from Germany, Netherlands, USA, Italy, Japan, Spain, Australia, France and Israel [1]. It describes a "paradigm change" away from a fatalistic approach in peritoneal cancer and toward a potentially curative approach using cytoreductive surgery (CRS) and hyperthermic intraperitoneal chemotherapy (HIPEC) as being "justified by the current state of the international data".

To many readers of this book, this statement might appear too optimistic. They do not believe this claim that a potential curative approach is being developed in a UICC stage IV cancer with an expected median survival of six months. Overall, very promising long-term survival has been shown in a subset of patients with a limited extent of peritoneal disease before treatment. Whether randomised controlled trials are needed to definitively show the magnitude of benefit, if any, of this approach is an important question [2]. On the one hand, it is the responsibility of the medical community to give encouragement to pursue novel techniques so that medical science can advance. On the other hand, it is the responsibility of the researcher to be cautious with the diffusion of early research results to prevent the generation of unrealistic hope. Implementing novel therapies in peritoneal carcinomatosis is a tightrope between promising research results and wishful thinking. This caveat has to govern further development of new forms of therapy in peritoneal cancer, including Pressurized IntraPeritoneal Aerosol Chemotherapy (PIPAC).

2.1 An unmet medical need

Peritoneal carcinomatosis is a common metastatic pattern in ovarian, gastric, colorectal and appendiceal cancer with about 167,940 new cases per year in Europe. In Germany alone, about 60 patients per day are diagnosed with peritoneal cancer, half of them being women with ovarian cancer (Table 2.1).

Life expectancy in peritoneal carcinomatosis is limited due to the aggressiveness of the tumor and poor therapeutic response. For example, many patients with gastric cancer (now the second most frequent malignancy in the world) are typically diag-

Table 2.1. Incidence of peritoneal carcinomatosis (PC) in Europe

	Ovarian cancer	Gastric cancer	Colorectal cancer	Appendix cancer
Annual incidence [3]	66,000	146,000	432,000	11,700
% PC [4]	60–80%	20–40%	15–20% [5]	20%
Incidence of PC	46,200	43,800	75,600	2,340

nosed at advanced stages and have a poor prognosis. Approximately 84% of patients will have advanced disease at the time of first diagnosis and the median time of survival of these patients without chemotherapy is only 3–4 months. Most of them will die of metastatic bowel involvement, anorexia and cachexia due to peritoneal carcinomatosis.

Resistance of peritoneal carcinomatosis to systemic chemotherapy is explained by molecular mechanisms of resistance [6] but also by limited drug distribution within peritoneal carcinomatosis nodules [7]. Thus, in spite of modern chemotherapy, gastric cancers remain highly lethal malignancies. Survival rates are among the worst reported for any malignancy. According to data from the US National Cancer Institute, the five-year survival for patients with gastric cancer improved only modestly over the last 50 years, from 12% in the years 1950 to 1954, to 22% during the period 1996 to 2003 [8]. Obviously, these survival rates did not increase during the last decades, at least not as much as we would have expected.

Novel therapies such as combining cytoreductive surgery (CRS) with intraperitoneal chemotherapy [9] are currently gaining acceptance worldwide. However, this combined therapy can only be recommended to a minority of highly selected patients, and is hampered by significant risks and side effects.

At present, peritoneal carcinomatosis remains an unmet medical need. Thus, there is an obvious and urgent need for innovative therapies in peritoneal cancer.

2.2 Role of the physician in provision of care in advanced peritoneal cancer

Surveys indicate considerable variation regarding the provision of cancer treatment at the end of life. The variation cannot be fully explained by differences concerning the clinical situation or patients' preferences. When experiences of medical oncologists with advanced cancer were explored, these physicians reported that a number of nonmedical factors influence professional decisions about the offering or limiting of cancer treatment in advanced cancer in addition to medical criteria. Physicians' individual judgments about the benefit of treatment, as well as the amount of their clinical experience, were cited as such factors [10].

In practice, oncologists are challenged to make tough treatment decisions. Many patients cannot tolerate side effects of chemotherapy, especially the combination regimens. As a rule, the decision to treat a patient with aggressive concepts should take into account the impact upon his quality of life. Against this framework, it might appear surprising that many patients continue to receive chemotherapy even in the last month of their lives. The effect of referral to palliative care on health-related outcome especially for patients with poor quality of life is still not very clear [11].

Many patients with platinum-resistant peritoneal carcinomatosis who searched for support in our tertiary center were not satisfied with the therapeutic options offered by their oncologist. Continuation of systemic chemotherapy was not desired by some patients; others were not satisfied with purely symptomatic therapy. In some cases, the patient's request for a second opinion was not supported by the oncologist. Isolated patients even reported fierce opposition of their oncologist to evaluation for PIPAC therapy, although this physician was probably aware about the limited efficacy of systemic chemotherapy in the platinum-resistant stage of peritoneal carcinomatosis. Interestingly, in our experience, general practitioners were more supportive for such a referral.

For evaluating these patients' referrals, we applied the strategy recommended by the German Cancer Society in this situation [12], namely the systematic collection of relevant clinical data regarding the outcomes of different treatment approaches in advanced peritoneal cancer, and discussion of the best option for a particular patient on an individual basis within an interdisciplinary tumor board. Of course, making decisions about offering or not offering PIPAC therapy based on the scarce evidence available was, and remains, challenging. However, this decision-making process was facilitated by interdisciplinary team discussions. The team gathered broad information on the various therapeutic options available, including ongoing phase-1 and phase-2 studies. Moreover, these discussions provided the opportunity to exchange different views and opinions on a particular case. With increasing experience, some standardized decisional criteria were determined, including:

- No priority was given to PIPAC, which was handled as an experimental therapy.
- Evidence-based therapy options were systematically recommended when they had not been exhausted.
- PIPAC was not offered to patients with extraperitoneal metastases.
- Small bowel obstruction, nasogastric tube and need for parenteral nutrition were considered exclusion criteria for PIPAC therapy.

This decisional process resulted into the refusal of the vast majority of patient referrals for PIPAC therapy. Each recommendation was documented in written form and transmitted to the treating physician.

2.3 Palliative care in peritoneal carcinomatosis

In recent years more attention has been paid to better symptom control in patients with advanced cancer diseases, in particular by earlier referral to specialized palliative care services. In a hallmark study in patients with advanced lung cancer, earlier referral to palliative care with standard oncological treatment resulted in improvement in quality of life and survival [13]. By analogy, in peritoneal carcinomatosis, much of the management is focused upon palliation and symptom management, and the time point of referral to a palliative care service is an important decision. However, there is a problem of definition of such palliative care.

According to the WHO definition [14], palliative care is an approach that improves the quality of life of patients and their families facing the problem associated with life-threatening illness, through the prevention and relief of suffering by means of early identification and impeccable assessment and treatment of pain and other problems, physical, psychosocial and spiritual. Palliative care:

- provides relief from pain and other distressing symptoms;
- affirms life and regards dying as a normal process;
- intends neither to hasten or postpone death;
- integrates the psychological and spiritual aspects of patient care;
- offers a support system to help patients live as actively as possible until death;
- offers a support system to help the family cope during the patients illness and in their own bereavement;
- uses a team approach to address the needs of patients and their families, including bereavement counseling, if indicated;
- will enhance quality of life, and may also positively influence the course of illness;
- is applicable early in the course of illness, in conjunction with other therapies that are intended to prolong life, such as chemotherapy or radiation therapy, and includes those investigations needed to better understand and manage distressing clinical complications.

However, standardized application of WHO criteria is difficult in everyday practice. In a recent survey on medical practice in patients with advanced cancer, the physicians distinguished approaches of active treatment from those of palliative care. Both labels covered a spectrum of treatment scenarios. The term active treatment, for example, was not limited to curative treatment but was also used for treatment that alters, at least in the interim, the natural course of the disease. This analysis suggested that the framing of a treatment approach as "active" or "palliative" has both clinically and ethically relevant implications concerning the focus of care and the perceived role in the decision-making process. Using this definition, PIPAC would be defined as an active, but neither curative nor palliative therapy in patients with peritoneal cancer [15].

The need for further research in palliative care research has been recognized by the European Commission in the recent FP7 call, with the focus in cancer to improving the patients' and survivors' quality of life and treatment with fewer side effects [16]. Against this framework, it is important to consider that many patients with advanced peritoneal carcinomatosis do not only complain about disease-related symptoms. Most of them have received platinum-based systemic chemotherapy and experience debilitating long-term side effects, including in particular peripheral neuropathy and chronic renal failure. With this previous experience, many patients are reluctant to accept further toxic systemic combination chemotherapy or to go for a major procedure such as CRS and HIPEC. Most patients are looking for an active therapy with a low side-effect profile, with the hope of both prolonging life and maintaining a good quality of life. In this respect, PIPAC has significant potential since it is a minimally-invasive procedure with limited systemic side effects.

Bibliography

[1] Brucher BL, Piso P, Verwaal V et al. Peritoneal carcinomatosis: cytoreductive surgery and HIPEC–overview and basics. Cancer Invest. 2012;30(3):209–224.
[2] Sugarbaker PH, Ryan DP. Cytoreductive surgery plus hyperthermic perioperative chemotherapy to treat peritoneal metastases from colorectal cancer: standard of care or an experimental approach? Lancet Oncol. 13, 8 (Aug 2012) e362–e369.
[3] http://www.iarc.fr, consulted on 27.09.2012
[4] Piso P et al. Dtsch Arztebl Int 108, 47 (2011) 802–808.
[5] Segelmann J et al. Br J Surg. 99, 5 (May 2012) 699–705.
[6] Kelland. L Nat Rev Cancer. 7, 8 (Aug 2007) 573–584.
[7] Minchinton AI, Tannock IF. Nat Rev Cancer. 6, 8 (Aug 2006) 583–592.
[8] SEER Cancer Statistics http://www.seer.cancer.gov/statistics/ (Accessed on 13.4.2014).
[9] Macrì A et al. World J Gastrointest Oncol. 3, 12 (Dec 15, 2011) 169–174.
[10] Schildmann J, Tan J, Salloch S, Vollmann J. “Well, I think there is great variation...”: a qualitative study of oncologists’ experiences and views regarding medical criteria and other factors relevant to treatment decisions in advanced cancer. Oncologist. 18, 1 (2013) 90–96.
[11] Shahrokni A, Saif MW. Metastatic pancreatic cancer: the dilemma of quality vs. quantity of life. JOP. 14, 4 (Jul 10 2013) 391–394.
[12] http://www.krebsgesellschaft.de/wub_zertifizierte_zentren_info,120896.html, consulted on 25.4.2014
[13] Temel JS, Greer JA, Muzikansky A, et al. Early palliative care for patients with metastatic non-small-cell lung cancer. N Engl J Med. 363 (2010) 733–742.
[14] http://www.who.int/cancer/palliative/definition/en/, consulted on 25.4.2014
[15] Schildmann J, Tan J, Salloch S, Vollmann J. “Well, I think there is great ariation...”: a qualitative study of oncologists’ experiences and views regarding medical criteria and other factors relevant to treatment decisions in advanced cancer. Oncologist. 18, 1 (2013) 90–96.
[16] http://ec.europa.eu/research/fp7/index_en.cfm?pg=health, consulted on 25.4.2014

W. Solass and M. A. Reymond

3 Normal and diseased peritoneum

The peritoneum is a semi-permeable, serous membrane that lines the abdominal wall (parietal peritoneum) and covers the abdominal organs (visceral peritoneum). The size of the peritoneum approximates the body surface area (1.5–2 m^2), about 30% being parietal peritoneum and 70% visceral peritoneum. It covers most of the intraabdominal organs. The peritoneum supports the abdominal organs and serves as a conduit for their vessels (arteries, veins and lymphatics). The organs within the intraperitoneal space are called "intraperitoneal" (e.g. the small bowel), the organs and structures (vessels, nerves) in the abdominal cavity that are located behind the peritoneum are called "retroperitoneal" (e.g. the aorta). The peritoneum is a closed sac in males. The fallopian tubes and ovaries open into the peritoneal cavity in females.

3.1 Ontology

Human tissues and organs derive from the ectoderm, mesoderm and endoderm. Parietal and visceral peritoneum are serosal membranes developing from the lateral plate mesoderm (somatopleural and splanchnopleural layers). Thus, the peritoneum is radically different from muscle, mucosa and vessels and is a significant exchange barrier between anatomical body compartments. The peritoneum is ontogenetically related to the ovarian epithelium, and it too has an increased risk of malignant disease [1].

3.2 Anatomy

Mesothelial cells provide an effective anti-adhesive surface and a protective barrier against physical damage [2]. Mesothelial cells are highly specialized, polarized squamous epithelial cells, measuring up to 45 µm (Figure 3.1).

There is an association between microvillar formation and surface charge, the former protecting the healing mesothelium by enhancing entrapment of serosal fluid and its contents [3].

Mesothelial cells produce and secrete large quantities of phosphatidylcholines (glycolipids), glycosaminglycans and proteoglycans, forming a resistant glycocalix [4]. These glycosaminoglycans and surfactants allow the parietal and visceral serosa to slide over each other. Mesothelial cells are sentinel cells that can sense and respond to signals within their microenvironment. They actively transport fluids, cells and particulates across the serosal membrane and between serosal cavities. They synthesise and secrete a diverse array of mediators in response to external signals which play important roles in regulating inflammatory, immune and tissue repair responses. In

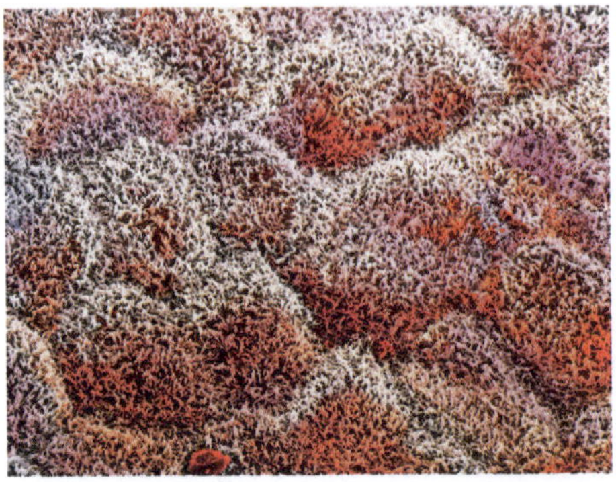

Fig. 3.1. The luminal membrane of mesothelial cells is covered with numerous microvilli increasing the peritoneal surface up to 40 m^2.

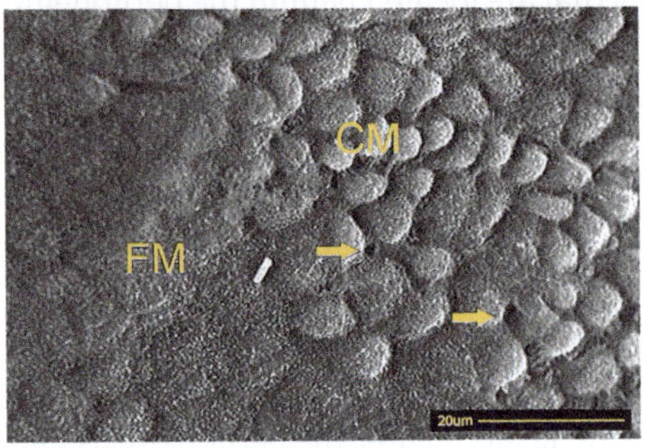

Fig. 3.2. Scanning electron microscopic view to show the two kinds of mesothelial cells: flat mesothelial cells (FM) and cubic mesothelial cells (CM). The round and oval lymphatic stomata are indicated by arrows (reproduced with permission from [5]).

addition, they are likely to protect from peritoneal dissemination of tumors until the integrity of the mesothelium is breached. Although the importance of mesothelial cells is being realised, we still do not understand the mechanisms regulating many of their functions. How the cells communicate with each other and surrounding cells, whether mesothelial cells differentiate into different cell types or if a mesothelial stem cell exists, the mechanisms regulating mesothelial repair and the role mesothelial cells play in serosal pathologies, all need further study.

The mesothelium usually forms a continuous surface, but in some areas may be fenestrated. Neighbouring cells are joined by junctional complexes, but probably permit the passage of macrophages (Figure 3.2).

The submesothelial connective tissue may also contain macrophages, lymphocytes and adipocytes (in some regions). Mesothelial cells may transform into fibroblasts, which may play an important role in the formation of peritoneal adhesions after surgery or inflammation of the peritoneum.

3.2.1 Blood supply

The parietal peritoneum derives its blood supply from the arteries in the abdominal wall. This blood drains into the systemic circulation. The visceral peritoneum is supplied by blood from the mesenteric and coeliac arteries which drain into the portal vein. The parietal peritoneum is therefore supplied by somatic blood vessels of the abdominal and pelvic walls and its lymphatics join those in the body wall and drain into parietal lymph nodes. The visceral peritoneum is best considered as an integral part of the viscera which it overlies; it derives its blood supply from the viscera, and its lymphatics join the visceral vessels to drain into the regional lymph nodes.

3.2.2 Lymphatics

The lymphatics are often not recognized as a third circulation in the body and a separate entity in the tissue space from the intenstitium; they play a major role in protein and lipid transport from the tissue to the blood. Subdiaphragmatic lymphatics are responsible for 80% of the drainage from the peritoneal cavity. The drainage is then absorbed into the venous circulation through the right lymph duct and the left thoracic lymph duct. A balance of solutes and fluid in the interstitial tissue is maintained by absorption of fluid from the peritoneal cavity. The average lymphatic rate of absorption in the peritoneal dialysis patient is 0.5–1.0 ml per minute. Factors that affect the rate of absorption are respiratory rate, posture, and intraabdominal pressure. Lymphatics play only a minor role in the short-term transfer of fluid and macromolecules from the cavity.

3.2.3 Lymphatic stomata

Lymphatic stomata are small openings of lymphatic capillaries on the free surface of the mesothelium (Figure 3.3). The peritoneal cavity, pleural cavity, and pericardial cavity are connected with the lymphatic system via these small openings, which have the function of active absorption. The lymphatic stomata play an important role in the physiological and pathological conditions, including peritoneal carcinomatosis and pathogenesis of malignant ascites.

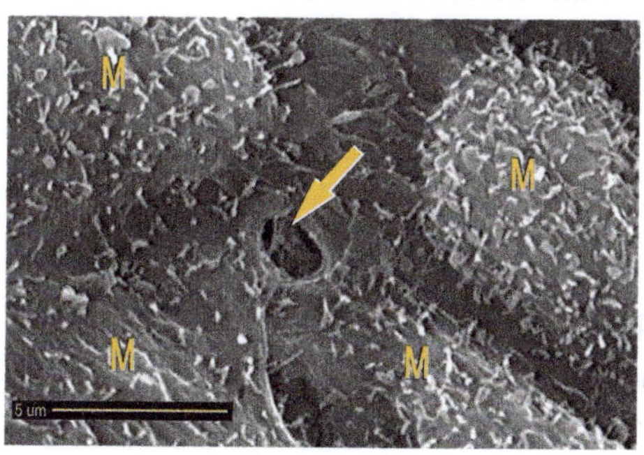

Fig. 3.3. Scanning electron microscopic view to show the lymphatic stomata (arrow) located at the junction of the four mesothelial cells (M). An endothelial cell process crosses the space below the lymphatic stomata (reproduced with permission from [5]).

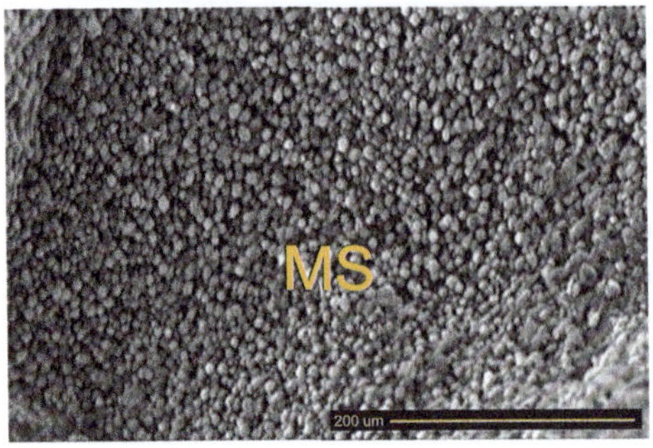

Fig. 3.4. Scanning electron micoscopic view showing the milky spots (MS) (reproduced with permission from [5]).

Anatomical regions in the peritoneal cavity with a high density of lymphatic stomata are the greater omentum, appendices epiploicae of the colon, inferior surface of the diaphragm, falciform ligament, Douglas pouch and small bowel mesentery. These locations are characterized by the presence of another lymphatic structure which is involved in the translymphatic peritoneal dissemination of free cancer cells, namely the milky spots [6].

3.2.4 Milky spots

Milky spots are very small structures, and mainly consist of macrophage and lymphocyte aggregation, while peritoneal milky spots are the first immune barrier in the peritoneal cavity, acting as a source of free macrophages. Abundant milky spots are distributed around lymphatic stomata (Figure 3.4). The exact role of these particular organs is still not clear, but they are similar to lymphatic structures and they play a role in peritoneal cancer dissemination [7]. Lymphatic stomata are found in the milky spots and peritoneal macrophages mobilize into the peritoneal cavity through the lymphatic orifices.

The peritoneum layering the Douglas pouch, for example, is rich in subperitoneal lymphatic vessels and milky spots. The intraperitoneal fluid containing free cancer cells, once reaching the pelvic subperitoneal lymphatics, goes toward the rectum and finally flows into the lymph nodes around the iliac artery. On the other hand the peritoneum covering the liver and the serosal surface of small bowel and spleen are devoid of lymphatic stomata as well as milky spots.

3.2.5 Greater omentum

The greater omentum (in Greek "epipleein" float or sail on) is a sheath of protective tissue overlying the stomach, the intestines and the pancreas, reaching in some women up to the ovaries. It extends from the greater curvature of the stomach, passing in front

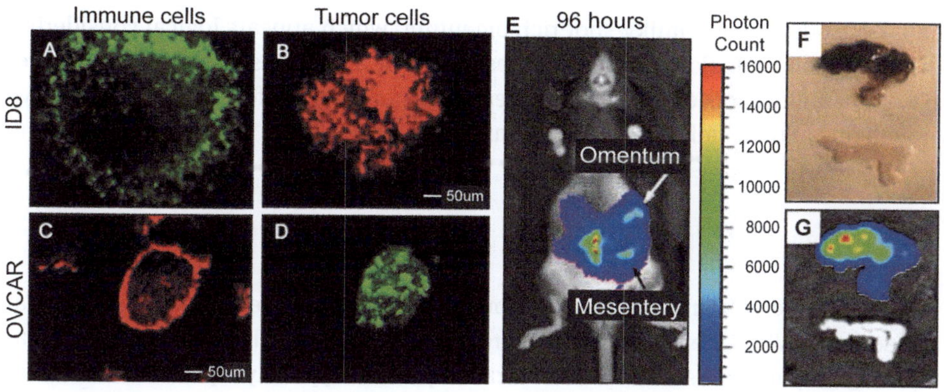

Fig. 3.5. Role of the omentum in intraperitoneal tumor cell dissemination. Both mouse (ID8/Cherry: a, b) and human ovarian tumor cells (OVCAR-3: c, d) bind selectively to the lymphatic stomata of the omentum when injected intraperitoneally in C57BL/6 mice. The omentum was removed six hours later and stained for CD45 to label immune cells (a, c). For each tumor, images from the same field illustrate a lymphatic stomata (a or c) that contains numerous tumor cells. Tumor cells were not found elsewhere on the omentum. The same mouse was then monitored for tumor growth 96 hours later (e). After this time, the omentum with a tumor was removed along with an omentum from an uninjected mouse (f) and both samples compared (g). Clearly, the tumor grows initially on the omentum and mesentery as illustrated in (g). Bars represent 50 µm (a, b) and 100 µm (c, d) (reproduced from [9]).

of the small intestines and reflects on itself to ascend to the transverse colon before reaching to the posterior abdominal wall.

In surgery, the omentum is used as a very potent transplantation tissue for encouraging wound healing. This suggests, besides a good vascularization pattern, an important immunological function in which lymphatic stomata and milky spots appear to be involved. Milky spots must be regarded as strongly reactive structures originating from perivascular effusions in the omentum. Moreover, they can firstly be a local source of potent immune effector cells i.e. peritoneal macrophages and secondly can, after specific immunization, be qualified as a lymphoid organ, that is, produce a specific (lymphocyte) mediated response. This may shed new light on the reason why the omentum works so well in wound healing (reviewed in [8].)

The omentum plays an important role in intraperitoneal tumor cell dissemination and collection (reviewed in [9]). Although tumor cells may attach to any intraperitoneal surface, the omentum appears to be a selective site of attachment of the initial disseminated cells and aggressive tumor growth and subsequent seeding to the rest of the peritoneal cavity (Figure 3.5).

As we have seen above, “milky spots” are clusters of immune cells originally and filter peritoneal fluid providing protection from infection. When tumor cell lines are injected intraperitoneally into the mouse, they bound preferentially to the milky spots. This matches the situation in the human patient where tumor cells appear to preferentially localize on the milky-spot-rich omentum, which appears logical considering the normal physiological function of these immune aggregates. It has been hypothesized that milky spots empower peritoneal metastases by conferring them aggressive growth due to their unique, proangiogenic vasculature [9].

3.2.6 Peritoneal nerves

Peritoneal innervation is warranted though two different afferent systems: visceral and somatic. When the visceral organs are threatened, e.g. via inflammation or dilatation, vague symptoms such as discomfort and pain are typically reported. In contrast, when the parietal peritoneum is concerned, localization and characterization of pain are distinct and the pain is called somatic.

True visceral afferents innervate the gut, and most run temporarily together with either the sympathetic or parasympathetic nerves to enter the spinal cord. During inflammation, silent afferents may become activated and contribute to the sensory response. Visceral afferents from the peritoneum that mediate conscious sensations run predominantly together with sympathetic nerves that reach the central nervous system (CNS), although some afferents join parasympathetic and parallel pathways. Most of the visceral afferents converge with lamina- and spino-thalamic tract (STT) neurons, which receive input from both superficial and deep somatic tissue as well as other visceral organs. Although the neuronal mechanisms are more complex, this convergence leads to referred somatic pain as well as viscero-visceral hyperalgesia. Most visceral organs exhibit spinal representation overlapping multiple segmental levels. This widespread and low-density nature of visceral sensory innervation explains why large areas of the gut appear to be relatively insensitive to pain stimuli. In the visceral nerve pathway, the N-methyl-D-aspartate (NMDA) receptor can be easily activated by short-lasting and low intensity stimuli. The resulting amplification of nociceptive processing may also explain the diffuse and unpleasant nature of visceral pain. In somatic peritoneal pain, the peritoneum and parietal serous membranes of the lungs and heart possess their own parietal nerve supply, which is organized like the skin. Hence, pain from these structures gives a distinct, intense and localized pain, which is comparable to the pain evoked by skin lesions. In the somatic system, prolonged or summated stimuli such as during inflammation are necessary to activate the N-methyl-D-aspartate (NMDA) receptor. The different neuroanatomical structures of the two systems explain to some degree why visceral pain is more challenging to diagnose than its somatic counterpart (reviewed in [10]).

The parietal serous membranes of the thorax and heart have their own nerve supply, which is organized like that of the somatic structures, explaining why heart attacks can generate shoulder and left arm pain.

3.3 Physiology of peritoneum

The anatomic peritoneum is highly permeable to water, small solutes, and proteins and therefore is not a physical barrier [11]. However, the presence of the so-called "peritoneum-plasma barrier" [12] results in a peritoneal drug clearance that is much slower than the plasma clearance. This allows the peritoneal tumor tissue to be exposed to much higher drug concentrations compared with those achieved by systemic delivery. The peritoneum-plasma barrier determines also the effect of intraperitoneal chemotherapy, depending on underlying physiological mechanisms of transport between the blood and the peritoneal cavity.

3.3.1 Peritoneum-plasma barrier

The normal peritoneum-plasma barrier consists of five layers. The first layer is made up of endothelial cells that line the intravascular space of capillaries. These cells have an extracellular glycocalyx and fixed anionic charge that makes it difficult for large blood plasma proteins, such as albumin, to pass through. Intracellular pores provide transport through this layer. The endothelial cell basement membrane provides the second layer. The interstitial space is the third layer and contains fibroblasts, collagen and hyaluronic acid, and it can block the diffusion of macromolecules before the submesothelial basement membrane (the fourth layer). The final layer consists of mesothelial cells, bound by tight junctions and secreting surface glycosaminoglycans (hyaluronan) into the abdominal space [13].

The early models of peritoneal membrane transport included multiple sites of resistance to the flow of solutes across the blood-peritoneum barrier. These included the

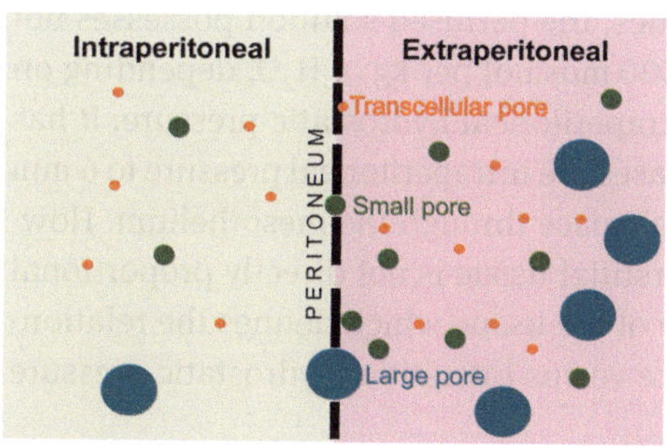

Fig. 3.6. Large pores (100–200 Å) exist in small numbers and constitute < 0.1% of all pores. They transport macromolecules and anatomically are identified as clefts between endothelial cells. Small pores (40–60 Å) are more numerous and believed to transport small solutes and water. Ultra-small or transcellular pores (4–6 Å) are water channels or aquaporin-1. They are numerous and resemble the water channels present in red blood cells and renal proximal tubules. They transport water only (sieving) and are present in the endothelial cells of the peritoneal capillaries.

capillary fluid film overlying the capillary endothelium, the capillary endothelium per se, the endothelial basement membrane, the interstitium, the mesothelial cells and the fluid overlying the peritoneal membrane. Transport actually occurs between the peritoneal cavity and blood which is contained in the retroperitoneal interstitium [14].

The modern model of the "peritoneal membrane" is a complex heterogeneous, semi-permeable membrane with multiple pores [15]. This "Pore Theory" is a theoretical model validated by clinical observations [16]. It suggests that the major resistance to peritoneal transport is in the capillary endothelium and its basement membrane. Solute and water transport across the peritoneal capillary is mediated by pores of three different sizes (Figure 3.6).

3.3.2 Intraperitoneal Hydrostatic Pressure

Studies in rodents and in dialysis patients have demonstrated that protein leaves the peritoneal cavity at rates 5–10 times the rate in which it appears in the blood. Since the only route of protein transfer from the cavity to the central circulation is via lymphatics, there must be some other mechanism responsible for the disappearance of protein from the peritoneal cavity. Through dissection of rodent tissues, it was shown that all of the protein that left the cavity but did not reach the blood was contained in the surrounding peritoneal tissues. In subsequent experiments, it was shown that the concentration in abdominal wall tissue was dependent on the *intraperitoneal hydrostatic pressure* in the rate of transfer. The rate of protein transfer was quantitatively the same as the rate of fluid transfer from an isotonic solution placed in the cavity. This means that the protein acts as a marker of fluid transport from the peritoneal cavity into the surrounding tissues and implies that the peritoneum is a very loose barrier to albumin and immunoglobulin (reviewed in [11]).

In intraperitoneal drug delivery techniques, the perfused solution possesses not only large initial osmotic pressures (300 to 500 mosmol per kg of H_2O, depending on the solution) but also exerts a significant intraperitoneal hydrostatic pressure. It has been shown that 2 L of dialysis solution increases the intraperitoneal pressure to 6 mm Hg. This pressure is exerted on the interstitial space through the mesothelium. However, the pressure in the retroperitoneal interstitial tissue is not directly proportional to the intraperitoneal pressure. The property of the tissue which defines the relationship between changes in the interstitial space versus interstitial hydrostatic pressure is called tissue compliance.

As we have seen, transport of solutes and water between the blood and the peritoneal cavity occurs across the blood capillary wall, through the interstitium, and across the mesothelium. The distributed model approach permits the integration of the properties of each of these entities. The capillary membrane is the primary barrier which determines the amount of a particular solute (sieving) which transports to the interstitium and has been successfully modelled as a three pore membrane for peritoneol transport. The interstitium can be represented as a two-phase gel which excludes large and small molecules from much of its volume and which effectively retards transport between the pericapillary region and the cavity.

Interstitial transport of small solutes is generally diffusion-dominated. However, convective forces appear to be increased in the parietal tissue and dominate in the transport of macromolecules. Net ultrafiltration depends on the opposing forces of the osmotic and hydrostatic pressures in the cavity. Under normal conditions, the interstitium has a hydrostatic pressure of near 0 mm Hg and significant edema can occur without increases above 1 mm Hg. As with any volume greater than 500 mL in the cavity, the i.p. hydrostatic pressure is usually greaten than 2 mm Hg, there exists a pressure gradient which drives fluid and solutes from the peritoneal cavity into the intenstitium. In the early portion of dialysis, the osmotic force which draws fluid into the cavity supersedes the hydrostatic force, and the peritoneal volume increases. After the effect of the high peritoneal osmolality is lost, the hydrostatic force is dominant and the volume decreases. On the basis of indirect evidence from protein absorption studies, the mesothelium does not present a significant barrier to solutes of clinical interest. The rate of protein solution absorption is directly proportional to hydrostatic pressure. Increased intra-abdominal pressure leads to an increased number of open lymphatic stomata [17]. Fluid absorbed into the interstitium from the cavity is taken up by blood and lymphatic capillaries. The protein is slowly returned to the venous circulation via the lymphatic vessels.

3.4 Pathophysiology of peritoneal carcinomatosis

Several gastrointestinal and gynecological malignancies have the potential to disseminate and grow in the peritoneal cavity. The occurrence of peritoneal carcinomatosis has been shown to significantly decrease overall survival in patients with liver and/or extraperitoneal metastases from gastrointestinal cancer. During the last three decades, the understanding of the biology and pathways of dissemination of tumors with intraperitoneal spread, and the understanding of the protective function of the peritoneal barrier against tumoral cell dissemination, has prompted the concept that peritoneal carcinomatosis is a loco-regional disease [18].

3.4.1 Epithelial-mesenchymal transition

The reaction of the peritoneum to aggression has been extensively studied in patients receiving peritoneal dialysis. Following exposition to bioincompatible solutions, denudation of mesothelial cells is observed and, ultimately, tissue fibrosis [19]. Reactive modified or regenerating mesothelial cells can undergo, under defined conditions, a transdifferentiation from an epithelial phenotype to a mesenchymal phenotype with

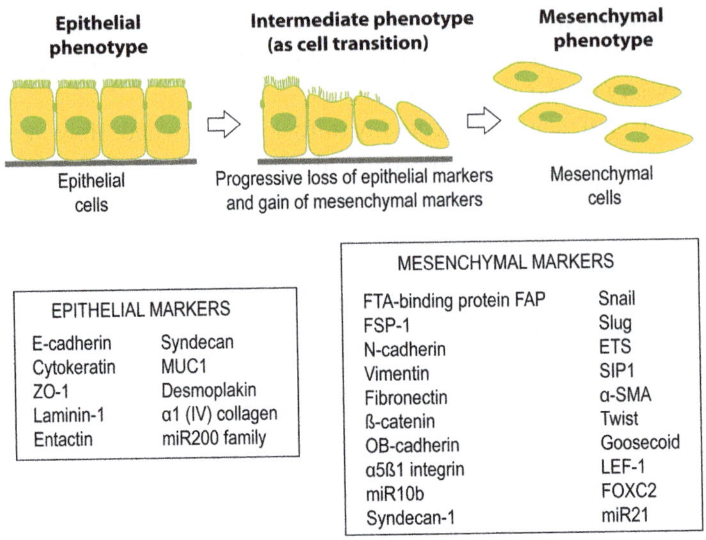

Fig. 3.7. Overview of epithelial-mesenchymal transition (EMT). An EMT involves a functional transition of polarized epithelial cells into mobile and ECM component-secreting mesenchymal cells. The epithelial and mesenchymal cell markers commonly used by EMT researchers are listed. Colocalization of these two sets of distinct markers defines an intermediate phenotype of EMT. ZO-1, zona occludens 1; MUC1, mucin 1, cell surface associated; miR200, microRNA 200; SIP1, survival of motor neuron protein interacting protein 1; FOXC2, forkhead box C2 (reproduced with permission from [21]).

a progressive loss of epithelial morphology and a decrease in the expression of cytokeratins and E-cadherin through an induction of the transcriptional repressor snail.

The biological process of epithelial-mesenchymal transition (EMT) is described as follows (Figure 3.7):
- epithelial cells are tightly integrated in their cellular environment by tight junctions or desmosomes;
- under the influence of different EMT mediators (such as growth factors or cytokines, discussed in detail below) epithelial cells gain a mesenchymal status;
- EMT is associated with different biological properties, particularly the ability to invade and metastasize.

EMT refers to a collective series of transcriptional and post-translational events that cause epithelial cells to take on mesenchymal features, thus allowing the cells to separate from the tissue context, lose baso-apical polarity and gain motility. It is of central importance that EMT processes are reversible so that mesenchymal cells can undergo MET to differentiate back to epithelial phenotypes. This reverse transition plays a key role in the formation of macroscopic metastases in different organs (reviewed in [20] and [21]).

3.4.2 Interstitial intratumoral fluid pressure

Both experimental and theoretical studies have shown that tumors may present elevated interstitial fluid pressure, which can be a formidable physical barrier for delivery of cell nutrients and small molecules into the tumor [22]. This barrier is an obstacle in tumor treatment, as it results in inefficient uptake of therapeutic agents. The flow of interstitial fluid and the associated interstitial fluid pressure in solid tumors and surrounding host tissues have been identified as critical elements in cancer growth and vascularization. Elevated interstitial fluid pressure may also exacerbate gradients of biochemical signals such as angiogenic factors released by tumors into the surrounding tissues. There are a number of factors that contribute to increased interstitial fluid pressure in the tumor, such as vessel abnormalities, fibrosis and contraction of the interstitial matrix [23].

Tumor angiogenesis generates abnormal vessels [24] that demonstrate several anomalies including an incomplete or absent endothelial cell layer and basement membrane which makes them hyperpermeable [25]. These vessels exhibit a high resistance to capillary blood flow and a low resistance to transcapillary flow, resulting in a net efflux of fluid into the surrounding interstitial space where a lack of functional lymphatics allows it to accumulate, distending the elastic extracellular matrix and increasing the interstitial pressure [26, 27]. An equilibrium is established where the capillary and interstitial pressures are equivalent resulting in reduced fluid movement through the interstitium [27]. In addition, the tumor interstitium itself is thought to be abnormal, comprising a dense network of collagen fibres, as well as increased fibroblasts, macrophages and other cells involved in inflammation, which further contribute to elevated intertstitial fluid pressure values [23]. It is clear from these previous studies that high intertstitial fluid pressure in tumors arises because of the complex interplay between the abnormal vasculature and the abnormal interstitium. However, the pathophysiologic mechanisms underlying widely varying intertstitial fluid pressure values in human and experimental tumors of the same and differing types, and the influence of growth site and the host, is less well understood. Elevated tumor intertstitial fluid pressure plays a role in the pathophysiological microenvironment that characterises solid tumors contributing to disease progression and chemotherapeutic resistance [23]. The mechanisms involved remain to be fully elucidated but several experimental animal studies have shown an improved uptake of therapeutic agents in response to a reduction in tumor intertstitial fluid pressure suggesting that high tumor intertstitial fluid pressure acts as a barrier to drug delivery (reviewed in [28]). Furthermore, there are clinical data showing that tumor intertstitial fluid pressure correlates with response to treatment [29, 30], with strong evidence for high intertstitial fluid pressure as an adverse prognostic indicator in cervix cancer patients treated with radiotherapy [31, 32]. Patients in the latter study were significantly more likely to develop distant recurrence if they presented with a tumor intertstitial fluid pressure value above the group median (19 mm Hg), which suggests a role for intertstitial fluid pressure in metastatic spread. A relationship has also been observed between tumor intertstitial fluid pressure values and metastasis in experimental melanoma xenografts [33].

These data, coupled with the breadth of data demonstrating elevated intertstitial fluid pressure in a wide range of human tumors [30, 31, 34–39], designate high tumor intertstitial fluid pressure as an important therapeutic problem.

3.4.3 Ascites

Ascites is defined as a pathological liquid collection within the peritoneal cavity, caused by a dysbalance between plasma inflow and outflow over the lymphatics vessels (Figure 3.8). In about 10% of patients, ascites is caused by a malignant disease. Primary tumors are in 80% of these patients ovarian or gastrointestinal cancers, in 20% other sources such as breast, lung, uterus or cervical cancer. Peritoneal invasion through tumor cells impairs flow regulation by and through the peritoneum, by various mechanisms.

The normal peritoneal cavity contains merely a thin film of fluid, with only few millilitres of transsudate in normal individuals. The movement of water across a semipermeable membrane from an area of low solute concentration to an area of high solute concentration is called osmosis. The hydrostatic pressure gradient and the osmotic gradient between the blood and the dialysis solution influence osmosis. The peritoneal membrane, when compared with the artificial kidney, appears tight to urea but leaky to protein. Thus, there is a significant amount of protein lost into an intraperitoneal (e.g. dialysis) solution. Protein loss increases if the patient develops a peritonitis. In the presence of hypoalbuminemia and of significant amounts of protein in the peritoneal cavity, the patients will develop ascites. Thus, it is of utmost importance that protein intake is adequate in peritoneal carcinomatosis patients undergoing intraperitoneal chemotherapy, since this therapy induces a chemical peritonitis. Minimal daily protein requirements are 1.2–1.5 g/kg of body weight.

Intraperitoneal tumor cells thus increase the production and reduce the reabsorption of intraperitoneal fluid. Vascular endothelial growth factor (VEGF) – formerly named vascular permeability factor – plays an essential role in generating such peritoneal hypersecretion. VEGF secretion by the tumor cells favored the accumulation of fluid in the peritoneal cavity in the animal model and was able to cause a reversible increase microvascular permeability without degranulation of mast cells, endothelial cells or further associated lesions [40]. Thus, production of VEGF alone was sufficient to increase capillary protein permeability. In humans, VEGF levels were higher in malignant ascites than in cirrhotic ascites and thus confirm the preclinical observations [41, 42]. Other studies have established the pro-angiogenic role of VEGF and specifically its central role in growth and cell migration of endothelial cells, increased permeability of the endothelial barrier to plasma proteins and alteration of the extra-

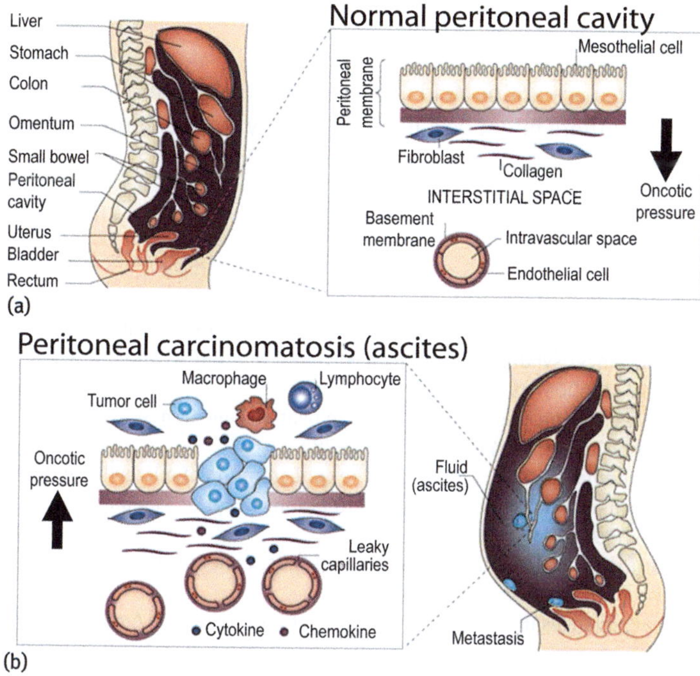

Fig. 3.8. Pathophysiology of ascites. (a) In physiological conditions, the difference in oncotic pressure across the peritoneal membrane (high at the endothelial layer and low at the mesothelial layer) limits capillary fluid filtration and prevents oedema that is due to water reabsorption into the capillaries from the interstitial space. (b) In patients with tumors in the abdominal cavity, the cross-sectional area of microvessels lining the peritoneal cavity is increased, and this results in an increased filtration surface for fluid. In addition, malignant ascites has a high protein concentration that is secondary to increased capillary permeability. Inflammatory cytokines and chemokines, as well as reduced lymphatic flow, all contribute to alterations of the peritoneal membrane. These changes decrease the plasma to peritoneal oncotic pressure difference, so the direction of flow of fluid is into the peritoneal cavity. This leads to the buildup of pathological volumes of fluid in the peritoneal cavity (reproduced with permission from [2]).

cellular matrix [43]. Neovascularization not only increases permeability capillary but also increases the surface of the capillary filter, thus facilitating protein extravasation and modifying oncotic pressure. Thus, VEGF acts on the majority of the factors intervening in the Starling's equation, resulting in an increase of the fluid outflow and accumulation thereof within the peritoneal cavity.

A further historical explanation for tumor ascites is the obstruction of lymphatic vessels by tumor cells, interrupting protein transport and creating an osmotic imbalance.

3.4.4 Hormonal changes

Other substances lost in ascites are amino acids, water-soluble vitamins, hormones and some medications, so that there might be a need for dietary supplements or even hormonal substitution.

Bibliography

[1] Casey MJ, et al. Intra-abdominal carcinomatosis after prophylactic oophorectomy in women of hereditary breast ovarian cancer syndrome kindreds associated with BRCA1 and BRCA2 mutations. Gynecol Oncol 97, 2 (2005) 457–467.

[2] Kipps E, Tan DS, Kaye SB. Meeting the challenge of ascites in ovarian cancer. new avenues for therapy and research. Nat Rev Cancer. 13, 4 (Apr 2013) 273–282.

[3] Mutsaers SE, Whitaker D, Papadimitriou JM. Changes in the concentration of microvilli on the free surface of healing mesothelium are associated with alterations in surface membrane charge. J Pathol. 180, 3 (Nov 1996) 333–339.

[4] Mutsaers SE, Wilkosz S. Structure and function of mesothelial cells. Cancer Treat Res 134 (2007) 1–19. Review.

[5] Wang ZB, Li M, Li JC. Recent advances in the research of lymphatic stomata. The Anatomical Record 293 (2010) 754–76.

[6] Yonemura Y, Kawamura T, Bandou E, Tsukiyama G, Endou Y, Miura M. The natural history of free cancer cells in the peritoneal cavity. In: Gonzalez-Moreno S (ed). Advances in Peritoneal Surface Oncology. Berlin, Germany: Springer-Verlag Berlin Heidelberg, 11–23, 2007.

[7] Sacchi G, DiPaolo N, Venezia F, Rossi A, Nicolai GA, Garosi G. Possible role of milky spots in mesothelial transplantation. Int J Artif Organs 30 (2007) 520–526.

[8] Beelen RH. The greater omentum: physiology and immunological concepts. Neth J Surg. 43, 5 (Oct 1991) 145–149.

[9] Sorensen EW, Gerber SA, Sedlacek AL, Rybalko VY, Chan WM, Lord EM. Omental immune aggregates and tumor metastasis within the peritoneal cavity. Immunol Res. 45, 2–3 (Dec 2009) 185–194.

[10] Brock C, L Arendt-Nielsen, Wilder-Smith O, Drewes AM. Sensory testing of the human gastrointestinal tract. World J Gastroenterol. 15, 2 (Jan 14 2009) 151–159. Review.

[11] Flessner MF. The transport barrier in intraperitoneal therapy. Am J Physiol Renal Physiol. 288, 3 (Mar 2005) F433–F442. Review.

[12] Dedrick RL, Myers CE, Bungay PM, Devita VT. Pharmacokinetic rationale for peritoneal drug administration in the treatment of ovarian cancer. Cancer Treat. Rep. 62 (1978) 1.

[13] Kipps E, Tan DS, Kaye SB. Meeting the challenge of ascites in ovarian cancer: new avenues for therapy and research. Nat Rev Cancer. 13 4 (Apr 2013) 273–282.

[14] Flessner MF. Peritoneal Transport Physiology: Insights from Basic Research. J Am Soc Nephrol 2 (1991) 122–135.

[15] http://www.advancedrenaleducation.com/PeritonealDialysis/BasicPrinciplesofPD/PhysiologyofthePeritoneum/tabid/151/Default.aspx, consulted on 18.3.2014.

[16] Rippe B. A three-pore model of peritoneal transport. Perit Dial Int 13 Suppl 2 (1993) S35–S38.

[17] Li JC, Lu ZL, Wu N, Zhou JL, Shi Y. A scanning microscopy and computer image processing morphometric study of the pharmacological regulation of patency of the peritoneal stomata. Ann Anat 178 (1996) 443–447.

[18] Coccolini F, Gheza F, Lotti M, et al. Peritoneal carcinomatosis. World J Gastroenterol; 19, 41 (2013) 6979–6994.

[19] Yáñez-Mó M, Lara-Pezzi E, Selgas R et al. Peritoneal dialysis and epithelial-to-mesenchymal transition of mesothelial cells. N Engl J Med. 348, 5 (Jan 30 2003) 403–413. Erratum in: N Engl J Med. 353, 26 (Dec 29 2005) 2827.

[20] Kiesslich T, Pichler M, Neureiter D. Epigenetic control of epithelial-mesenchymal-transition in human cancer. Mol Clin Oncol. 1 (Jan 1 2013) 3–11. Epub 2012 Sep 25. Review.

[21] Kalluri R, Weinberg RA. The basics of epithelial-mesenchymal transition. J Clin Invest. 2009 Jun;119(6):1420–1428.

[22] Wu M, Frieboes HB, McDougall SR, Chaplain MA, Cristini V, Lowengrub J. The effect of interstitial pressure on tumor growth: coupling with the blood and lymphatic vascular systems. J Theor Biol. 7, 320 (Mar 2013) 131–151.

[23] Heldin CH, Rubin K, Pietras K, Ostman A. High interstitial fluid pressure – an obstacle in cancer therapy. Nat Rev Cancer. 4 (Oct 2004) 806–813. Review.

[24] Jain RK. Transport of molecules in the tumor interstitium: a review. Cancer Res 47 (1987) 3039–3305.

[25] Baluk P, Morikawa S, Haskell A, Mancuso M, McDonald DM. Abnormalities of basement membrane on blood vessels and endothelial sprouts in tumors. Am J Pathol. 163 (2003) 1801–1815.

[26] Baxter LT, Jain RK. Transport of fluid and macromolecules in tumors I. Role of interstitial pressure and convection. Microvasc Res. 37 (1989) 77–104.

[27] Milosevic M, Fyles A, Hedley D, Hill R. The human tumor microenvironment: invasive (needle) measurement of oxygen and interstitial fluid pressure. Semin Radiat Oncol. 14 (2004) 249–258.

[28] Lunt SJ, Kalliomaki TM, Brown A, Yang VX, Milosevic M, Hill RP. Interstitialfluid pressure, vascularity and metastasis in ectopic, orthotopic and spontaneoustumors. BMC Cancer. 7, 8 (Jan 2008) 2.

[29] Roh HD, Kalnicki S, Buchsbaum R, Bloomer WD, Jain RK. Interstitial hypertension in carcinoma of uterine cervix in patients: Possible correlation with tumor oxygenation and radiation response. Cancer Res. 51 (1991) 6695–6698.

[30] Curti BD, Urba WJ, Alvord WG, Janik JE, Smith JW, Madara K, Longo DL. Interstitial pressure of subcutaneous nodules in melanoma and lymphoma patients: changes during treatment. Cancer Res. 53 (1993) 2204–2207.

[31] Milosevic M, Fyles A, Hedley D, Pintilie M, Levin W, Manchul L, Hill R. Interstitial fluid pressure predicts survival in patients with cervix cancer independent of clinical prognostic factors and tumor oxygen measurements. Cancer Res. 61 (2001) 6400–6405.

[32] Fyles A, Milosevic M, Pintilie M, Syed A, Levin W, Manchul L, Hill RP. Long-term performance of interstial fluid pressure and hypoxia as prognostic factors in cervix cancer. Radiother Oncol. 80 (2006) 132–137.

[33] Rofstad EK, Tunheim SH, Mathiesen B, Graff BA, Halsor EF, Nilsen K, Galappathi K. Pulmonary and lymph node metastasis is associated with primary tumor interstitial fluid pressure in human melanoma xenografts. Cancer Res. 62 (2002) 661–664.

[34] Roh HD, Kalnicki S, Buchsbaum R, Bloomer WD, Jain RK. Interstitial hypertension in carcinoma of uterine cervix in patients: Possible correlation with tumor oxygenation and radiation response. Cancer Res. 51 (1991) 6695–6698.

[35] Less JR, Posner MC, Boucher Y, Borochovitz D, Wolmark N, Jain RK. Interstitial hypertension in human breast and colorectal tumors. Cancer Res. 52 (1992) 6371–6374.

[36] Taghian AG, Abi-Raad R, Assaad SI, Casty A, Ancukiewicz M, Yeh E, Molokhia P, Attia K, Sullivan T, Kuter I, Boucher Y, Powell SN. Paclitaxel decreases the interstitial fluid pressure and improves oxygenation in breast cancers in patients treated with neoadjuvant chemotherapy: clinical implications. J Clin Oncol. 23 (2005) 1951–1961.

[37] Nathanson SD, Nelson L. Interstitial fluid pressure in breast cancer, benign breast conditions, and breast parenchyma. Ann Surg Oncol. 1 (1994) 333–338.

[38] Boucher Y, Kirkwood JM, Opacic D. Interstitial hypertension in superficial metastatic melanomas in humans. Cancer Res. 51 (1991) 6691–6694.

[39] DiResta GR, Lee J, Larson SM, Arbit E. Characterization of neuroblastoma xenograft in rat flank. I. Growth, interstitial fluid pressure, and interstitial fluid velocity distribution profiles. Microvasc Res. 46 (1993) 158–177.

[40] Senger DR, Galli SJ, Dvorak AM, Perruzzi CA, Harvey VS, Dvorak HF. Tumor cells secrete a vascular permeability factor that promotes accumulation of ascites fluid. Science 219 (1983) 983–985.

[41] Zebrowski BK, Liu W, Ramirez K, Akagi Y, Mills GB, Ellis LM. Markedly elevated levels of vascular endothelial growth factor in malignant ascites. Ann Surg Oncol 6 (1999) 373–378.

[42] Kraft A, Weindel K, Ochs A, et al. Vascular endothelial growth factor in the sera and effusions of patients with malignant and non-malignant disease. Cancer 85 (1999) 178–187.

[43] Dvorak HF, Brown LF, Detmar M, Dvorak AM. Vascular permeability factor/vascular endothelial growth factor, microvascular hyperpermeability, and angiogenesis. Am J Pathol 146 (1995) 1029–1039.

W. Solass and M. A. Reymond

4 Diagnosis and staging of peritoneal carcinomatosis

Preoperative diagnosis of peritoneal carcinomatosis is difficult. Imaging techniques (mainly based upon CT scanning and magnetic resonance imaging), could assist in planning surgery but also in preventing unwarranted laparotomy in patients with unresectable disease. However, they are limited in their ability to visualize localized peritoneal carcinomatosis, having low sensitivity for small volume disease. The gold standard in diagnosing peritoneal carcinomatosis continues to be the direct peritoneal visualization, either by laparotomy or laparoscopy [1].

4.1 Diagnostic workup

In order to decide the best possible therapy in a particular patient suffering pertioneal carcinomatosis, obligate investigations include:
- physical examination;
- nephrological investigation;
- evaluation of the hepatic function;
- evaluation of nutritional state;
- body mass index, albuminemia and pro-albuminemia;
- extent of disease and staging;
- contrast-enhanced multisliced computed tomography (CT) of the abdomen with intravenous, oral and rectal enhancement.

In addition, in patients with pleural carcinomatosis, lung function testing is helpful but is not performed routinely.

4.2 Imaging studies

Imaging studies are essential in the evaluation of patients with suspected or known peritoneal malignancy. Despite major advances in imaging technology in the last few years, the early and adequate detection of a peritoneal dissemination remains challenging because of the great variety in size, morphology and location of the peritoneal lesions.

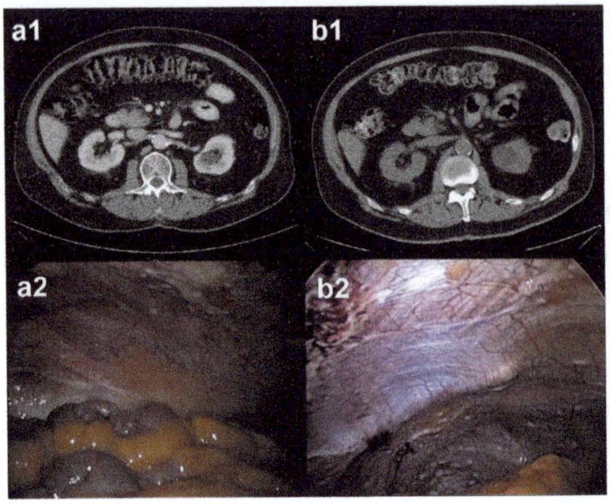

Fig. 4.1. 74-year-old patient with peritoneal carcinomatosis of gastric origin. CT scans immediately before first PIPAC (a1) and third PIPAC (b1) six weeks later. There is no radiological evidence for peritoneal carcinomatosis. However, laparoscopy at first PIPAC (a2) and third PIPAC (b2) showed peritoneal metastases, with a PCI of 12 at first PIPAC and 17 at third PIPAC. Peritoneal carcinomatosis was confirmed by histology in both instances. This exemplifies the poor value of CT scanning for visualizing low-volume peritoneal carcinomatosis (staging) and for follow up (therapy response assessment).

4.2.1 Computer tomography (CT scan)

Despite its known limited accuracy in detecting small peritoneal lesions and the involvement of the small bowel/mesentery, contrast-enhanced CT remains the standard imaging modality in the assessment of peritoneal carcinomatosis. CT scanning is the mainstay of tumor staging and plays a major role in everyday assessments of hepatic metastasis, ascites and lymphadenopathy. However, CT scans miss 30–45% of peritoneal nodules or lesions, in particular if these are smaller than 5 mm [2]. Computed tomography or magnetic resonance imaging may be used in particular cases, e.g. for differential diagnosis between ovarian cancer and a primary gastrointestinal tumor [3]. However, both procedures tend to underestimate peritoneal and mesenteric carcinomatosis, which are common in advanced ovarian and gastric cancer (Figure 4.1).

Contrast-enhanced CT scans will show or exclude the presence of liver and/or lung metastases, which are usually an exclusion criteria for cytoreductive surgery and HIPEC [4, 5].

4.2.2 Magnetic Resonance Imaging (MRI)

Magnetic Resonance Imaging (MRI), especially with diffusion-weighted images, is a promising method for the evaluation of peritoneal carcinomatosis with superior results in recent studies [6]. However, the use of MRI remains a complex issue. MRI has excellent contrast, spatial and temporal resolution; however, there are many image acquisition variables involved in MRI, which greatly impact image quality, lesion conspicuity and measurement. MRI still has a limited role in selected cases because of high costs and limited availability. As with CT, if an MRI is performed, the technical specifications of the scanning sequences used should be optimised for the evaluation of the type and site of disease. Furthermore, as with CT, the modality used at follow up should be the same as was used at baseline and the lesions should be measured and assessed on the same pulse sequence [7].

4.2.3 Ultrasound

Ultrasound examinations should not be used in clinical trials to measure tumor regression or progression of lesions because the examination is necessarily subjective and operator dependent. The reasons for this are several. Entire examinations cannot be reproduced for independent review at a later date. Furthermore, if, for example, the only measurable lesion is in the para-aortic region of the abdomen and if gas in the bowel overlies the lesion, the lesion will not be detected because the ultrasound beam cannot penetrate the gas [7]. However, of all imaging procedures used to diagnose ovarian cancer, transvaginal ultrasound is the most valuable in determining whether lesions are benign or malignant [8].

4.2.4 FDG-Positron emission tomography (PET)

Optional radiological investigations include FDG-positron emission tomography (PET) and magnetic resonance imagery [9]. FDG-PET/CT can be considered as a useful tool for the selection of patients for HIPEC treatment in the absence of distant metastasis. In ovarian cancer for example, FDG-PET/CT showed excellent results for the positive diagnosis and tumor burden for lesions more than 1 cm (positive predictive value PPV 93–100%). However, the sensitivity was low in the presence of millimetric disease with or without prior chemotherapy. When the diagnostic performance of (18)FDG-PET/CT, MRI with and without diffusion-weighted imaging, and contrast-enhanced CT were compared for the detection of peritoneal dissemination of malignant tumors, the sensitivity of PET/CT (94%) was significantly higher than that of MRI without diffusion-weighted imaging (70%). The specificities of the three modalities were not significantly different. The positive predictive value of PET/CT (93%) was significantly higher than that of the other three modalities (contrast-enhanced CT, 73%; MRI without diffusion-weighted imaging, 70%; MRI with diffusion-weighted imaging, 72%). Thus, PET/CT is the most useful technique for staging of patients with peritoneal carcinomatosis [10], but it has limitations for small-sized nodules, is not widely available and is expensive.

4.3 Diagnostic laparoscopy

Thus, the extent of peritoneal carcinomatosis is difficult to evaluate preoperatively, and precise evaluation is most often performed during surgical exploration [11]. Staging by conventional imaging techniques has limitations and often results in understaging and unnecessary laparotomy. In many cases diagnostic laparoscopy can be helpful to gain more detailed information on the intraperitoneal tumor or histological confirmation of the suspicion of peritoneal carcinosis [12–15] In particular, staging laparoscopy can be considered to exclude peritoneal carcinomatosis in patients without radiological evidence of metastatic disease when a neoadjuvant chemotherapy protocol is recommended [16]. A standardized technique minimizes the risk of tumor contamination of the trocars insertion sites [17]; this method minds the complications of diagnostic laparotomy and allows staging during the follow up. Moreover, exploratory laparoscopy can be used in order to evaluate the efficacy of neoadjuvant chemotherapy [18].

4.3.1 Peritoneal Cancer Index

Four quantitative assessments have been proposed to determine the extent of peritoneal carcinomatosis: the Gilly staging, Japanese gastric cancer P score, peritoneal cancer index (PCI), and the simplified peritoneal cancer index (SPCI) [19]. The Peritoneal Cancer Index is the most common scoring system for determining and standardizing the extent of peritoneal carcinomatosis. The PCI combines size and distribution parameters to determine a numerical score [20].

For determining the Peritoneal Cancer Index, two transverse planes and two sagittal planes divide the abdomen into nine regions (Figure 4.2). The upper transverse plane is located at the lowest aspect of the costal margin and the lower transverse plane is placed at the anterior superior iliac spine. The sagittal planes divide the abdomen into three equal sectors. The lines define the nine regions which are numbered in a clockwise direction with zero at the umbilicus and one defining the space beneath the right hemidiaphragm. Regions 9–12 divide the small bowel. The lesion size is used to define the size of peritoneal nodules (Table 4.1).

The lesion size (LS) score is determined after complete lysis of all adhesions and complete inspection of all parietal and visceral peritoneal surfaces within the abdominopelvic regions. LS-0 indicates no implants seen. LS-1 indicates implants less than 0.25 cm. LS-2 indicates implants between 0.25 and 2.5 cm. LS-3 indicates implants greater than 2.5 cm. It refers to the greatest diameter of tumor implants that are distributed on the peritoneal surfaces. Primary tumors or localized recurrences at the primary site that can be removed definitively are excluded from the assessment. If there is a confluence of disease matting abdominal or pelvic structures together, this is automatically scored as LS-3 even if it is a thin layer of cancerous implants.

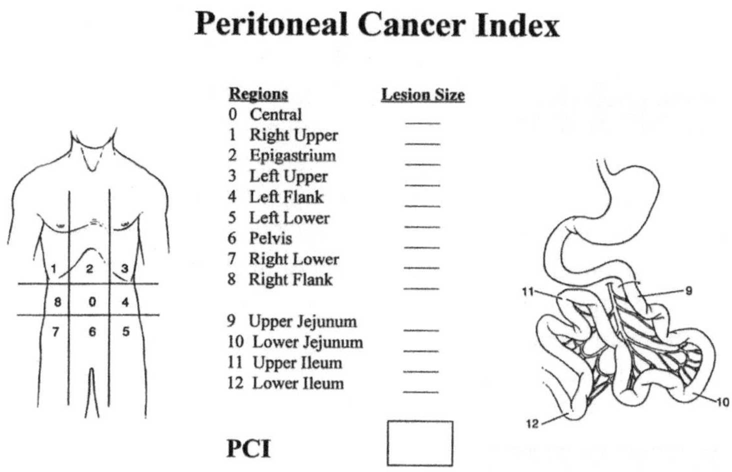

Fig. 4.2. Peritoneal cancer index (PCI) (modified from [20]). The extent of the disease within all regions of abdomen and pelvis is indicated by a numerical score from 0 to 39.

Table 4.1. Peritoneal Cancer Index. Definition of lesion size.

Lesion Size	Definition
LS0	No tumor seen
LS1	Tumor up to 0.5 cm
LS2	Tumor up to 2.5 cm
LS3	Tumor 2.5 cm or confluence

An exception to the utility of the PCI is found in treating patients with pseudomyxoma peritonei and minimally aggressive mesothelioma. Because the disease is noninvasive, a PCI of 39 can be converted to 0 by cytoreductive surgery. There is a low probability of recurrence after complete cytoreduction with perioperative intraperitoneal chemotherapy and therefore the PCI has no prognostic implication [21].

Another caveat that must be observed when using the PCI occurs in cases in which a low PCI score is recorded in the presence of invasive cancer at a crucial anatomic site. For example, at exploration one may find invasive tumors in and around the common bile duct with little disease elsewhere. Another example is diffuse small bowel involvement, which is not amenable to complete cytoreduction. Even though the PCI is low, a complete cytoreduction may not be possible. In these cases, invasive cancer at a crucial anatomic site places the patient into the same category as would systemic metastasis in the lungs or bone. Only palliative surgery is indicated if residual disease post-cytoreduction will be present [22].

The preoperative CT scan is an excellent tool in locating and quantifying mucinous adenocarcinoma within the peritoneal cavity [23]. Unfortunately, accuracy of CT scanning in other histologies is not satisfying [24]. In colorectal cancer, CT detection of peritoneal carcinomatosis is moderate and imaging of individual peritoneal tumor deposits poor. Interobserver differences are statistically significant. When CT scanning was compared with intraoperative findings, the accuracy of tumor detection varied widely per anatomic site. Statistically significant interobserver differences were noted, Therefore, preoperative CT scanning seems not to be a reliable tool for detection of presence, size, and location of peritoneal tumor implants in view of treatment planning in patients with colorectal cancer [25]. However, CT scanning can give some useful hints for excluding patients for cytoreductive surgery, such as:

- segmental obstruction of the small bowel;
- tumor nodules greater than 5 cm;
- invasive character small bowel infiltration;
- large tumor nodules on small bowel or its mesentery;
- invasion of the hepatoduodenal ligament.

There are some special demands on CT scanning to optimize diagnostic accuracy. First, oral contrast enhancement is helpful to distinguish bowel loops cut in cross section from cancer nodules. Second, a delay of 60–120 seconds after intravenous contrast injection will optimize contrast of superficial solid tumors deposits on the peritoneal surfaces. Third, solid or semi-solid tumors may mimic ascites on the CT scan so that an ultrasound might be useful to complement the analysis.

4.4 Peritoneal or pleural cytology

Peritoneal lavage cytology has been proposed as a complementary staging parameter in patients at risk for developing peritoneal carcinomatosis, e.g. patients with newly-diagnosed gastric tumors, with perforated colorectal tumors, or with locally advanced ovarian cancer. However, the clinical value of peritoneal cytology is not yet established. Analysis of current guidelines show different recommendations for different organs, and also differences between Asia and Europe.

4.4.1 Gastric cancer

Cytology from ascites or peritoneal lavage can help to establish the diagnosis. Peritoneal lavage cytology during laparotomy is included as a staging process in the thirteenth edition of Japanese Classification of Gastric Carcinoma [26]. However, the usefulness of peritoneal lavage cytology during staging laparoscopy for gastric cancer is controversial, since clinical benefit is only marginal [27–29].

4.4.2 Ovarian cancer

In ovarian cancer, the current German S3-guideline recommends peritoneal lavage and cytology as a part of the routine staging during surgical resection [30].

4.4.3 Colorectal cancer

The current German S3-guideline does not mention peritoneal cytology in colorectal cancer so that it use cannot be recommended for therapeutic decisions [31].

Bibliography

[1] Coccolini F, Gheza F, Lotti M et al. Peritoneal carcinomatosis. World J Gastroenterol 19, 41 (2013) 6979–6994.

[2] Angelelli G, Ianora AA, Scardapane A, Pedote P, Memeo M, Rotondo A. Role of computerized tomography in the staging of gastrointestinal neoplasms. Semin Surg Oncol 20 (2001) 109–121.

[3] Burges A, Schmalfeldt B. Ovarian cancer: diagnosis and treatment. Dtsch Arztebl Int. 108, 38 (Sep 2011) 635–641.

[4] Elias D, Benizri E, Vernerey D, et al. Preoperative criteria of incomplete resectability of peritoneal carcinomatosis from non-appendiceal colorectal carcinoma. Gastroenterol Clin Biol. 29 (2005) 1010–1013.

[5] Glehen O, Kwiatkowski F, Sugarbaker PH, et al. Cytoreductive surgery combined with perioperative intraperitoneal chemotherapy for the management of peritoneal carcinomatosis from colorectal cancer: a multi-institutional study. J Clin Oncol. 22 (2004) 3284–3292.

[6] Pfannenberg C, Schwenzer NF, Bruecher BL. [State-of-the-art imaging of peritoneal carcinomatosis]. Rofo. 184, 3 (Mar 2012) 205–213.

[7] Eisenhauer EA, Therasse P, Bogaerts J et al. New response evaluation criteria in solid tumors: revised RECIST guideline (version 1.1). Eur J Cancer. 45, 2 (Jan 2009) 228–247.

[8] Kinkel K, et al. Indeterminate ovarian mass at US: incremental value of second imaging test for characterization – meta-analysis and Bayesian analysis. Radiology 236, 1 (2005) 85–94.

[9] Berthelot C, Morel O, Girault S, et al. Use of FDG-PET/CT for peritoneal carcinomatosis before hyperthermic intraperitoneal chemotherapy. Nucl Med Commun 32 (2011) 23–29.

[10] Satoh Y, Ichikawa T, Motosugi U, Kimura K, Sou H, Sano K, Araki T. Diagnosis of peritoneal dissemination: comparison of 18F-FDG PET/CT, diffusion-weighted MRI, and contrast-enhanced MDCT. AJR Am J Roentgenol. 196, 2 (Feb 2011) 447–453.

[11] Cotte E, Passot G, Gilly FN, Glehen O. Selection of patients and staging of peritoneal surface malignancies. World J Gastrointest Oncol 2, 1 (2010) 31–35.

[12] Yan TD, Morris DL, Shigeki K, et al. Preoperative investigations in the management of peritoneal surface malignancy with cytoreductive surgery and perioperative intraperitoneal chemotherapy: Expert consensus statement. J Surg Oncol 98 (2008) 224–227.

[13] Lowy AM, Mansfield PF, Leach SD, Ajani J. Laparoscopic staging for gastric cancer. Surgery 119 (1996) 611–614.

[14] Nieveen van Dijkum EJ, de Wit LT, van Delden OM et al. The efficacy of laparoscopic staging in patients with upper gastrointestinal tumors. Cancer 79 (1997) 1315–1319.

[15] Shelat VG, Thong JF, Seah M, Lim KH. Role of staging laparoscopy in gastric malignancies – our institutional experience. World J Gastrointest Surg. 4, 9 (Sep 27 2012) 214–219.

[16] Chua YJ, Cunningham D. The UK NCRI MAGIC trial of perioperative chemotherapy in resectable gastric cancer: implications for clinical practice. Ann Surg Oncol. 14, 10 (Oct 2007) 2687–2690.

[17] Balli JE, Franklin ME, Almeida JA, Glass JL, Diaz JA, Reymond M. How to prevent port-site metastases in laparoscopic colorectal surgery. Surg Endosc. 14, 11 (Nov 2000) 1034–1036. Review.

[18] A. Okines, M. Verheij,W. Allum, D. Cunningham, and A. Cervantes, "Gastric cancer: ESMO clinical practice guidelines for diagnosis, treatment and follow up," Annals of Oncolog 21 (2010) v50–v54.

[19] Harmon RL, Sugarbaker PH. Prognostic indicators in peritoneal carcinomatosis from gastrointestinal cancer. Int Semin Surg Oncol. 2, 1 (Feb 8 2005) 3.

[20] Jacquet P, Sugarbaker PH. Clinical research methodologies in diagnosis and staging of patients with peritoneal carcinomatosis. In: Sugarbaker PH (ed). Peritoneal carcinomatosis: principles of management. Boston: Kluwer Academic publishers, 1996. pp. 359–374.

[21] Sugarbaker PH. Management of peritoneal surface malignancy: The surgeon's role. Langenbeck's Arch Surg. 384 (1999) 576–587.

[22] Harmon RL, Sugarbaker PH. Prognostic indicators in peritoneal carcinomatosis from gastrointestinal cancer. Int Semin Surg Oncol. 2, 1 (Feb 8 2005) 3.

[23] Jacquet P, Jelinek JS, Chang D, Koslowe P, Sugarbaker PH. Abdominal computed tomographic scan in the selection of patients with mucinous peritoneal carcinomatosis for cytoreductive surgery. J Am Coll Surg. 181 (1995) 530–538.

[24] Jacquet P, Jelinek JS, Steves MA, Sugarbaker PH. Evaluation of computer tomography in patients with peritoneal carcinomatosis. Cancer. 72 (1993) 1631–1636.

[25] de Bree E, Koops W, Kröger R, van Ruth S, Witkamp AJ, Zoetmulder FA. Peritoneal carcinomatosis from colorectal or appendiceal origin: correlation of preoperative CT with intraoperative findings and evaluation of interobserver agreement. J Surg Oncol. 86, 2 (May 1 2004) 64–73. Review.

[26] Japanese Gastric Cancer Association. Japanese Classification of Gastric Carcinoma – 2nd English edn. – Gastric Cancer 1 (1998) 10–24.

[27] Sotiropoulos GC, Kaiser GM, Lang H, Treckmann J, Brokalaki EI, Pottgen C, Gerken G, Paul A, Broelsch CE. Staging laparoscopy in gastric cancer. Eur J Med Res 10 (2005) 88–91.

[28] van Dijkum EJM, Sturm PD, de Wit LT, Offerhaus J, Obertop H, Gouma DJ. Cytology of peritoneal lavage performed during staging laparoscopy for gastrointestinal malignancies: is it useful? Ann Surg 228 (1998) 728–733.

[29] Nakagawa S, Nashimoto A, Yabusaki H. Role of staging laparoscopy with peritoneal lavage cytology in the treatment of locally advanced gastric cancer. Gastric Cancer 10 (2007) 29–34.

[30] Leitlinienprogramm Onkologie (Deutsche Krebsgesellschaft, Deutsche Krebshilfe, AWMF): S3-Leitlinie Diagnostik, Therapie und Nachsorge maligner Ovarialtumoren, Langversion 1.1, 2013, AWMF-Registernummer: 032/035OL, http://leitlinienprogramm-onkologie.de/Leitlinien.7.0.html, [Stand: 12.4.2014].

[31] Leitlinienprogramm Onkologie (Deutsche Krebsgesellschaft, Deutsche Krebshilfe, AWMF): S3-Leitlinie Kolorektales Karzinom, Langversion 1.0, AWMF Registrierungsnummer: 021–007OL, http://leitlinienprogramm-onkologie.de/Leitlinien.7.0.html [Stand: 12.4.2014].

C. Demtröder, U. Giger-Pabst, W. Solass, and M. A. Reymond

5 Therapy of peritoneal carcinomatosis

Peritoneal and pleural carcinomatosis are two examples of situations where therapeutic options were not available until recently that might improve life expectation and quality of life. However, even though the disease from which the patients suffer remains, for most of them, incurable, novel systemic and locoregional therapies are now emerging that might change this paradigm.

The following therapeutic options can be considered for patients with peritoneal carcinomatosis:

1. Systemic palliative chemotherapy (pre-, peri- or postoperative) including combination therapies.
2. Systemic administration of biologicals, including angiogenesis inhibitors
3. combined cytoreductive surgery (CRS) with Hyperthermic IntraPEritoneal Chemotherapy (HIPEC).
4. Early Postoperative Intraperitoneal Chemotherapy (EPIC).
5. Pressurized IntraPeritoneal Aerosol Chemotherapy (PIPAC).
6. Intraperitoneal immunotherapy, including catumaxomab and radioimmunotherapy.
7. Palliative surgery.
8. Endoscopic procedures.
9. Radio(chemo)therapy.
10. Intraperitoneal cytolytic virotherapy (GL-ONC1).

Thus, there are at least ten different active therapies available in peritoneal carcinomatosis patients, plus all possible combinations. The physician must determine the optimal treatment individually in each case, by discussing the options with the patient. Due to the challenges and complexity of therapy of peritoneal carcinomatosis patients, this can be best achieved by a multi-professional board. Scientific progress creates new treatment options that are now available and change the historical nihilistic, fatalistic paradigm in peritoneal carcinomatosis. As the number of options rises, the need for discussion to pick the best option rises as well. Technical progress does not obviate the need for specialized medical care, but rather increases it, as only specialists have the requisite knowledge of all therapeutic options to be able to discuss them with patients.

5.1 Systemic palliative chemotherapy

Systemic therapy with combination chemotherapy, including the use of so-called biologicals, has significantly improved prognosis for patients with metastasized cancer. Therefore, palliative systemic chemotherapy is considered the standard of care for most patients with metastatic cancer.

Palliative systemic chemotherapy is the current standard of care for peritoneal and pleural metastatic disease, and has documented, evidence-based effects. For example, in peritoneal carcinomatosis from colorectal cancer, median overall survival increased from 12.6 months [1] for patients treated with 5-FU/folinic acid alone to to 24 months [2] when using modern chemotherapy (oxaliplatin). In other origins of peritoneal carcinomatosis such as gastric cancer, results are not so good. First-line chemotherapy regimens include mainly CF (cisplatin plus infusional 5-FU) and ECF (cisplatin plus infusional 5-FU plus epirubicin). They obtain responses in 20–40% of patients and improve quality of life. Median time to tumor progression is about 4–5 months and median survival does not exceed 7–10 months [3].

However, in a subset of patients with peritoneal carcinomatosis, the beneficial effect of systemic chemotherapy remains questionable [4]. It appears that systemic chemotherapy has only a limited effect on peritoneal carcinomatosis due to drug resistance in advanced tumor stages and to poor bioavailability within the abdominal cavity after systemic drug application [5].

5.2 Intraperitoneal chemotherapy

In patients with tumors confined to the peritoneal cavity, there is established pharmacokinetic and tumor biology-related evidence that intraperitoneal drug administration is advantageous [6]. Intraperitoneal delivery of anticancer drugs for abdominal malignancy is not a new concept. The earliest intraperitoneal "drug therapy" was reported in 1744 by the English surgeon Christopher Warrick, who injected a mixture of "Bristol water" and "claret" (a Bordeaux wine) into the peritoneal cavity of a woman suffering from intractable ascites [7]. Since the discovery of the antineoplastic potential of nitrogen mustard during World War II, intraperitoneal chemotherapy has been studied in clinical trials for more than 50 years [8]. The results from recent randomized trials in ovarian and colorectal cancer patients have led to a renewed interest in the concept of intraperitoneal cytotoxic drug therapy [9–11].

The aim of intraperitoneal chemotherapy is not to treat the peritoneum itself or the retroperitoneal interstitial tissue, but to destroy tumor nodes implemented onto the peritoneum, or invading visceral organs. Therefore, it is important to take into account specific tumor-related factors that would influence local drug uptake and therefore drug efficacy. In order to exert their anticancer effects, drugs have to gain access to tumor cells by penetrating into tissue. The available data on tumor tissue distribution of cytotoxic drugs and their relation with antitumor efficacy are limited, and mainly stem from in vitro multicellular models such as tumor spheroids (spherical tumor aggregates; diameter approximately 1 mm) and multilayered cell cultures [12]. Tissue penetration in these models is studied following incubation in a medium containing anticancer drugs, and generally the results show a very limited cytotoxic drug penetration [13].

5.3 Drug uptake into tumoral tissue

Drug uptake into tumoral tissue is a function of pharmacokinetic parameters such as dose, concentration, and exposure time and convection (Figure 5.1). The periphery of the tumor is entered by diffusion (concentration gradients) or convection (motion of interstitial fluid). The convective and diffusive transport may be in the same direction or in opposite directions depending upon the pressure and concentration gradients [14].

The extent of penetration will depend on drug properties and properties related to the tumor.

5.3.1 Diffusion

The semi-permeable "peritoneal membrane" allows solutes and water to be transported from the vascular system to the peritoneal cavity and vice versa. This process of solutes moving from an area of higher concentration to an area of lower concen-

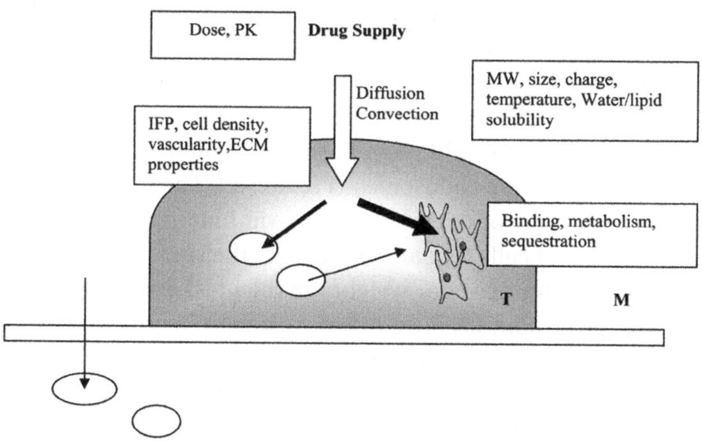

Fig. 5.1. Schematic representation of drug penetration into peritoneal metastatic tumors. The periphery of the tumor is entered by diffusion and convection. Once intracellular, the drug will accumulate in tumor cells by binding to target structures, nonspecific binding, and sequestration in cellular organelles. A fraction of the drug will be altered by metabolic pathways. Systemic drug absorption occurs both in submesothelial tissue and in tumor tissue. T, tumor nodule; M, mesothelium; PK, pharmacokinetics; IFP, interstitial tissue pressure; ECM, extracellular matrix; MW, molecular weight (reproduced from: [13]).

tration is called diffusion. Eventually, the concentrations become equal on both sides of the membrane. This is termed equilibrium. The movement of solute molecules is random and driven by thermal energy. This thermal energy is transferred to kinetic energy which is the multiple of mass and velocity. Since this energy is the same for different sized molecules at the same temperature, the larger molecules move more slowly. Thus, the rate of diffusion depends on molecular weight.

Solute transport is influenced by the membrane permeability and size, characteristics of the solute, the volume of dialysate instilled, and blood flow to the membrane. Solute transport can be increased by maximizing the contact of intraperitoneal solution with the membrane e.g. by increasing the exchange surface.

Substances that are absorbed from intraperitoneal solution into the systemic circulation include electrolytes, glucose and others (e.g. drugs). The increased concentration of glucose in some chemotherapy solutions (e.g. oxaliplatin-based HIPEC) can lead to hyperglycemia and hyponatremia.

Parameters of diffusion through tissue

The physicochemical properties of drugs (for example, molecular weight, shape, charge and aqueous solubility) determine the rate of diffusion through tissue (reviewed in [12]). The *penetration* of a drug is also dependent on its consumption, which functions to remove free drug, thereby inhibiting further permeation. Water-soluble drugs distribute most readily in the extracellular matrix, and therefore efficiently diffuse around and between cells. Lipid-soluble drugs penetrate lipid membranes, and so can be transported through cells. *Consumption* includes the effects of metabolism, binding to tissue elements (both specific to the target receptor and nonspecific), and uptake and retention in tumor cells. *Retention* in tumor cells can be due to binding at the site of lethal activity (usually DNA), although basic drugs can be sequestered in acidic organelles such as perinuclear endosomes (Figure 5.2). For example, the poor penetration through tissue of doxorubicin is due to avid binding to DNA and sequestration in acidic endosomes of cells that are proximal to the vasculature.

Thus, low lipophility and a high molecular weight are the ideal drug characteristics for intraperitoneal administration, because drugs with these features allow a favorable ratio to be achieved between peritoneal and plasma concentrations, due to the reduced tendency to diffuse through the plasma-peritoneal barrier, even after extensive removal of the peritoneum. Moreover, a low rate of diffusion through the tumor capillaries implies a low rate of drug clearance, with a higher intratumoral drug accumulation.

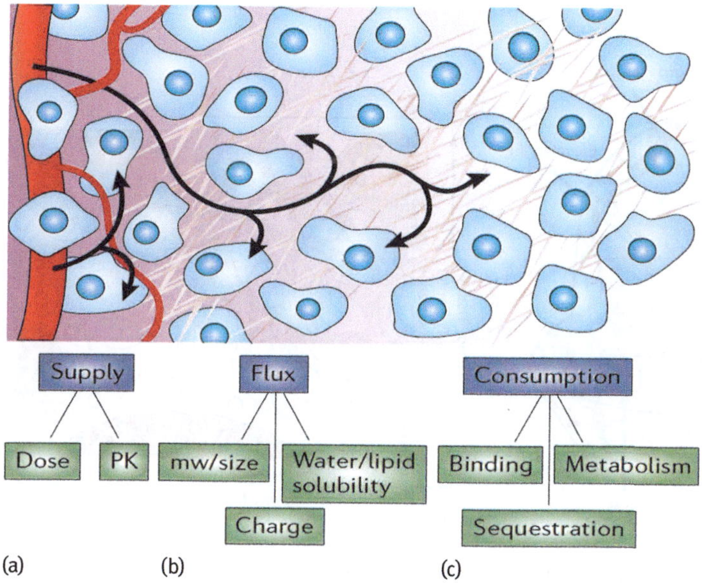

Fig. 5.2. Drug distribution in tissue occurs in three consecutive steps: supply, flux and consumption. (a) Supply. The supply of a drug to the tissue will depend on its dose and pharmacokinetics (PK). (b) Flux. After leaving the vasculature, flux through tissue can occur through extracellular or transcellular pathways, depending on relative solubility in water and lipids. Although diffusion through water will vary with size or molecular weight (mw), movement will be hindered by interactions with extracellular and cellular components, and the barrier posed by the cell membrane. (c) Consumption. Tissue penetration will be determined by the balance between delivery (supply and flux) and consumption. Cellular metabolism will reduce drug penetration and buildup within the tissue, and binding and sequestration can increase net tissue levels of a drug but limit its penetration (Reproduced with permission from [12]).

5.3.2 Convection

Convection is the second mechanism of supply, and plays an important role in the adsorption of macromolecules and lipids. Absolute rates of convection into and out of the peritoneal cavity cannot yet be accurately predicted, but the physiological forces can be specified (Figure 5.3).

In recent years an increased interest in macromolecular vehicles and other modulations of chemotherapeutic agents as a means of exploiting the regional dose intensity has emerged (reviewed in [16]). The results of this research are conflicting. Contrary to intuitive thinking, macromolecules may penetrate more deeply in the subperitoneal space despite their lower diffusivity. The nature of the capillary permeability is probably the major factor responsible for this higher concentration in the subperitoneal space together with an increased role of convection [17]. One should be cautious to conclude that this increased penetration into the subperitoneal space results in increased drug absorption into tumor nodules. One should not assume that

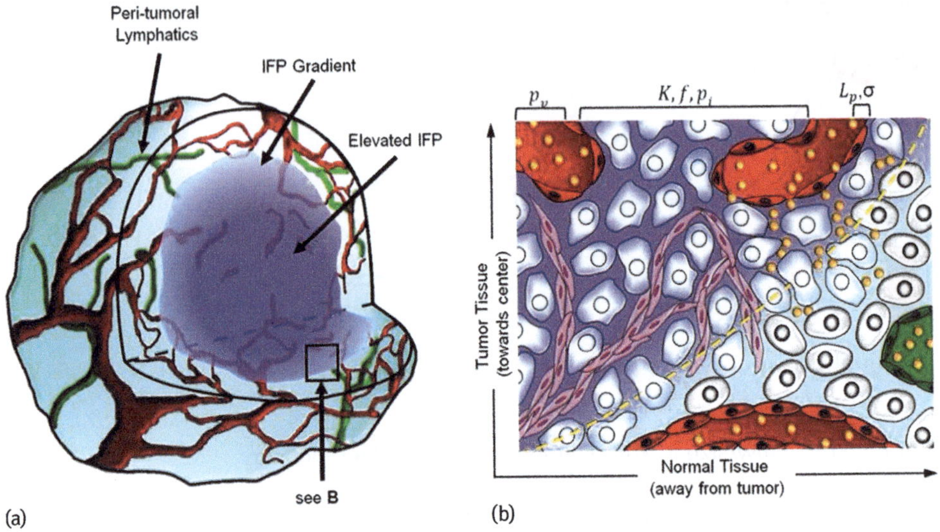

Fig. 5.3. An illustration of convective transport. (a) Tumors experience elevated central intratumoral fluid pressure due to an increased transvascular fluid transport (L_p), decreased interstitial fluid transport (K), and lack of functional lymphatic vessels. Peri-tumoral lymphatics drain excess fluid at the tumor periphery, resulting in a gradient in intratumoral fluid pressure. (b) An illustration of the peri-tumoral region where the yellow dashed line indicates the border between tumor and healthy tissue. Transvascular ($p_v - p_i$) and interstitial (∇p_i) pressure gradients drive the convective transport across blood vessels and through the tumor interstitium. This process occurs predominantly along the tumor periphery where significant transvascular and interstitial pressure gradients are present. Convection transports lipids and liposomes through large endothelial pores (σ) and through the extracellular matrix (f) where they accumulate due to a lack of lymphatic clearance. In normal tissue, tight endothelial junctions limit liposome extravasation and functional lymphatics contribute to the clearance of the agent from the interstitium (reproduced from: [15]).

the neovascularity of tumor nodules has the same selectivity for macromolecules as normal capillaries [18]. A second obstacle to cancer chemotherapy penetration into tumor nodules concerns the interstitial pressures in tumor nodules. It is significantly higher than that of the surrounding tissue space [19]. Convection may reduce tumor penetration by macromolecules.

5.4 Effect of peritonectomy on drug clearance

The effect of peritonectomy on drug clearance has been reviewed by Flessner [20]. A number of studies of eviscerated animals have reported relatively little reduction in the rate of clearance of low-molecular-weight substances from the peritoneal cavity, despite the removal of a large fraction of the peritoneal surface area. This is not explained by a disproportionately large role of the liver surface, but by a discrepancy between the geometric peritoneal surface area and the effective functional surface area available for transport. Thus, the anatomic peritoneum (mesothelium and associated connective tissue) is not a significant barrier to small solutes or macromolecules and elimination of the peritoneum does not alter transport significantly. This leaves the blood vessel wall and the surrounding interstitium as the major barriers to transport.

5.5 Influence of intraperitoneal drug concentration

Drug concentration in the peritoneum is an important determinant of intraperitoneal chemotherapy efficacy for several reasons (reviewed in [6]). First, small (that is, less than 1 mm) peritoneal tumor nodules are characterized by pronounced hypoxia and a poorly developed or absent vasculature that compromises intravenous drug delivery [21]. Any increase in the concentration gradient between the peritoneal compartment and the tumor stroma will theoretically enhance drug delivery. Second, most cytotoxic drugs exhibit a steep (near exponential) dose-effect relationship, which is even more pronounced in small, rapidly growing tumor deposits that have not yet reached the plateau phase [22]. Preclinical data with cisplatin showed an exponential dose-related reduction in survival of human ovarian cancer cells [23] Also, higher intracellular drug concentrations can partially help to overcome platinum resistance [24].

5.6 Tissue penetration of various drugs

The physicochemical properties of drugs (for example, molecular weight, shape, lipophility, etc.) determine their suitability for intraperitoneal chemotherapy.

A rational choice of a cytotoxic agent for intraperitoneal chemotherapy should consider the following elements:

- activity against the disease process;
- cell cycle specificity;
- relation between dose / exposure time and response;
- pharmacokinetic advantage (peritoneal/plasma AUC ratio);
- pharmacodynamic properties;
- local and systemic toxicity;
- thermal enhancement ratio (when used in combination with hyperthermia).

Table 5.1 summarizes the dose, Area Under the Curve (AUC) ratio and drug penetration distance of the most common intraperitoneal chemotherapy agents.

Among the drugs used so far for HIPEC, the combination of cisplatin and doxorubicin appears to be one of the most effective available regimens with acceptable locoregional toxicity. Pharmacological aspects of intraperitoneal administration of these drugs are well known so that we can rely on solid state-of-the-art. Doxorubicin showed

Table 5.1. Pharmacokinetic and pharmacodynamic properties of cytotoxic agents used during intraoperative or early postoperative intraperitoneal chemotherapy (reproduced from [13]).

Drug	MW (Da)	Ip dose (Mg/m^2)	AUC Ratio*	Drug penetration distance	TE
Alkylating agents					
Mitomycin C	334.3	35	10–23.5	2 mm	+
Platinum compounds					
Cisplatin	300.1	90–120	1.9–5.3	1–3 mm	+
Carboplatin	371.3	350–800	1.9–53	0.5 mm	+
Oxaliplatin	397.3	460	3.5	1–2 mm	+
Antimicrotubule agents					
Paclitaxel	853.9	20–175	NA	> 80 cell layers	?
Docetaxel	861.9	40–156	207	NA	+
Topoisomerase Interactive Agents					
Topocetan	457.9		NA	NA	?
Itinotecan	677.2		NA	NA	±
Mitoxantrone	517.4	28	15.2	5–6 cell layers	±
Doxorubicin	543.5	60–75	162	4–6 cell layers	+
Antimetabolites					
5-Fluorouracil	130.1	650	NA	0.2 mm	–

MW, molecular weight; ip, intraperitoneal; TE, thermal enhancement; NA, not available; AUC, area under the conentration-time curve; *only data referring to clinical studies with hyperthermic chemoperfusion

a much more advantageous plasma/peritoneal AUC ratio than cisplatin (162 ± 113 and 20 ± 6, respectively). On the other hand, very high intraperitoneal concentrations of cisplatin can be achieved without incurring significant systemic toxicity. Penetration of the tumor mass by cisplatin is greater than doxorubicin. This phenomenon is enhanced by hypotonic solutions of sodium chloride used as the perfusate (reviewed in [25]).

5.6.1 Doxorubicin (see also page 199)

Doxorubicin is an antitumor antibiotic and is one of the earliest intraperitoneal chemotherapeutic agents used in clinical trials. Its molecular weight is 543 g/mol and the AUC ratio of intraperitoneal to intravenous concentration time is 230. It is metabolized as a single pass through the liver so there is a low likelihood of systemic toxicities. Doxorubicin efficacy is augmented with heat and tissue penetration through at least five cell layers. This drug is ideally suited for intraperitoneal administration after a maximal attempt of cytoreduction. It can also be used effectively with other intraperitoneal drugs, such as cisplatin and mitomycin C without pharmacological incompatibility. Recent pharmacokinetic studies demonstrated that the doxorubicin content in small mesothelioma nodules far surpassed that measured in the peritoneal fluid. An active uptake of doxorubicin by mesothelioma tumor nodules was proposed and would be expected to result in a maximal response (reviewed in [26]).

5.6.2 Cisplatinum (see also page 198)

Cisplatinum is an alkylating agent. It has been used by intraperitoneal administration for treating gastric cancer, ovarian cancer and diffuse malignant peritoneal mesothelioma. Its molecular weight is 300 g/mol and the AUC ratio of intraperitoneal concentration to plasma concentration times time is approximately 10. Cisplatin can be used synchronously with many other agents. Its cytotoxicity is augmented by heat up to 3 times at 41.5 °C. It can effectively penetrate tumor nodules up to 3 mm (reviewed in [26]).

5.6.3 Oxaliplatinum

Oxaliplatinum is a third generation platinum complex and has become the standard of care in first-line intravenous chemotherapy of metastatic colorectal cancer. In vitro, hyperthermia enhanced the cytotoxicity and DNA adduct formation of oxaliplatin, although less so than that of cisplatin [27]. In peritoneal carcinomatosis patients treated with HIPEC (30 minutes at 43 °C) using oxaliplatin in increasing doses, half of the dose was absorbed after the perfusion, and at the highest dose level (460 mg/m^2) the maximal drug concentration was 25 times higher in the perfusate than in plasma. Oxaliplatinum concentrations were significantly higher in tumor tissue (339 ng/mg) compared to unbathed normal muscle (19 ng/mg) although plasma AUC values were higher than those commonly obtained during intravenous administration of oxaliplatin [28]. The peritoneal/plasma AUC ratio as estimated from the published data is low (approximately 3.5). Since oxaliplatin can only be administered intraperitoneally in a dextrose 5% solution, severe hyperglycaemia and hyponatriemia develops during chemoperfusion (reviewed in [13]).

5.6.4 Taxanes (Paclitaxel, Docetaxel)

Paclitaxel is well studied in the context of intraperitoneal therapy of advanced ovarian cancer. In this setting, the large molecular weight of the agent resulted in prolonged exposure of the peritoneal cavity and a very high peritoneal/plasma AUC ratio (996 [29] to 1350 [30]). A study in histiocultures showed that paclitaxel penetration is limited to the tumor periphery in the first 24 hours; later, however, increasing apoptosis resulted in more extensive penetration of the xenografts (at least 1 mm or 80 cell layers). Paclitaxel is heat stable, but thermal enhancement of its cytotoxicity is not clearly defined and likely dependent on the cell type under scrutiny (reviewed in [26]). Intraperitoneal administration of paclitaxel showed excellent clinical results for peritoneal carcinomatosis of ovarian cancer [31, 32] as well as gastric cancer [33, 34]. Docetaxel was reported to be effective against peritoneal carcinomatosis of gastric cancer [35, 36].

5.7 Perioperative intraperitoneal chemotherapy

This kind of chemotherapy aims at delivering drugs directly into the abdominal cavity using the intraperitoneal route of administration. Theoretically, this route of administration has several advantages. The drugs can be delivered at a high dose concentration to the site of recurrence (i.e. peritoneum) with decreased systemic toxicity. Several methods have been described for distributing intraperitoneal chemotherapy in the perioperative phase. They include CHPP, NIPS, HIPEC, EIPL and EPIC (Table 5.2).

Table 5.2. Intraperitoneal chemotherapy strategies [37].

Abbrevation	***Definition***
CHPP	Continuous hyperthermic peritoneal perfusion
NIPS	Neoadjuvant intraperitoneal-systemic chemotherapy
HIPEC	Hyperthermic intraperitoneal chemoperfusion
EIPL	Extensive intraoperative peritoneal lavage
EPIC	Early postoperative intraperitoneal chemotherapy

5.7.1 CHPP

CHPP (Continuous hyperthermic peritoneal perfusion) is a technique proposed 30 years ago by the team of the University of Fukui in Japan, with a focus on gastric cancer therapy. CHPP can be used as a prophylaxis for preventing development of peritoneal cartcinomatosis [38], or as a therapy for established peritoneal carcinomatosis. The authors claim that prophylactic CHPP improves prognosis, and that therapeutic CHPP induces survival benefit for gastric cancer patients with slight to moderate peritoneal dissemination [39]. For treating pseudomyxoma peritonei, CHPP following incomplete tumor resection is effective even without peritonectomy [40]. However, only small retrospectives have been published on CHPP.

5.7.2 NIPS

NIPS is the abbreviation for Neoadjuvant IntraPeritoneal-Systemic chemotherapy and has been proposed by Yonemura et al [41]. Usually, NIPS is combined with cytoreductive surgery (Figure 5.4).

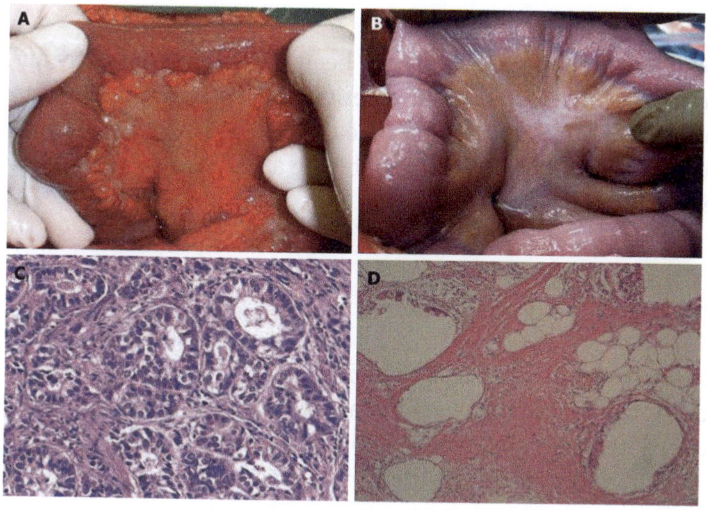

Fig. 5.4. A 48-year-old male patient with PC from gastric cancer treated with NIPS. (a) Macroscopic finding of peritoneal carcinomatosis on bowel mesentery; (b) After 2 courses of NIPS, peritoneal carcinomatosis nodules show fibrotic changes; (c) Histologic findings of peritoneal carcinomatosis nodule obtained at the first operation; (d) Complete degeneration of cancer cells in a peritoneal carcinomatosis nodule obtained at second look operation after NIPS (Reproduced from [37]).

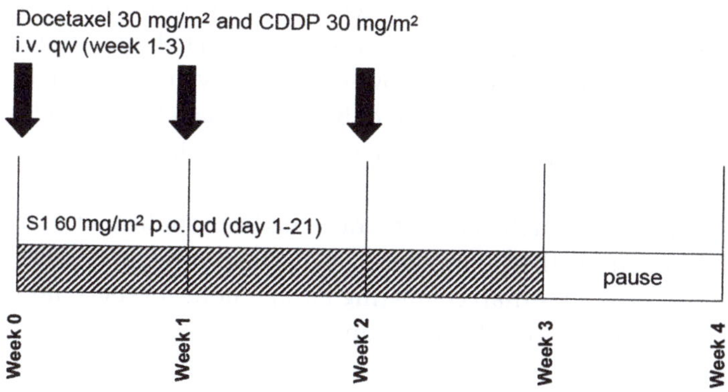

Fig. 5.5. Bidirectional chemotherapy for peritoneal carcinomatosis from gastric cancer (adapted from [37]).

NIPS is a bidirectional chemotherapy protocol aimed at treating peritoneal tumor nodules by direct access through the abdomen and by systemic administration. A possible combination therapy is described in Figure 5.5.

5.7.3 EIPL

EIPL (Extensive intraoperative peritoneal lavage) has been proposed recently by another surgical team from Japan [42] for preventing peritoneal recurrence in patients with peritoneal free cancer cells without overt peritoneal metastasis. A dilution effect is achieved with saline solution that has been found by the authors to be effective in preventing development of peritoneal metastases.

5.7.4 EPIC

For EPIC (Early postoperative intraperitoneal chemotherapy), a catheter is implemented into the peritoneal cavity and connected to a subcutaneous chamber (port-catheter), allowing the repeated application of chemotherapy.

EPIC is relatively common in Asia for gastric cancer, and in North America for ovarian cancer.

For gastric cancer, a meta-analysis summarizing 13 randomized controlled trials has been published. Ten reports were judged to be of fair quality. A significant improvement in survival was associated with hyperthermic intraoperative intraperitoneal chemotherapy (HIPEC) alone or HIPEC combined with early postoperative intraperitoneal chemotherapy (EPIC). There was a trend towards survival improvement with normothermic intraoperative intraperitoneal chemotherapy ($p = 0.06$), but this was not significant with either EPIC alone or delayed postoperative intraperitoneal chemotherapy. Intraperitoneal chemotherapy was also found to be associated with higher risks of intraabdominal abscess [43]. However, disparity in methodology (drugs, dosage, duration of the treatment, addition of hyperthermia, etc.) precludes the adoption of a shared protocol to be used in the clinical practice in high risk patients [44].

For ovarian cancer, IntraPeritoneal (IP) chemotherapy has been studied for years to improve the survival of patients with ovarian cancer. A US prospective randomized trial (Gynecologic Oncology Group 172 trial) comparing intraperitoneal versus intravenous administration of cisplatin-based chemotherapy demonstrated survival benefit for the intraperitoneal arm. This trial was the third randomized controlled trial showing a survival advantage of intraperitoneal chemotherapy in this indication, and on the basis of the meta-analysis of these results, the National Cancer Institute (NCI) released a clinical announcement encouraging the gynecological oncology community to consider intraperitoneal chemotherapy as the standard treatment for optimally debulked advanced ovarian cancer patients. However, there still are controversial issues regarding the use of intraperitoneal chemotherapy (reviewed in [45]) and this therapy is not widely used in Europe, mainly because of the risk of local toxicity, catheter complications and because of the high number of patients interrupting such therapy because of side effects.

ICARuS is the first prospective randomized controlled trial comparing the effectiveness of Early Post-operative Intraperitoneal Chemotherapy (EPIC) and Hyperthermic IntraPEritoneal Chemotherapy (HIPEC) after optimal cytoreductive surgery for neoplasms of the appendix, colon or rectum with isolated peritoneal metastasis [46].

5.8 Intraperitoneal chemotherapy for ascites

This therapeutic approach, directly targeting peritoneal tumor cells, aims at regulating the permeability of the peritoneal membrane and at minimizing systemic toxicities. The best ascites control has been obtained so far with platinum salts, in particular in the management of malignant ascites of ovarian and colorectal origin [47], as well as in peritoneal mesothelioma [48]. Moreover, recent evidence suggests that targeting VEGF may have the potential to suspend the ascites production resulting from peritoneal metastasis (reviewed in [49]) but further clinical studies are necessary. Application of the trivalent antibody catumaxomab is detailed elsewhere in Chapter 5.

5.9 Limitations of intraperitoneal chemotherapy

The rationale for intraperitoneal administration of cytotoxic drugs as an adjunct to surgery is based on theoretical and pharmacokinetic principles. Intraoperative intraperitoneal cytotoxic therapy results in a definite pharmacological advantage, since high peritoneal concentrations are achieved with limited systemic absorption. At present, however, it is not clearly established to what extent this pharmacokinetic advantage results in enhanced anticancer activity and in particular, in a survival benefit [13].

Limitations of intraperitoneal chemotherapy have been reviewed in a seminal article by Flessner [20]. Two pharmacokinetic problems appear to limit the effectiveness of intraperitoneal therapy: poor tumor penetration by the drug and incomplete irrigation of serosal surfaces by the drug-containing solution.

5.9.1 Poor drug penetration

Both theoretical predictions and experimental measurements suggest very limited penetration of drugs into tissues, including tumors, adjacent to the peritoneal cavity

(Table 5.1). This limited penetration may limit the antitumor effect, but it may also protect sensitive normal cells on the mucosal side of the gastrointestinal tract. These problems have been examined in the context of a very simple, spatially distributed model. If D is the diffusivity of the drug in a tissue adjacent to the peritoneal cavity and k is the rate constant for removal of the drug from the tissue by capillary blood, the model predicts that (for slowly reacting drugs) the characteristic penetration distance is $(D/k)^{1/2}$ and the apparent permeability of the surface of a peritoneal structure is $(Dk)^{1/2}$. The permeability area product used in classical pharmacokinetic calculations for the peritoneal cavity as a whole is the sum of the products of the tissue-specific permeabilities and the relevant superficial surface areas. Since the model is mechanistic, it provides insight into the expected effect of procedures such as pharmacologic manipulation or physical mixing.

5.9.2 Poor surface exposition

Various observations in experimental animals suggest limited exposure of the peritoneal surface under conditions of peritoneal dialysis. Adequate quantitative data are not available in human subjects, but the experimental studies predict a major problem. In fact, cancer patients may present additional problems because of their altered peritoneal anatomy with adhesions and postsurgical scarring. Simulated peritoneal dialysis experiments were carried out in anesthetized, supine rats with Evans' blue dye and bovine serum albumin in the dialysis solution [6]. Large parts of the visceral and parietal peritoneum displayed no stain or very little stain. These include one side of the coecum and stomach as well as portions of the small and large intestines and of the diaphragm. These results imply that much of the peritoneal surface has little or no contact with dialysis fluid during quiescent dialysis.

Large changes in tissue penetration may be difficult to achieve but there is little information on the transport characteristics within tumors in this setting or their response to vasoactive drugs. Enhanced mixing is likely to offer significant potential for improved therapy; however, procedures easily applicable to the clinical setting have not been adequately investigated and should be given high priority. The solution of these two problems, poor drug penetration and poor surface exposition, could potentially improve, perhaps dramatically, the efficacy of intraperitoneal chemotherapy.

5.9.3 Local toxicity

Despite the local application of chemotherapy, intraperitoneal chemotherapy is not free of systemic side effects and can be associated with serious complications. The benefits of intraperitoneal chemotherapy should be weighed against its potential harm to maximize efficacy and to minimize morbidity and mortality as much as possible. In nine randomised controlled trials studying 2,119 women receiving primary treatment for ovarian cancer, combined intraperitoneal/intravenous component chemotherapy prolonged the disease-free survival (five studies, 1,311 women) but there was greater serious toxicity with regard to gastrointestinal effects, pain, fever and infection but less totoxicity with the intraperitoneal than the intravenous route [50]. The most frequent grade 3/4 toxicities were neutropenia (48%), gastrointestinal (9%), metabolic (9%), and infection (5%) [51]. In the GOG prospective randomized trial comparing intravenous paclitaxel plus cisplatin with intravenous paclitaxel plus intraperitoneal cisplatin and paclitaxel in patients with stage III ovarian cancer [11], grade 3 and 4 pain, fatigue, and hematologic, gastrointestinal, metabolic, and neurologic toxic effects were more common in the intraperitoneal therapy group than in the intravenous therapy group ($P \leq 0.001$). Only 42% of the patients in the intraperitoneal therapy group completed six cycles of the assigned therapy. In gastric cancer, a recent meta-analysis including ten randomized controlled trials with various forms of intraperitoneal chemotherapy (Hyperthermic intraperitoneal chemotherapy, HIPEC plus postoperative intraperitoneal chemotherapy and normothermic intraoperative intraperitoneal chemotherapy) showed a significant increase in the incidence of bone marrow depression, a significantly higher incidence of fever and intraabdominal abscess. There were no significant differences between intraperitoneal chemotherapy and control for perioperative mortality, anastomotic leakage, ileus, bowel perforation and pancreatic fistula [52]. Thus, the potential for catheter-related complications and toxicity needs to be considered when deciding on the most appropriate treatment for each individual patient.

5.9.4 Peritoneal sclerosis

Exposition of the peritoneal membrane to chemotherapeutic agents causes a chemical peritonitis. It is well known from peritoneal dialysis (PD) patients that repeated peritoneal exposition to bioincompatible solutions induces progressive fibrosis, angiogenesis, ultrafiltration failure and ultimately, peritoneal sclerosis.

Peritoneal fibrosis (or sclerosis) is a term that comprises a wide spectrum of peritoneal structural alterations, ranging from mild inflammation to severe sclerosing peritonitis and its most complicated manifestation, encapsulating peritoneal sclerosis (EPS) (reviewed in [53]). Simple sclerosis (SS), an intermediate stage of peritoneal fibrosis, is the most common peritoneal lesion found in the patients after few months on PD, and could represent the initial phase of sclerosing peritonitis syndrome (SPS). The peritoneum has a normal thickness of 20 μm, but after a few months on peritoneal dialysis could reach up to 40 μm. The sclerosing peritonitis (SP) is a progressive sclerosis that is characterized by a dramatic thickening of the peritoneum (up to 4,000 μm) and is accompanied by inflammatory infiltrates, calcification, neovascularization and dilatation of blood and lymphatic vessels, the thickening being the most commonly used pathological criterion for differential diagnosis.

Peritoneal sclerosis is a severe disease with no effective therapy that can lead to bowel obstruction [54, 55] and, eventually, to death [56]. The development of peritoneal fibrosis is not recognized so far as a significant problem in peritoneal carcinomatosis patients, probably because this problem appears as a "luxury" question in patients with a short life expectation. Such an attitude might be acceptable in advanced, palliative situations but the problem will gain in importance when intraperitoneal chemotherapy might be applied earlier in the natural course of disease, for example as a prophylaxis of peritoneal carcinomatosis in high-risk patients.

By analogy, the intrapleural application of chemotherapy might induce a pleural fibrosis potentially inducing secondary restrictive lung disease. So far, there is a single report of interstitial pneumonia after Hyperthermic IntraThOracic Chemotherapy (HITOC) [57].

5.10 Intraperitoneal immunotherapy

Intraperitoneal immunotherapy is a promising concept for treatment of peritoneal carcinomatosis for several reasons. The use of a specifically engineered therapy in terms of antibodies or stimulated T-lymphocytes against epithelial tumor antigens offers an elegant way to attack tumors on the peritoneal surface, as peritoneal cells have a mesenchymal origin (reviewed in [58]).

5.10.1 Catumaxomab

Catumaxomab is a trifunctional bispecific monoclonal antibody with two binding sites directed to the epithelial cell adhesion molecule (EpCAM) and the T-cell antigen CD3. With its Fc-fragment, catumaxomab additionally binds accessory cells, including dendritic cells, macrophages, and natural killer cells. The trifunctional approach thus leads to a major histocompatibility complex-unrestricted but specific killing of epithelial tumor cells without the need for preactivation or external costimulation. Catumaxomab has been approved in Europe for the intraperitoneal treatment of malignant ascites in patients with EpCAM-positive epithelial tumors where standard therapy is not available or no longer feasible [59]. Because EpCAM is expressed in most solid tumors, but not in tissue of mesothelial origin, intraperitoneal treatment with catumaxomab is tumor-specific. Intraperitoneal treatment with catumaxomab resulted in a significant prolongation of puncture-free survival in patients with malignant ascites due to epithelial cancer. Puncture-free survival was significantly longer in the catumaxomab group (median 46 days) than the control group (median 11 days) as was median time to next paracentesis (77 versus 13 days) [60]. In addition, catumaxomab patients had fewer signs and symptoms of ascites than control patients. Treatment with catumaxomab significantly delayed deterioration in patient quality of life [61]. However, adverse events associated with catumaxomab were frequent: 58% patients experienced serious adverse events, of whom 15% were considered to be treatment related. The most common adverse events were fever, nausea, vomiting and abdominal pain. These events were generally mild to moderate in intensity and reversible.

5.10.2 Bevacizumab

Vascular endothelial growth factor A (VEGF-A) is a key mediator of angiogenesis, and bevacizumab, a humanized variant of an anti-VEGF antibody, has shown significant efficacy in combination with chemotherapy and is now widely used for metastatic colorectal cancer [62]. VEGF is markedly elevated in malignant ascites, where it worsens the condition by increasing endothelial cell permeability [63]. Therefore, VEGF inhibition in the peritoneal cavity is considered beneficial, not only as an inhibitor of tumorigenesis but also as an inhibitor of malignant ascites formation [49], although no clinical trials addressing the use of bevacizumab with intraperitoneal chemotherapy have been reported. However, bevacizumab might be administered systemically, because it is rapidly absorbed from the peritoneum and enters the systemic circulation when administered by intraperitoneal injection [64, 65].

5.10.3 Immunoradiotherapy

Immunoradiotherapy has been proposed to treat intraperitoneal disease (reviewed in [66]. Due to the generally slow and incomplete transit of intraperitoneally infused agents into the circulation, treating disease confined to the peritoneal cavity with radionuclides provides a pharmacologic advantage. A higher intraperitoneal concentration can be achieved than could be tolerated by systemic administration. Non-targeted intraperitoneal 32P radionuclide therapy has been used in the treatment of ovarian cancer for more than three decades, but side effects have been problematic. Efforts to improve specificity have used a number of antigens expressed on ovarian cancer cells as targets for selective delivery of radionuclide-conjugates. Targeted therapy using radionuclides such as α-, β- and Auger emitters coupled to antibodies seems a promising option. Although β-emitters have shown promising results in preclinical and clinical Phase I/II studies, these results could not be confirmed in randomized controlled trials studies. Because α-particles very efficiently eradicate small tumor cell nodules, they represent a promising option for treatment of micrometastatic disease characteristic of peritoneal carcinomatosis. Although confirmation of these results in clinical trials is missing and problems still exist concerning worldwide availability, α-emitters could contribute to optimizing strategies for therapy of peritoneal carcinomatosis [67].

5.11 Intraperitoneal cytolytic virotherapy

A novel approach for treating therapy-resistant peritoneal carcinomatosis is locoregional administration of viruses exhibiting oncolytic properties. Oncolytic viruses and gene therapy have been actively investigated as a new way of treating cancer [68]. After extensive investigations in cell lines and animal models, a phase I/II study [69] was designed in patients with refractory peritoneal carcinomatosis to assess the activity and safety of GL-ONC1, a recombinant vaccinia virus (VACV) genetically engineered to selectively replicate in and destroy cancer cells. GL-ONC1 was administered intraperitoneally up to four times every 28 days under a standard 3+3 dose escalation design. Antitumor activity was determined by "fluid biopsies" obtained via repetitive paracenteses and by serial PET-CT scans. Four patients have received ten doses of GL-ONC1 ranging from 10^7 to 10^8 infectious viral particles per application. Adverse events have generally been limited to grade 1/2, being mostly transient flu-like symptoms as well as increased abdominal pain resulting from treatment-induced peritonitis. In one gastric cancer patient, effective intraperitoneal replication of GL-ONC1 was demonstrated for more than three weeks. Of note, VACV-positive cancer cells morphologically showed significant degenerative changes. These preliminary data demonstrate that GL-ONC1 is well tolerated when infused intraperitoneally. Importantly, a single intraperitoneal delivery of GL-ONC1 was found to be sufficient to cause a dramatic decline in the number of malignant cells in the ascitic fluid, suggesting that GL-ONC1 effectively removes tumor cells in the ascites of patients with peritoneal carcinomatosis [70]. Vascularization of peritoneal nodes appear to play an important role in such intraperitoneal oncolytic viral therapy [71].

5.12 Nanodrugs

Nanodrugs are a new type of drug formulation, 20–100 nm in molecular diameter, significantly smaller than conventional drugs (reviewed in [72]). Nanodrugs effectively accumulate in tumor tissue due to enhanced permeability and retention (EPR) [73], which results in enhanced antitumor effects and less toxicity in normal tissues. The EPR effect is based on the particular characteristics of solid tumor tissues, such as incomplete vascular architecture, hyperpermeability of tumor vessel walls, and immature lymphatic drainage. Based on this concept, various kinds of nanodrugs have been developed for cancer treatment [74–77]. For example, Abraxane®, an albumin-bound paclitaxel, is currently in clinical use for breast, lung, and gastric cancer [78, 79]. NK105 is a paclitaxel-incorporating "core-shell-type" polymeric micellar nanoparticle formulation [80, 81]. PMB-30W is a water-soluble, amphiphilic polymer composed of 2-methacryloxyethyl phosphorylcholine and N-butyl methacrylate enables the construction of paclitaxel-containing nanoparticles of approximately 50 nm diameter [82]. Intraperitoneal administration of paclitaxel formulated with PMB-30W resulted in deeper tissue penetration into peritoneal nodules and exhibited enhanced antitumor effects against peritoneal xenografts of human gastric cancer as compared to conventional cremophor-conjugated paclitaxel in a murine model [83, 84]. In the same model, intraperitoneal administration of NK105 was also shown to enhance antitumor effects, compared with intraperitoneal taxotere [85]. Intraperitoneal chemotherapy with nanoparticulate drugs might be a promising strategy for the treatment of peritoneal carcinomatosis.

5.13 Combined CRS with HIPEC

Cytoreductive surgery followed by hyperthermic intraperitoneal chemotherapy has developed as a treatment for patients with peritoneal carcinomatosis during the last 20 years [86, 87]. A comprehensive, evidence-based review [88] of CRS and HIPEC has recently been published by the British NHS and these guidelines are largely cited in this chapter [89].

5.13.1 Cytoreductive surgery (CRS)

The cytoreductive procedure involves removal of the maximum amount of the visible (macroscopic) tumor through a series of peritonectomy procedures (greater and lesser omentectomies, right and left upper quadrant peritonectomies, and anterior parietal and pelvic peritonectomies) with resection of involved nonessential organs as required. The exact scope of the surgery depends on the visible spread of the tumor and must be determined individually in each patient [90, 91].

Completeness of Cytoreduction Score

In peritoneal carcinomatosis, it is difficult to apply the R-classification of the UICC, since microscopic determination of tumor involvement of resection margins is virtually impossible when hundreds of peritoneal nodes are resected.

Therefore, in peritoneal cancer, a "Completeness of Cytoreduction Score" (CC) has been proposed to assess the success of a cytoreductive surgery, by determining the size of the residual tumor (Table 5.3). The CC score is useful for standardizing surgical cytoreduction within clinical studies, and to compare results from different studies. Moreover, it has been shown to have prognostic value in pseudomyxoma peritonei, peritoneal carcinomatosis from colon cancer, sarcomatosis, peritoneal mesothelioma, and ovarian cancer [92].

Although no formal statement in the literature is available, it is thought that the definition of complete versus incomplete cytoreduction varies with the histologic type of the malignancy. For example, mucinous tumors by diffusion are well penetrated with intraperitoneal chemotherapy solutions. With minimally invasive mucinous tumors such as pseudomyxoma peritonei, complete cytoreduction may occur in the combined treatment plan with tumor nodules up to a full centimeter in size. In contrast, hard fibrotic nonmucinous colon cancer is poorly penetrated by a chemotherapy solution. Only cytoreduction down to no visible evidence of disease would be expected to result in long-term survival with a sclerotic malignant process. Also, some cancers may be remarkably more responsive to chemotherapy than others. This is likely the case with a majority of ovarian cancers. Their complete response to systemic chemotherapy is also frequently seen with intraperitoneal chemotherapy solutions or a bidirectional (intraperitoneal combined with intravenous chemotherapy) approach. In both these situations the definition of a complete cytoreduction scored by a CC-1 designation would vary with the clinical situation [93].

The evidence suggests that the completeness of cytoreduction is an important determinant of effectiveness, and therefore this parameter should be monitored where the procedure is undertaken [89]

5.13.2 Hyperthermic IntraPEritoneal Chemotherapy (HIPEC)

Hyperthermic intraperitoneal chemotherapy involves flushing the abdominal cavity with a chemotherapy agent. This can be performed either as an open or closed procedure. The therapeutic aim is to achieve a high local concentration of chemotherapy in the peritoneal cavity and absorption of the substance into the superficial cell layers and therefore cause only minimal systemic toxic side effects from the cytostatic medication. Heating the chemotherapy agent increases its therapeutic effect by improving penetration of the tissue [90, 94].

Patient selection for the treatment of peritoneal carcinomatosis associating cytoreductive surgery and HIPEC depends on three conditions. First, physical and health status of the patient should be good enough to tolerate an aggressive combination therapy with surgery and chemotherapy. Second, tumors have to be completely resectable, which in practice excludes patients with diffuse small bowel involvement. Third, a progression of peritoneal carcinomatosis under systemic chemotherapy should be a contraindication (with the exception of pseudomyxoma peritonei and

Table 5.3. Completeness of cytoreduction (CC) score.

Score	Residual tumor
CC-0	No residual disease
CC-1	Residual disease < 0.25 cm
CC-2	0.25 cm < Residual disease < 2.5 cm
CC-3	Residual disease > 2.5 cm

peritoneal mesothelioma, which are primitive carcinomatosis and frequently not sensitive to systemic chemotherapy).

5.13.3 Colorectal cancer

In April 2014, the NHS published a literature search revealing a cohort study considering the outcomes of those patients with disease of colorectal origin [95].

The review of the literature also yielded two randomised controlled trials each comparing different hyperthermic intraperitoneal chemotherapeutic agents [96, 97].

Also found were a number of studies including a consecutive case-series [98], case-series [99], and case-series from registries [100, 101], the results of which are in accord with the other studies. One trial registration filing [102] for a randomised control trial comparing cytoreduction surgery plus hyperthermic intraperitoneal chemotherapy to standard care was identified. This trial is not expected to report until 2017.

The international consensus statement on peritoneal carcinomatosis produced by representatives from Germany, Netherlands, USA, Italy, Japan, Spain, Australia, France and Israel [103] describes a "paradigm change" away from a fatalistic approach and toward a potentially curative approach using cytoreduction surgery and hyperthermic intraperitoneal chemotherapy as being "justified by the current state of the international data". Specifically they note the high quality randomised controlled trial (evidence grade 1b) that shows a clear survival benefit [1, 104]. In an intention-to-treat analysis in August 2007, after a median follow up of 94 months, patients in the standard arm had a median survival of 12.6 months compared to the median survival of patients in the experimental arm of 22.2 months ($p = 0.028$). The six-year survival was 5% in the standard arm and 20% in the experimental arm.

The meta-analysis by Cao et al. [105] showed little difference between cytoreduction and early postoperative intraperitoneal chemotherapy. It only included the first three years of the Verwaal [104] study where much clearer benefits are shown in the longer term data [1]. These longer term data show a five-year survival of 45%. Criteria for entry into the trial were under 71 years of age and fit for major abdominal surgery. Compared, indirectly, with the five-year stage-specific relative survival rates for ovarian cancer from the Anglia Cancer Network for the period 2004–2008 survival is improved. In this registry for adults (15–99 years) the more usual five-year survival for patients with peritoneal carcinomatosis would be between 6% (stage IV disease) and 22% (Stage III disease) [106]. A large multicentre cohort [95] also showed five-year survival of 27% (evidence grade 2b).

When delivered by surgeons and units with the experience and expertise in achieving high rates of complete cytoreduction, it provides a significant survival benefit in peritoneal carcinomatosis secondary to colorectal carcinoma.

5.13.4 Ovarian Cancer

The review of the literature of the NHS [89] found three reviews [50, 107, 108], one randomised controlled trial of chemotherapy versus primary surgery (EORTC-NCIC) [109], and one trial that replicated the protocol of the EORTC-NCIC randomised trial [110]. Also found were: one retrospective case-control study of cytoreduction surgery plus hyperthermic intraperitoneal chemotherapy versus cytoreduction surgery [111], one retrospective case series [112], one large consecutive-case series [113] and one nonrandomised phase II efficacy trial of cytoreduction surgery plus hyperthermic intraperitoneal chemotherapy [114].

Two of the systematic reviews [107, 108] identified only low quality evidence in the form of retrospective studies with significant risk in their design of bias. The third systematic review found much higher quality evidence but compared systematic chemotherapy with a range of regimes using intraperitoneal chemotherapy at some point in their care pathway [50]. The meta-analysis with this review showed a clear benefit of treatment regimes that included intraperitoneal chemotherapy. The randomised controlled trial of chemotherapy versus primary surgery by Vergote et al. [109] showed no difference between chemotherapy and cytoreduction surgery HR 0.98 (90% confidence interval [CI], 0.84 to 1.13). However, this trial had a very low proportion of patients who had residual disease less than 1 cm (41.6%). This is much lower than most trials in this area report, so applicability may be limited. Retrospective case analysis following the same protocol as this randomised trial [110] had 71% of patients with residual disease of less than 1 cm, and a significant survival benefit in the uncontrolled treatment arm with median overall survival of 50 months. This proportion of patients with complete cytoreduction is much more in keeping with that more generally published, and given the strongly identified link between completeness of cytoreduction and survival this calls into question the possible extrapolation of the results (no difference in outcomes between chemotherapy and cytoreduction surgery) made by Vergote et al. [109].

Thus, success rates of CRS and HIPEC in ovarian cancer appear to depend on careful patient selection. When delivered by surgeons and units with the experience and expertise in achieving high rates of complete cytoreduction it provides a significant survival benefit in peritoneal carcinomatosis secondary to ovarian carcinoma.

5.13.5 Gastric Cancer

Since the NICE review [90] of cytoreduction surgery there have been randomised control trials published of its use in peritoneal carcinomatosis secondary to gastric carcinoma. However the randomised controlled trials [115, 116] only considered the additional benefits of hyperthermic intraperitoneal chemotherapy when added to cytoreduction surgery. These trials showed positive benefits to the combination of cytoreduction surgery and hyperthermic intraperitoneal chemotherapy compared to cytoreduction surgery alone, in keeping with the retrospective multicenter cohort series [117].

These studies do not consider the primary question of the effects of cytoreduction surgery plus hyperthermic intraperitoneal chemotherapy compared to systemic chemotherapy. However, they do provide evidence that there are additional benefits of hyperthermic intraperitoneal chemotherapy when used with cytoreduction surgery in peritoneal carcinomatosis secondary to gastric carcinoma. There is also clear evidence of the survival benefits with improving completeness of the cytoreduction procedure [115, 117–120].

Thus, cytoreduction surgery plus hyperthermic intraperitoneal chemotherapy is more effective than cytoreduction surgery alone in gastric carcinoma, but the literature has not yet explored its specific benefit over systemic chemotherapy.

5.13.6 Learning curve and expertise

There was a clear theme within all the available literature relating to what might loosely be called “expertise”. The cytoreduction surgery places heavy demand on the surgical team [31] with the operations lasting 8–12 hours [121–123] and requiring a meticulous approach. There is a clearly described learning curve in performing these procedures [94, 124, 125].

A prognostic factor repeatedly reported across the literature for peritoneal carcinomatosis secondary to colorectal, ovarian and gastric carcinomas, is completeness of cytoreduction [89]. So if we can take completeness of cytoreduction as a marker of surgical technique then there is a clear correlation between surgical technique and outcome. Institutional experience is specifically noted as an important factor in toxicity and being an independent prognostic factor [118].

This is an important policy consideration that has not yet come to prominence in the reviews of the evidence. It is a consideration of particular importance in the interpretation of the randomised controlled trial of chemotherapy versus primary surgery in ovarian carcinoma (EORTC-NCIC) [109], as is clearly shown by the trial that replicated its protocol [110].

5.13.7 Evidence of cost effectiveness

No cost or cost effectiveness studies were published for cytoreductive surgery and HIPEC.

5.13.8 Safety

The NHS review also reported on the safety characteristics of cytoreduction surgery and hyperthermic intraperitoneal chemotherapy. The 11 papers reporting safety characteristics identified cover colorectal, gastric, and ovarian carcinomas and include all the most recent paper reporting morbidity [89]. In general 30-day mortality is less than 5% with some trials and series showing 0% 30-day mortality. Major complications occurred between 15–40% (and might commonly include paralytic ileus and more rarely some of the following: pneumonia, pancreatitis, pneumothorax, intraabdominal abscess, renal failure, urine bladder dysfunction, wound infection, pleural effusion, thrombosis, cardiac arrhythmia, pulmonary embolism, and re-operation). These are generally in line with other major abdominal operations.

5.13.9 Indications for CRS and HIPEC

A stringent patient selection is a precondition to achieve clinical benefit, taking into consideration not only the expected postoperative mortality and morbidity, but also the long-term oncological results. Thus, CRS associated with HIPEC for the treatment of peritoneal carcinomatosis should be performed only in younger patients with limited and resectable carcinomatosis, and carried out only by specialized centers with enough expertise [126]. The best level of evidence for this guideline is given for colorectal cancer.

Bibliography

[1] Verwaal VJ, Bruin S, Boot H et al. 8-year follow up of randomized trial: cytoreduction and hyperthermic intraperitoneal chemotherapy versus systemic chemotherapy in patients with peritoneal carcinomatosis of colorectal cancer. Ann Surg Oncol 5 (2008) 2426–2432.

[2] Elias D, Lefevre JH, Chevalier J et al. Complete Cytoreductive Surgery Plus Intraperitoneal Chemohyperthermia With Oxaliplatinum for Peritoneal Carcinomatosis of Colorectal Origin. J Clin Oncol 7 (2 2009) 681–685.

[3] Rivera F, Vega-Villegas ME, López-Brea MF. Chemotherapy of advanced gastric cancer. Cancer Treat Rev. 33, 4 (Jun 2007) 315–324.

[4] Klaver YL, Lemmens VE, Creemers GJ, Rutten HJ, Nienhuijs SW, de Hingh IH. Population-based survival of patients with peritoneal carcinomatosis from colorectal origin in the era of increasing use of palliative chemotherapy. Ann Oncol. 22, 10 (Oct 2011) 2250–2256.

[5] Jacquet P, Sugarbaker PH. Peritoneal-plasma barrier. Cancer Treat Res. 82 (1996) 53–63.

[6] Ceelen WP, Flessner MF. Intraperitoneal therapy for peritoneal tumors: biophysics and clinical evidence. Nat Rev Clin Oncol. 7 (2010) 108–115.

[7] Warrick C. An improvement on the practice of tapping; whereby that operation, instead of a relief for symptoms, becomes an absolute cure for an ascites, exemplified in the case of Jane roman; and recommended to the consideration of the royal Society, by Christopher Warrick, of Truro, Surgeon. Philos. Trans. R. Soc. Lond. B. Biol. Sci 43, 12–19 (1744).

[8] Weisberger AS, Levine B, Storaasli JP. Use of nitrogen mustard in treatment of serous effusions of neoplastic origin. J. Am. Med. Assoc. 159, 1704–1707 (1955).

[9] Alberts DS et al. Intraperitoneal cisplatin plus intravenous cyclophosphamide versus intravenous cisplatin plus intravenous cyclophosphamide for stage III ovarian cancer. N. Engl. J. Med. 335 (1996) 1950–1955.

[10] Markman M et al. Phase III trial of standard-dose intravenous cisplatin plus paclitaxel versus moderately high-dose carboplatinum followed by intravenous paclitaxel and intraperitoneal cisplatin in small-volume stage III ovarian carcinoma: an intergroup study of the Gynecologic Oncology Group, Southwestern Oncology Group, and Eastern Cooperative Oncology Group. J. Clin. Oncol. 19, 1001–1007 (2001).

[11] Armstrong DK, Bundy B, Wenzel L, Huang HQ, Baergen R, Lele S, Copeland LJ, Walker JL, Burger RA, Gynecologic Oncology Group. Intraperitoneal cisplatin and paclitaxel in ovarian cancer. N Engl J Med. 354, 1 (Jan 5 2006) 34–43.

[12] Minchinton AI, Tannock IF. Drug penetration in solid tumors. Nat Rev Cancer 6 (2006) 583–592,.

[13] Ceelen WP, Påhlman L, Mahteme H. Pharmacodynamic aspects of intraperitoneal cytotoxic therapy. Cancer Treat Res. 134 (2007) 195–214. Review.

[14] Jain RK. Transport of molecules in the tumor interstitium: a review. Cancer Res. 47, 12 (Jun 15 1987) 3039–3051. Review.

[15] Stapleton S et al. A mathematical model of the enhanced permeability and retention effect for liposome transport in solid tumors. PLoS One. 8, 12 (Dec 2 2013) e7 (8115).

[16] Van der Speeten K, Stuart OA, Sugarbaker PH. Using pharmacologic data to plan clinical treatments for patients with peritoneal surface malignancy. Curr Drug Discov Technol. 6, 1 (Mar 2009) 72–81. Review.

[17] Rippe B, Haraldsson B. Transport of macromolecules across microvascular walls: the two-pore theory. Physiol. Rev. 74(1), 163–219, (1994).

[18] Yuan F, Dellian M, Fukumura D, Leunig M, Berk DA, Torchillin VP, Jain RK. Vascular permeability in a human tumor xenograft: molecular size dependence and cutoff size. Cancer Res. 55(17), 3752–3756, (1995).

[19] Flessner MF, Choi J, Credit K, Deverkadra R, Henderson K. Resistance of tumor interstitial pressure to the penetration of intraperitoneally delivered
antibodies into metastatic ovarian tumors. Clin. Cancer Res. 11(8), 3117–3125, (2005).

[20] Flessner MF. The transport barrier in intraperitoneal therapy. Am J Physiol Renal Physiol. 288, 3 (Mar 2005) F433–F442. Review.

[21] Li XF. et al. Visualization of hypoxia in microscopic tumors by immunofluorescent microscopy. *Cancer Res.* 67, 7646–7653 (2007).

[22] Jakobsen A, Mortensen LS. On the importance of sensitivity to the dose-effect relationship in chemotherapy. *Acta Oncol.* 36, 375–381 (1997).

[23] Alberts DS, Young L, Mason N, Salmon SE. In vitro evaluation of anticancer drugs against ovarian cancer at concentrations achievable by intraperitoneal administration. Semin. Oncol. 12, 38–42 (1985).

[24] Andrews PA, velury S, Mann SC, Howell SB. Cis-Diamminedichloroplatinum(Ii) accumulation in sensitive and resistant human ovarian carcinoma sells. *Cancer Res.* 48 (1988) 68–73.

[25] Rossi CR, Mocellin S, Pilati P, Foletto M, Quintieri L, Palatini P, Lise M. Pharmacokinetics of intraperitoneal cisplatin and doxorubicin. Surg Oncol Clin N Am. 12, 3 (Jul 2003) 781–794. Review.

[26] Yan TD, Cao CQ, Munkholm-Larsen S. A pharmacological review on intraperitoneal chemotherapy for peritoneal malignancy. World J Gastrointest Oncol. 2, 2 (Feb 15 2010) 109–116.

[27] Rietbroek RC, vandeVaart PJM, Haveman J, Blommaert FA, Geerdink A, Bakker PJM, Veenhof CHN. Hyperthermia enhances the cytotoxicity and platinum-DNA adduct formation of lobaplatinum and oxaliplatin in cultured SW 1573 cells. J Cancer Res Clin Oncol 123, 1 (1997) 6–12.

[28] Elias D, Bonnay A, Puizillou JM, Antoun S, Demirdjian S, El Otmany A, Pignon JP, Drouard-Troalen L, Ouellet JF, Ducreux M. Heated intraoperative intraperitoneal oxaliplatin after complete resection of peritoneal carcinomatosis: pharmacokinetics and tissue distribution. Ann Oncol 13, 2 (2002) 267–272.

[29] Markman M, Reichman B, Hakes T, Lewis JL, Jones W, Rubin S, Barakat R, Curtin J, Almadrones L, Hoskins W. Impact on Survival of Surgically Defined Favorable Responses to Salvage Intraperitoneal Chemotherapy in Small-Volume Residual Ovarian-Cancer. J Clin Oncol 10, 9 (1992) 1479–1484.

[30] Hofstra LS, Bos AME, de Vries EGE, van der Zee AGJ, Willemsen ATM, Rosing H, Beijnen JH, Mulder NH, Aalders JG, Willemse PHB. Kinetic modeling and efficacy of intraperitoneal paclitaxel combined with intravenous cyclophosphamide and carboplatinum as first-line treatment in ovarian cancer. Gynecol Oncol 85, 3 (2002) 517–523.

[31] Rufian S, Munoz-Casares FC, Briceno J, Diaz CJ, Rubio MJ, Ortega R, et al. Radical surgery-peritonectomy and intraoperative intraperitoneal chemotherapy for the treatment of peritoneal carcinomatosis in recurrent or primary ovarian cancer. *J Surg Oncol.* 94 (2006) 316–324.

[32] Armstrong DK, Fleming GF, Markman M, Bailey HH. A phase I trial of intraperitoneal sustained-release paclitaxel microspheres (Paclimer) in recurrent ovarian cancer: a Gynecologic Oncology Group study. *Gynecol Oncol.* 103 (2006) 391–396.

[33] Ishigami H, Kitayama J, Kaisaki S, Hidemura A, Kato M, Otani K, et al. Phase II study of weekly intravenous and intraperitoneal paclitaxel combined with S-1 for advanced gastric cancer with peritoneal metastasis. *Ann Oncol – Off J Eur Soc Med Oncol/ESMO.* 21 (2010) 67–70.

[34] Kitayama J, Ishigami H, Yamaguchi H, Yamashita H, Emoto S, Kaisaki S, et al. Salvage gastrectomy after intravenous and intraperitoneal paclitaxel (PTX) administration with oral S-1 for peritoneal dissemination of advanced gastric cancer with malignant ascites. *Ann Surg Oncol.* 21, 2 (Feb 2014) 539–546.

[35] Fushida S, Kinoshita J, Kaji M, Hirono Y, Goda F, Yagi Y, et al. Phase I/II study of intraperitoneal docetaxel plus S-1 for the gastric cancer patients with peritoneal carcinomatosis. *Cancer Chemother Pharmacol.* 71 (2013) 1265–1272.

[36] Fujiwara Y, Takiguchi S, Nakajima K, Miyata H, Yamasaki M, Kurokawa Y, et al. Neoadjuvant intraperitoneal and systemic chemotherapy for gastric cancer patients with peritoneal dissemination. *Ann Surg Oncol.* 18 (2011) 3726–3731.

[37] Yonemura Y et al. Multidisciplinary therapy for treatment of patients with peritoneal carcinomatosis from gastric cancer. World J Gastrointest Oncol. 2 (2010) 85–97.

[38] Yonemura Y, Ninomiya I, Kaji M, Sugiyama K, Fujimura K, Sawa T, Katayama K, Tanaka S, Hirono Y, Miwa K et al. Prophylaxis with intraoperative chemohyperthermia against peritoneal recurrence of serosal invasion-positive gastric cancer. World J Surg. 19, 3 (May/Jun 1995) 450–454.

[39] Hirono Y, Katayama K, Murakami M, Iida A, Yamaguchi A. [Intraperitoneal chemotherapy in gastric cancer patients with peritoneal dissemination]. Gan To Kagaku Ryoho. 32, 10 (Oct 2005) 1404–1409.

[40] Katayama K, Yamaguchi A, Murakami M, Koneri K, Nagano H, Honda K, Hirono Y, Goi T, Iida A, Ito H. Chemo-hyperthermic peritoneal perfusion (CHPP) for appendiceal pseudomyxoma peritonei. Int J Clin Oncol. 14, 2 (Apr 2009) 120–124.

[41] Yonemura Y, Elnemr A, Endou Y, Ishibashi H, Mizumoto A, Miura M, Li Y. Effects f neoadjuvant intraperitoneal/systemic chemotherapy (bidirectional chemotherapy) or the treatment of patients with peritoneal metastasis from gastric cancer. Int Surg Oncol. 2012 (2012) 148420.
[42] Kuramoto M, Shimada S, Ikeshima S, Matsuo A, Kuhara H, Eto K, Baba H. A proposal of a practical and optimal prophylactic strategy for peritoneal recurrence. J Oncol. 2012 (2012) 340380.
[43] Yan TD, Black D, Sugarbaker PH, Zhu J, Yonemura Y, Petrou G, Morris DL. A systematic review and meta-analysis of the randomized controlled trials on adjuvant intraperitoneal chemotherapy for resectable gastric cancer. Ann Surg Oncol. 14, 10 (Oct 2007) 2702–2713.
[44] Bozzetti F, Yu W, Baratti D, Kusamura S, Deraco M. Locoregional treatment of peritoneal carcinomatosis from gastric cancer. J Surg Oncol. 98, 4 (Sep 15 2008) 273–276.
[45] Fujiwara K, Armstrong D, Morgan M, Markman M. Principles and practice of intraperitoneal chemotherapy for ovarian cancer. Int J Gynecol Cancer. 17, 1 (Jan/Feb 2007) 1–20. Review.
[46] www.clinicaltrials.gov, NCT9 (0181535) consulted on 30.4.2014.
[47] Schilsky RL, Choi KE, Grayhack J et al. Phase I clinical and pharmacologic study of intraperitoneal cisplatin and fluorouracil in patients with advanced intraabdominal cancer. J Clin Oncol 8 (1990) 2054–2061.
[48] Markman M, Kelsen D. Efficacy of cisplatin-based intraperitoneal chemotherapy as treatment of malignant peritoneal mesothelioma. J Cancer Res Clin Oncol 118 (1992) 547–550.
[49] Kobold S, Hegewisch-Becker S, Oechsle K, Jordan K, Bokemeyer C, Atanackovic D. Intraperitoneal VEGF inhibition using bevacizumab: a potential approach for the symptomatic treatment of malignant ascites? Oncologist. 14, 12 (Dec 2009) 1242–1251.
[50] Jaaback K, Johnson N, Lawrie TA. Intraperitoneal chemotherapy for the initial management of primary epithelial ovarian cancer. Cochrane Database Syst Rev. 9, 11 (Nov 2011) CD005340.
[51] Teefey P, Bou Zgheib N, Apte SM, Gonzalez-Bosquet J, Judson PL, Roberts WS, Lancaster JM, Wenham RM. Factors associated with improved toxicity and tolerability of intraperitoneal chemotherapy in advanced-stage epithelial ovarian cancers. Am J Obstet Gynecol. 208, 6 (Jun 2013) 501.e1–.e7.
[52] Huang JY, Xu YY, Sun Z, Zhu Z, Song YX, Guo PT, You Y, Xu HM. Comparison of different methods of intraoperative and intraperitoneal chemotherapy for patients with gastric cancer: a meta-analysis. Asian Pac J Cancer Prev. 13, 9 (2012) 4379–4385.
[53] Aguilera A, Loureiro J, Gonzalez-Mateo G et al. The Mesothelial to Mesenchymal Transition: a Pathogeneioc and Therapeutic Key for Peritoneral Sclerosis. http://dx.doi.org/10.5772/56598, consulted on 26.4.2014.
[54] Chan WS, Bohmer R, McIntosh R, Blomfield P. Peritoneal fibrosis leading to small bowel obstruction two years after first-line intraperitoneal chemotherapy for optimally debulked ovarian cancer. Aust N Z J Obstet Gynaecol. 51, 1 (Feb 2011) 91–92.
[55] Vlasveld LT, Taal BG, Kroon BB, Gallee MP, Rodenhuis S. Intestinal obstruction due to diffuse peritoneal fibrosis at 2 years after the successful treatment malignant peritoneal mesothelioma with intraperitoneal mitoxantrone. Cancer Chemother Pharmacol. 29, 5 (1992) 405–408. Erratum in: Cancer Chemother Pharmacol 30, 3 (1992) 249.
[56] Minutolo V, Gagliano G, Angirillo G, Minutolo O, Morello A, Rinzivillo C. Intestinal obstruction due to idiopathic sclerosing encapsulating peritonitis. Clinical report and review of literature. G Chir. 29, 4 (Apr 2008) 173–176. Review.
[57] Zappa L, Savady R, Humphries GN, Sugarbaker PH. Interstitial pneumonitis following intrapleural chemotherapy. World J Surg Oncol. 7 (Feb 12 2009) 17.
[58] Ströhlein MA, Heiss MM. Immunotherapy of peritoneal carcinomatosis. Cancer Treat Res. 134 (2007) 483–491.

[59] Sebastian M. Review of catumaxomab in the treatment of malignant ascites. Cancer Manag Res. 2 (Nov 8 2010) 283–286.

[60] Heiss MM, Murawa P, Koralewski P et al. The trifunctional antibody catumaxomab for the treatment of malignant ascites due to epithelial cancer: Results of a prospective randomized phase II/III trial. Int J Cancer. 127, 9 (Nov 1 2010) 2209–2221.

[61] Wimberger P, Gilet H, Gonschior AK, Heiss MM, Moehler M, Oskay-Oezcelik G et al. Deterioration in quality of life (QoL) in patients with malignant ascites: results from a phase II/III study comparing paracentesis plus catumaxomab with paracentesis alone. *Ann Oncol – Off J Eur Soc Med Oncol/ESMO*. 23 (2012) 1979–1985.

[62] Hurwitz H, Fehrenbacher L, Novotny W, Cartwright T, Hainsworth J, Heim W, et al. Bevacizumab plus irinotecan, fluorouracil, and leucovorin for metastatic colorectal cancer. *N Engl J Med*. 350 (2004) 2335–2342.

[63] Zebrowski BK, Liu W, Ramirez K, Akagi Y, Mills GB, Ellis LM. Markedly elevated levels of vascular endothelial growth factor in malignant ascites. *Ann Surg Oncol*. 6 (1999) 373–378.

[64] Yagi Y, Fushida S, Harada S, Tsukada T, Kinoshita J, Oyama K, et al. Biodistribution of humanized anti-VEGF monoclonal antibody/bevacizumab on peritoneal metastatic models with subcutaneous xenograft of gastric cancer in mice. *Cancer Chemother Pharmacol*. 66 (2010) 745–753.

[65] Shah DK, Veith J, Bernacki RJ, Balthasar JP. Evaluation of combined bevacizumab and intraperitoneal carboplatinum or paclitaxel therapy in a mouse model of ovarian cancer. *Cancer Chemother Pharmacol*. 68 (2011) 951–958.

[66] Meredith RF, Buchsbaum DJ, Alvarez RD, LoBuglio AF. Brief overview of preclinical and clinical studies in the development of intraperitoneal radioimmunotherapy for ovarian cancer. Clin Cancer Res. 13, 18 Pt 2 (Sep 2007) 5643s–5645s.

[67] Seidl C, Essler M. Radioimmunotherapy for peritoneal cancers. Immunotherapy. 5, 4 (Apr 2013) 395–405.

[68] Parato KA, Senger D, Forsyth PA, Bell JC. Recent progress in the battle between oncolytic viruses and tumors. Nat Rev Cancer. 5 (2005) 965–976.

[69] www.clinicaltrials.gov (NCT01443260), consulted on 28.4.2014.

[70] Lauer U, Zimmermann M, Sturm J et al. Phase I/II clinical trial of a genetically modified and oncolytic vaccinia virus GL-ONC1 in patients with unresactable, chemotherapy-resistant peritoneal carcinomatosis. J Clin Oncol 31, (2013) (suppl abstr 3098).

[71] Ottolino-Perry K, Tang N, Head R, Ng C, Arulanandam R, Angarita FA, Acuna SA, Chen Y, Bell J, Dacosta RS, McCart JA. Tumor vascularization is critical for oncolytic vaccinia virus treatment of peritoneal carcinomatosis. Int J Cancer. 134, 3 (Feb 1 2014) 717–730.

[72] Kitayama J. Intraperitoneal chemotherapy against peritoneal carcinomatosis: Current status and future perspective. Surg Oncol. 2014 Mar 27. pii: S0960–7404(14)00027–00029. doi: 10.1016/j.suronc.2014.03.004. [Epub ahead of print].

[73] Matsumura Y, Maeda H. A new concept for macromolecular therapeutics in cancer chemotherapy: mechanism of tumoritropic accumulation of proteins and the antitumor agent smancs. *Cancer Res*. 46 (1986) 6387–6392.

[74] Maeda H, Wu J, Sawa T, Matsumura Y, Hori K. Tumor vascular permeability and the EPR effect in macromolecular therapeutics: a review. *J Control Release*. 65 (2000) 271–284.

[75] Peer D, Karp JM, Hong S, Farokhzad OC, Margalit R, Langer R. Nanocarriers as an emerging platform for cancer therapy. *Nat Nanotechnol*. 2 (2007) 751–760.

[76] Davis ME, Chen ZG, Shin DM. Nanoparticle therapeutics: an emerging treatment modality for cancer. *Nat Rev Drug Discov*. 7 (2008) 771–782.

[77] Matsumura Y, Kataoka K. Preclinical and clinical studies of anticancer agent-incorporating polymer micelles. *Cancer Sci*. 100 (2009) 572–579.

[78] Gradishar WJ, Tjulandin S, Davidson N, Shaw H, Desai N, Bhar P, et al. Phase III trial of nanoparticle albumin-bound paclitaxel compared with polyethylated castor oil-based paclitaxel in women with breast cancer. *J Clin Oncol – Off J Am Soc Clin Oncol*. 23 (2005) 7794–7803.

[79] Petrelli F, Borgonovo K, Barni S. Targeted delivery for breast cancer therapy: the history of nanoparticle-albumin-bound paclitaxel. *Expert Opin Pharmacother*. 11 (2010) 1413–1432.

[80] Hamaguchi T, Matsumura Y, Suzuki M, Shimizu K, Goda R, Nakamura I, et al. NK105, a paclitaxel-incorporating micellar nanoparticle formulation, can extend in vivo antitumor activity and reduce the neurotoxicity of paclitaxel. *Br J Cancer*. 92 (2005) 1240–1246.

[81] Kato K, Tahara M, Hironaka S, Muro K, Takiuchi H, Hamamoto Y, et al. A phase II study of paclitaxel by weekly 1-h infusion for advanced or recurrent esophageal cancer in patients who had previously received platinum-based chemotherapy. *Cancer Chemother Pharmacol*. 67 (2011) 1265–1272.

[82] Konno T, Watanabe J, Ishihara K. Enhanced solubility of paclitaxel using water-soluble and biocompatible 2-methacryloyloxyethyl phosphorylcholine polymers. *J Biomed Mater Res A*. 65 (2003) 209–214.

[83] Soma D, Kitayama J, Konno T, Ishihara K, Yamada J, Kamei T, et al. Intraperitoneal administration of paclitaxel solubilized with poly(2-methacryloxyethyl phosphorylcholine-co n-butyl methacrylate) for peritoneal dissemination of gastric cancer. *Cancer Sci*. 100 (2009) 1979–1985.

[84] Kamei T, Kitayama J, Yamaguchi H, Soma D, Emoto S, Konno T, et al. Spatial distribution of intraperitoneally administrated paclitaxel nanoparticles solubilized with poly (2-methacryloxyethyl phosphorylcholine-co n-butyl methacrylate) in peritoneal metastatic nodules. *Cancer Sci*. 102 (2011) 200–205.

[85] Emoto S, Yamaguchi H, Kishikawa J, Yamashita H, Ishigami H, Kitayama J. Antitumor effect and pharmacokinetics of intraperitoneal NK105, a nanomicellar paclitaxel formulation for peritoneal dissemination. *Cancer Sci*. 103 (2012) 1304–1310.

[86] Sugarbaker PH. Successful management of microscopic residual disease in large bowel cancer. Cancer Chemother Pharmacol. 43 (1999) Suppl:S15–25.

[87] Sugarbaker PH. Peritonectomy procedures. Ann Surg. 221, 1 (1995) 29–42.

[88] GRADE working group. Grading quality of evidence and strength of recommendations. BMJ. 328, 7454 (2004) 1490.

[89] http://www.england.nhs.uk/wp-content/uploads/2013/04/a08-p-a.pdf, consulted on 21.4.2014.

[90] NICE. Interventional procedure overview of cytoreduction surgery followed by hyperthermic intraoperative peritoneal chemotherapy for peritoneal carcinomatosis. IPG331. London: National Institute for Health and Clinical Excellence, 2009.

[91] Rout S, Renehan AG, Parkinson MF et al. Treatments and outcomes of peritoneal surface tumors through a centralized national service (United Kingdom). Dis Colon Rectum. 52, 10 (2009) 1705–1714.

[92] Sugarbaker PH. An Overview of Peritonectomy, Visceral resections, and Perioperative Chemotherapy for Peritoneal Surface Malignancy. In: Sugarbaker PH (ed). Cytoreductive Surgery & Perioperative Chenotherapy for Peritoneal Szrface Malignancy. Cine.Med, Woodbury, 2013. 1–29.

[93] Harmon RL, Sugarbaker PH. Prognostic indicators in peritoneal carcinomatosis from gastrointestinal cancer. Int Semin Surg Oncol. 2, 1 (Feb 8 2005) 3.

[94] Piso P, Glockzin G, von Breitenbuch P et al. Patient selection for a curative approach to carcinomatosis. Cancer J. 15, 3 (2009) 236–242.

[95] Elias D, Gilly F, Boutitie F et al. Peritoneal colorectal carcinomatosis treated with surgery and perioperative intraperitoneal chemotherapy: retrospective analysis of 523 patients from a multicentric French study. J Clin Oncol. 28, 1 (2010) 63–68.
[96] Li Y, Yang X, Yang G et al. An evaluation of cytoreductive surgery plus hyperthermic intraperitoneal chemotherapy on patients with peritoneal carcinomatosis: Final results of a phase II prospective and randomized clinical trial. J Clin Oncol. (2011), Conference (var. pagings).
[97] Quenet F, Goere D, Mehta SS et al. Results of two bi-institutional prospective studies using intraperitoneal oxaliplatin with or without irinotecan during HIPEC after cytoreductive surgery for colorectal carcinomatosis. Ann Surg. 254, 2 (2011) 294–301.
[98] Franko J, Ibrahim Z, Gusani NJ et al. Cytoreductive surgery and hyperthermic intraperitoneal chemoperfusion versus systemic chemotherapy alone for colorectal peritoneal carcinomatosis. Cancer. 116, 16 (2010) 3756–3762.
[99] Chua TC, Morris DL, Saxena A et al. Influence of modern systemic therapies as adjunct to cytoreduction and perioperative intraperitoneal chemotherapy for patients with colorectal peritoneal carcinomatosis: A multicenter study. Ann Surg Oncol. 18, 6 (2011) 1560–1567.
[100] Esquivel J, Chua TC, Stojadinovic A et al. Accuracy and clinical relevance of computed tomography scan interpretation of peritoneal cancer index in colorectal cancer peritoneal carcinomatosis: a multi-institutional study. J Surg Oncol. 102, 6 (2010) 565–570.
[101] Goere D, Tzanis D, Gava VG et al. Can patients be cured after cytoreductive surgery plus intraperitoneal chemotherapy for colorectal peritoneal carcinomatosis? J Clin Oncol. (2011), Conference (var. pagings).
[102] Ripley RT, Davis JL, Kemp CD et al. Prospective randomized trial evaluating mandatory second look surgery with HIPEC and CRS vs. standard of care in patients at high risk of developing colorectal peritoneal metastases. Trials. 11 (2010) 62.
[103] Brucher BL, Piso P, Verwaal V et al. Peritoneal carcinomatosis: cytoreductive surgery and HIPEC–overview and basics. Cancer Invest. 30, 3 (2012) 209–224.
[104] Verwaal VJ, van Tinteren H, van Ruth S, Zoetmulder FA. Predicting the survival of patients with peritoneal carcinomatosis of colorectal origin treated by aggressive cytoreduction and hyperthermic intraperitoneal chemotherapy. Br J Surg. 91, 6 (2004) 739–746.
[105] Cao C, Yan TD, Black D, Morris DL. A systematic review and meta-analysis of cytoreductive surgery with perioperative intraperitoneal chemotherapy for peritoneal carcinomatosis of colorectal origin. Ann Surg Oncol. 16, 8 (2009) 2152–2165.
[106] Cancer Research UK. Ovarian cancer survival statistics: 2012. [cited 2012 Aug 12]. London: Cancer Research UK, 2012.
[107] Ang C, Chan KK, Bryant A et al. Ultra-radical (extensive) surgery versus standard surgery for the primary cytoreduction of advanced epithelial ovarian cancer. Cochrane Database Syst Rev. 2011(4):CD007697.
[108] Dovern E, de Hingh IH, Verwaal VJ et al. Hyperthermic intraperitoneal chemotherapy added to the treatment of ovarian cancer. A review of achieved results and complications. Eur J Gynaecol Oncol. 31, 3 (2010) 256–261.
[109] Vergote I, Trope CG, Amant F et al. Neoadjuvant chemotherapy or primary surgery in stage IIIC or IV ovarian cancer. N Engl J Med. 363, 10 (2010) 943–953.
[110] Chi DS, Musa F, Dao F et al. An analysis of patients with bulky advanced stage ovarian, tubal, and peritoneal carcinoma treated with primary debulking surgery (PDS) during an identical time period as the randomized EORTC-NCIC trial of PDS vs neoadjuvant chemotherapy (NACT). Gynecol Oncol. 124, 1 (2012) 10–14.
[111] Leo F, Canonico G, Scaringi S et al. Cytoreductive surgery with or without hyperthermic intraperitoneal chemotherapy for synchronous or metachronous peritoneal carcinomatosis from ovarian cancer. European J Surg Oncol. (2010), Conference (var. pagings): 1028.

[112] Parson N, Shen P, Russell GB et al. Outcomes after cytoreductive surgery and hyperthermic intraperitoneal chemotherapy for peritoneal surface dissemination from ovarian neoplasms. Ann Surg Oncol. (2010), Conference (var. pagings): February.
[113] Fotopoulou C, Richter R, Braicu IE et al. Clinical outcome of tertiary surgical cytoreduction in patients with recurrent epithelial ovarian cancer. Ann Surg Oncol. 18, 1 (2011) 49–57.
[114] Deraco M, Kusamura S, Virzi S et al. Cytoreductive surgery and hyperthermic intraperitoneal chemotherapy as upfront therapy for advanced epithelial ovarian cancer: multi-institutional phase-II trial. Gynecol Oncol. 122, 2 (2011) 215–220.
[115] Yang XJ, Huang CQ, Suo T et al. Cytoreductive surgery and hyperthermic intraperitoneal chemotherapy improves survival of patients with peritoneal carcinomatosis from gastric cancer: final results of a phase III randomized clinical trial. Ann Surg Oncol. 18, 6 (2011) 1575–1581.
[116] Strohlein MA, Bulian DR, Heiss MM. Clinical efficacy of cytoreductive surgery and hyperthermic chemotherapy in peritoneal carcinomatosis from gastric cancer. Expert Rev Anticancer Ther. 11, 10 (2011) 1505–1508.
[117] Glehen O, Gilly FN, Arvieux C et al. Peritoneal carcinomatosis from gastric cancer: a multi-institutional study of 159 patients treated by cytoreductive surgery combined with perioperative intraperitoneal chemotherapy. Ann Surg Oncol. 17, 9 (2010) 2370–2377.
[118] Glehen O, Gilly FN, Boutitie F et al. Toward curative treatment of peritoneal carcinomatosis from nonovarian origin by cytoreductive surgery combined with perioperative intraperitoneal chemotherapy: a multi-institutional study of 1,290 patients. Cancer. 116, 24 (2010) 5608–5618.
[119] Gill RS, Al-Adra DP, Nagendran J et al. Treatment of gastric cancer with peritoneal carcinomatosis by cytoreductive surgery and HIPEC: a systematic review of survival, mortality, and morbidity. J Surg Oncol. 104, 6 (2011) 692–698.
[120] Glockzin G, Schlitt HJ, Piso P. Peritoneal carcinomatosis: patients selection, perioperative complications and quality of life related to cytoreductive surgery and hyperthermic intraperitoneal chemotherapy. World J Surg Oncol. 7 (2009) 5.
[121] Rout S, Renehan AG, Parkinson MF et al. Treatments and outcomes of peritoneal surface tumors through a centralized national service (United Kingdom). Dis Colon Rectum. 52, 10 (2009) 1705–1714.
[122] Tauceri F, Dipietrantonio D, Solfrini G et al. Cytoreduction and HIPEC in peritoneal carcinomatosis from ovarian cancer. Eur J Surg Oncol. (2010), Conference (var. pagings): 1028.
[123] Turner K, Hanna NN, Zhu Y et al. Assessment of neoadjuvant chemotherapy on operative parameters and outcome in patients with peritoneal dissemination from high grade appendiceal cancer. Ann Surg Oncol. (2012), Conference (var. pagings): February.
[124] Mohamed F, Moran BJ. Morbidity and mortality with cytoreductive surgery and intraperitoneal chemotherapy: the importance of a learning curve. Cancer J. 15, 3 (2009) 196–199.
[125] Moradi BN, III, Esquivel J. Learning curve in cytoreductive surgery and hyperthermic intraperitoneal chemotherapy. J Surg Oncol. 100, 4 (2009) 293–296.
[126] Cotte E, Passot G, Gilly FN, Glehen O. Selection of patients and staging of peritoneal surface malignancies. World J Gastrointest Oncol 2, 1 (2010) 31–35.

W. Solass and M. A. Reymond

6 Assessing tumor response in peritoneal carcinomatosis

6.1 Natural history of peritoneal carcinomatosis

The natural history of peritoneal carcinomatosis is a poorly investigated topic and has been reviewed recently by Van der Speeten et al. [1]. Little was done to clarify the impact of peritoneal seeding upon survival until the report of Chu and colleagues was published [2]. These investigators studied 100 patients with nongynecologic malignancy that had biopsy-proven peritoneal carcinomatosis. The mean survival of 45 colorectal cancer patients was 8.5 months, of 20 pancreatic cancer patients 2.4 months, and 6 gastric cancer patients 2.2 months. The presence of ascites was an important poor prognostic variable in all of these patients. In 2000 Sadeghi and coworkers reported on 370 patients with peritoneal carcinomatosis from non-gynecologic malignancies who were enrolled in a European prospective multicenter trial (Evolution of Peritoneal Carcinomatosis 1 [EVOCAPE 1]) [3]. These patients had the benefit of fluorouracil (5-FU)-based systemic chemotherapy, but the results were remarkably similar to those reported by Chu et al. a decade earlier. The mean survival of 118 patients with carcinomatosis from colorectal cancer was 6.0 months, of 58 patients with pancreatic cancer 2.9 months, and of 125 patients with gastric cancer 6.5 months. In 2002 Jayne and colleagues from Singapore used a database of 3,019 colorectal cancer patients to identify 349 (13%) with peritoneal carcinomatosis [4]. Of special interest were the 125 patients (58%) who had synchronous primary colorectal cancer and peritoneal implants. The median survival of those patients was only 7 months. The authors reported that survival was adversely affected by the extent of the peritoneal carcinomatosis and the stage of the primary cancer.

The availability of a gold standard is a precondition for determining therapy response in peritoneal carcinomatosis. The assessment of the change in tumor burden is an important feature of the clinical evaluation of cancer therapeutics: both tumor shrinkage (objective response) and disease progression are useful endpoints in clinical trials. Most clinical studies in oncology rely on the so-called RECIST criteria for determining therapy response.

6.2 RECIST criteria

RECIST criteria were published in 2000 and revised in 2009, with the following changes [5]:

- The number of lesions required to assess tumor burden for response determination was reduced from a maximum of ten to a maximum of five total (and from five to two per organ, maximum).
- Assessment of pathological lymph nodes is now incorporated. Nodes with a short axis of 15 mm are considered assessable as target lesions. Nodes that shrink to < 10 mm short axis are considered normal.
- Confirmation of response is required for trials with response primary endpoint but is no longer required in randomised studies.
- Disease progression is clarified in several aspects. In addition to the previous definition of progression in target disease of 20% increase in sum, a 5 mm absolute increase is now required as well to guard against over-calling PD when the total sum is very small.
- Finally, a section on detection of new lesions, including the interpretation of FDG PET-CT scan assessment is included. The revised RECIST includes a new imaging appendix with updated recommendations on the optimal anatomical assessment of lesions.

6.2.1 RECIST criteria in peritoneal carcinomatosis

Peritoneal metastases are difficult to detect by imaging techniques, and often classified as 'nonmeasurable disease' and considered ineligible for response evaluation. As a result, these patients are not included in randomised studies [6]. Obviously, the criteria defined above are most difficult or even impossible to apply in peritoneal carcinomatosis, because small lesions are poorly visualised on CT scans, and because it is a small-volumetric disease affecting large surfaces. In the revised RECIST criteria, guidance is offered on what constitutes 'unequivocal progression' of nonmeasurable or nontarget disease, a source of confusion in the original RECIST guideline. However, in our opinion, current RECIST criteria are clearly inadequate to assess therapy response in limited peritoneal carcinomatosis.

6.3 Laparoscopy in peritoneal carcinomatosis

The utilisation of laparoscopy for objective tumor evaluation is not advised in the current RECIST guidelines. However, the role of laparoscopy is recognized in confirming complete pathological response when biopsies are obtained or to determine relapse in trials where recurrence following complete response or surgical resection is an endpoint. The frequency of tumor re-evaluation while on treatment should be protocol-specific and adapted to the type and schedule of treatment. However, in the context of phase-2 studies where the beneficial effect of therapy is not known, follow up every 6–8 weeks (timed to coincide with the end of a cycle) is recommended [5] (Figure 6.1).

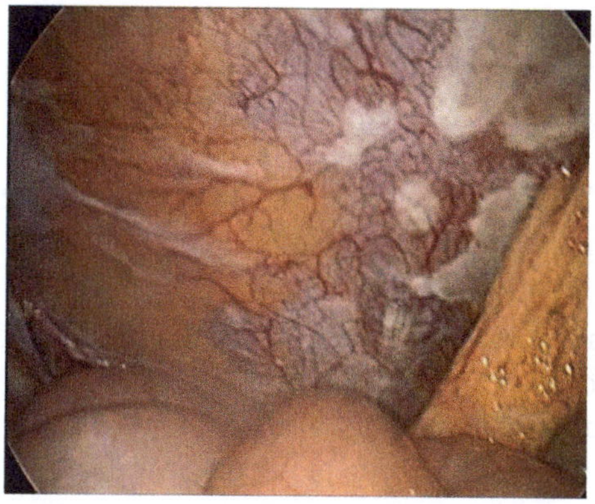

Fig. 6.1. Intraoperative PCI determination after PIPAC therapy. According to the Sugarbaker Index, these tumor manifestations should be classified LS3 (confluent lesions). However, histology showed only fibrosis without tumor cells. This example illustrates the difficulty of using PCI as a regression criteria in peritoneal carcinomatosis, since scars are difficult to distinguish from tumor nodes macroscopically.

6.4 Histology for determining tumor response

The histological response of colorectal cancer liver metastases to chemotherapy can be graded based on the extent of tumor regression. Tumor regression is characterized by fibrosis overgrowing on tumor cells, decreased necrosis, and tumor glands (if present) at the periphery of hepatic colorectal metastases. Classifying histological response based on tumor regression grades qualifies to predict the outcome of patients with colorectal cancer liver metastases. Tumor regression grading provides a

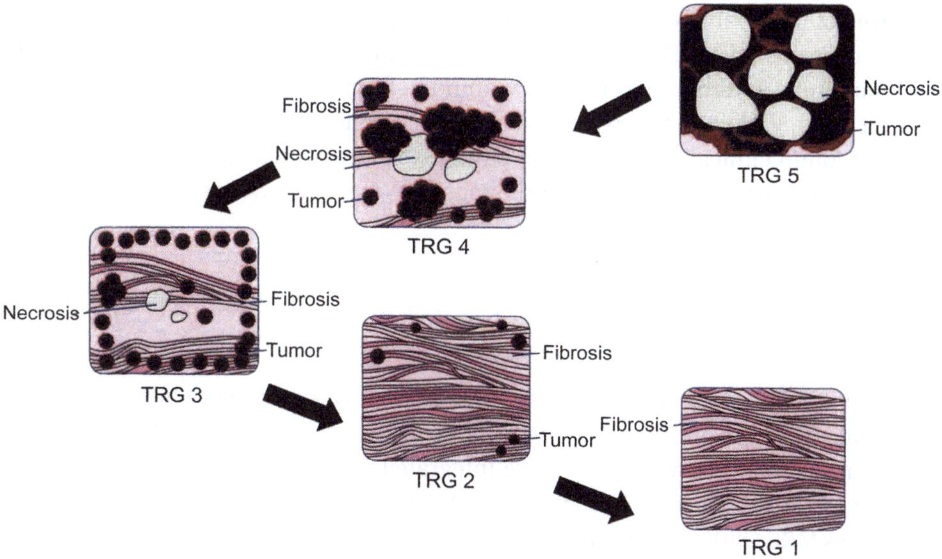

Fig. 6.2. Tumor regression grading (TRG). Major pathological response: fibrosis without tumor cells (TRG1) or isolated tumor cells within extensive fibrosis (TRG2). Partial/minor pathological response: tumor cell clusters within extensive fibrosis, some degree of necrosis (TRG3). No pathological response: tumor cells dominating in fibrotic reaction, necrosis (TRG4) or vital tumor without fibrosis (TRG5, no regression). (Adapted from [8]).

standardized pathological response evaluation [7] (Figure 6.2). By analogy, it appears reasonable to apply tumor regression grading to assess pathological tumor response in peritoneal carcinomatosis nodules from colorectal cancer.

6.5 Tumor markers for determining tumor response

Tumor markers alone cannot be used to assess objective tumor response. If markers are initially above the upper normal limit, however, they must normalise for a patient to be considered in complete response. Because tumor markers are disease specific, instructions for their measurement should be incorporated into protocols on a disease-specific basis.

6.5.1 Gastric cancer

The question of the significance of tumor markers in the primary diagnosis of gastric (and junctional) adenocarcinomas has been the object of numerous studies. Classical tumor markers (such as CEA, CA19-9 und CA72-4) as well as novel tests, including carcinogenetic, metabolic and pathophysiological biomarkers, have been investigated. As of today, the reported sensitivity and specificity are not high enough for clinical primary diagnosis. In particular, sensitivity is often under 60%. Moreover, most markers have not been validated prospectively in large patient cohorts, but retrospectively in case-control studies. Thus, at the present stage, no recommendation can be given for determining serum tumor markers within the framework of primary diagnosis of gastric cancer. Various biomarkers correlate with prognosis in gastric cancer, but so far have not found clinical application, in particular for therapeutic choices. No benefit of determining serum biomarkers for diagnosis of tumor recurrence or patient follow up has been documented so far [9].

6.5.2 Ovarian cancer

Specific guidelines for CA-125 response (in recurrent ovarian cancer) have been published [10, 15–17]. In addition, the Gynecologic Cancer Intergroup has developed CA-125 progression criteria which are to be integrated with objective tumor assessment for use in first-line trials in ovarian cancer [11]. However, in the meantime, results of the studies MRC OV05 and EORTC 55955 [12] showed unambiguously that the survival rates of patients in whom treatment is begun early when there is an increase in tumor markers are no better than those of patients in whom treatment is begun later following clinical symptoms and objective evidence of a tumor [13]. A rise of tumor marker serum values in asymptomatic patients without further evidence of tumor progression is no indication for starting a further chemotherapy [14]. The evidence for an association between detected tumor markers and prediction and prognosis has been insufficient in ovarian cancer and their use is not recommended by the current German S3 guideline.

6.5.3 Colorectal cancer

The Serum Carcino-Embryonic Antigen (CEA) level is elevated in about 30% of colorectal cancer patients at timepoint of diagnosis. In particular, CEA is helpful for diagnosis of recurrence, and is an independent prognostic factor in patients with liver metastases [15]. Therefore, CEA determination is recommended as a part of the initial diagnostic workup and for follow up. CA 19-9 does not increase the accuracy of CEA for diagnosis or recurrence and is therefore not recommended.

6.6 Determining clinical benefit rate in peritoneal carcinomatosis

In our experience, there are only two reliable outcome criteria for assessing therapy response in peritoneal carcinomatosis, namely overall survival and tumor regression grading, as assessed by repeated and multiple biopsies.

Since it has been shown that pathological tumor response correlates with survival in colorectal cancer patients with liver metastases [7, 17], it appears reasonable to apply the same regression criteria in peritoneal carcinomatosis of colorectal origin. For other histologies such as gastric or ovarian cancer, a specific tumor regression grading system still needs to be established and validated.

CT scans or, better, FGD PET-CT scans, are useful to determine therapy response in centimetric disease or in the presence of ascites or pleural effusion. Since RECIST criteria are the accepted international standard, and since laparoscopy and histological tumor response are not yet widely accepted as response criteria, we recommend performing an abdominal (and/or thoracic) CT scan immediately before each PIPAC (or PITAC) session.

Bibliography

[1] Van der Speeten K, Stuart OA, Sugarbaker PH. Using pharmacologic data to plan clinical treatments for patients with peritoneal surface malignancy. Curr Drug Discov Technol. 6, 1 (Mar 2009) 72–81. Review.

[2] Chu DZ, Lang NP, Thompson C, Osteen PK, Westbrook KC. Peritoneal carcinomatosis in nongynecologic malignancy. A prospective study of prognostic factors. Cancer 63, 2 (1989) 364–367.

[3] Sadeghi B, Arvieux C, Glehen O, Beaujard AC, Rivoire M, Baulieux J, Fontaumard E, Brachet A et al. Peritoneal carcinomatosis from nongynecologic malignancies: results of the EVOCAPE 1 multicentric prospective study. Cancer 88, 2 (2000) 358–363.

[4] Jayne DG, Fook S, Loi C, Seow-Choen F. Peritoneal carcinomatosis from colorectal cancer. Br. J. Surg. 89 (2002) 1545–1550.

[5] Eisenhauer EA, Therasse P, Bogaerts J et al. New response evaluation criteria in solid tumors: revised RECIST guideline (version 1.1). Eur J Cancer. 45, 2 (Jan 2009) 228–247.

[6] Klaver YL, Lemmens VE, Creemers GJ, Rutten HJ, Nienhuijs SW, de Hingh IH. Population-based survival of patients with peritoneal carcinomatosis from colorectal origin in the era of increasing use of palliative chemotherapy. Ann Oncol. 22, 10 (Oct 2011) 2250–2256.

[7] Klinger M, Tamandl D, Eipeldauer S et al. Bevacizumab improves pathological response of colorectal cancer liver metastases treated with XELOX/FOLFOX. Ann Surg Oncol. 17, 8 (Aug 2010) 2059–2065.

[8] Blazer DG 3rd, Kishi Y, Maru DM et al. Pathologic response to preoperative chemotherapy: a new outcome end point after resection of hepatic colorectal metastases. J Clin Oncol. 26, 33 (Nov 20 2008) 5344–5351.

[9] Moehler M, Al-Batran SE, Andus T et al. AWMF. [German S3-guideline “Diagnosis and treatment of esophagogastric cancer”]. Z Gastroenterol. 49 (2011) 461–531.

[10] Rustin GJ, Quinn M, Thigpen T et al. Re: New guidelines to evaluate the response to treatment in solid tumors (ovarian cancer). J Natl Cancer Inst 96 (2004) 487–488.

[11] Vergote I, Rustin GJ, Eisenhauer EA et al. Re: new guidelines to evaluate the response to treatment in solid tumors [ovarian cancer]. Gynecologic Cancer Intergroup. J Natl Cancer Inst 92 (2000) 1534–1535.

[12] Rustin GJ et al. Early versus delayed treatment of relapsed ovarian cancer (MRC OV05/EORTC 55955): a randomised trial. Lancet, 376, 9747 (2010) 1155–1163.

[13] Burges A, Schmalfeldt B. Ovarian cancer: diagnosis and treatment. Dtsch Arztebl Int. 108, 38 (Sep 2011) 635–641.

[14] Leitlinienprogramm Onkologie (Deutsche Krebsgesellschaft, Deutsche Krebshilfe, AWMF): S3-Leitlinie Diagnostik, Therapie und Nachsorge maligner Ovarialtumoren, Langversion 1.1, 2013, AWMF-Registernummer: 032/035OL, http://leitlinienprogramm-onkologie.de/Leitlinien.7.0.html [Stand: 12.04.2014].

[15] Levy M et al. Tumor markers in staging and prognosis of colorectal carcinoma. Neoplasma, 55, 2 (2008) 138–142.

[16] Lewis MR et al. Metastatic colorectal adenocarcinoma involving the ovary with elevated serum CA-125: a potential diagnostic pitfall. Gynecol Oncol, 105, 2 (2007) 395–398.

[17] Rubbia-Brandt L, Giostra E, Brezault C et al. Importance of histological tumor response assessment in predicting the outcome in patients with colorectal liver metastases treated with neo-adjuvant chemotherapy followed by liver surgery. Ann Oncol. 18, 2 (Feb 2007) 299–304.

M. A. Reymond, B. Hu, A. Garcia, T. Reck, F. Köckerling, J. Hess, and P. Morel

7 Principle of therapeutic capnoperitoneum

The automated carbon dioxide (CO_2) pneumoperitoneum, introduced by Semm et al. [1] in 1980, is now the accepted standard for exposing the abdominal cavity during laparoscopic procedures. In the meantime, it has been claimed that CO_2 pneumoperitoneum has several side effects. In particular, it has recently been documented that CO_2 stimulates tumor growth after laparoscopy for cancer [2], and that it increased bacterial translocation in peritonitis [3].

Gasless laparoscopy has been proposed as a solution for these side effects [4–6], but limited exposure might prevent the use of this technique for advanced laparoscopic procedures such as colonic resections. Alternative types of gas have been proposed for expanding the abdominal cavity. In particular, helium has inhibitory effects on tumor growth [7, 8], but this gas is not resorbable and therefore carries a potential risk of lethal gas embolisms in the case of venous lesions [9, 10].

We propose a different solution to prevent some side effects of CO_2 without increasing the technical difficulty of the surgical procedure nor the risks for the patient. The CO_2 might be used not only as an abdominal wall expander to expose peritoneal surfaces, but also as a drug carrier, introducing the novel concept of "therapeutic capnoperitoneum [11]. Thus, therapeutic capnoperitoneum might not only prevent the side effects of CO_2, but might also improve the results of minimally-invasive surgery in selected indications by allowing intraoperative multimodal therapy. Arguments for using a drug in aerosol form carried by the insufflation gas rather than as a peritoneal wash are a better distribution of the drug in the abdomen and better drug diffusion into the tissues by the pressurization of the peritoneal cavity (Figure 7.1).

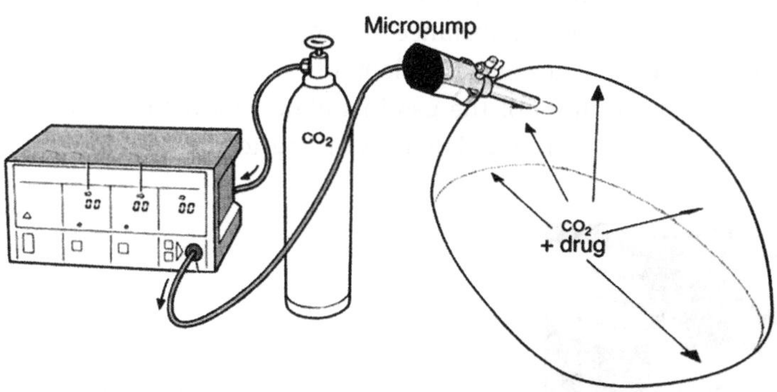

Fig. 7.1. Principle of therapeutic capnoperitoneum. CO_2 is loaded with an aerosolized therapeutic solution during laparoscopy.

To create such a therapeutic capnoperitoneum, an intracavitary drug delivery device suitable for minimally-invasive surgery procedures is necessary. After designing and manufacturing such a prototype, we performed in vitro experiments to determine the behavior of the micropump with various kinds of solutions and to assess the flow rate, the influence of viscosity, the optimal delivery rate, and the optimal droplet size. We then conducted in vivo experiments to test the intraabdominal delivery rate and the peritoneal coating uniformity, and to detect possible unexpected events caused by the device during surgical procedures. The results of these experiments are reported in the current feasibility study.

7.1 Material and methods

The current invention is an intracavitary drug delivery device suitable for minimally-invasive surgery procedures, allowing the creation of a therapeutic capnoperitoneum. The efficiency of the therapeutic capnoperitoneum depends on the activity of the substance (which depends on the composition), the place of impact (i.e. the place at which it may carry out its activity), dose repeatability (i.e. the fact that the volume of each dose remains constant), and, if indicated, the concentration repeatability (meaning that the drug flow remains constant with the gas flow).

7.1.1 Design of the prototype

The device consists of two elements: a micropump and a monitor. The micropump delivers the drug (in liquid form) as a dispersion of atomized droplets, thanks to the incorporated monodispersive spray device. The device is located between a gas insufflator and the body cavity where surgery is performed, which allows the device to aerosolize microdroplets of the therapeutic substance into the capnoperitoneum. The liquid is aerosolized by excitation of a piezoelectric element.

The monitor is placed in the vicinity of the gas insufflator. Flow rate, concentration, and amount of drug delivery are regulated according to the gas flow in a

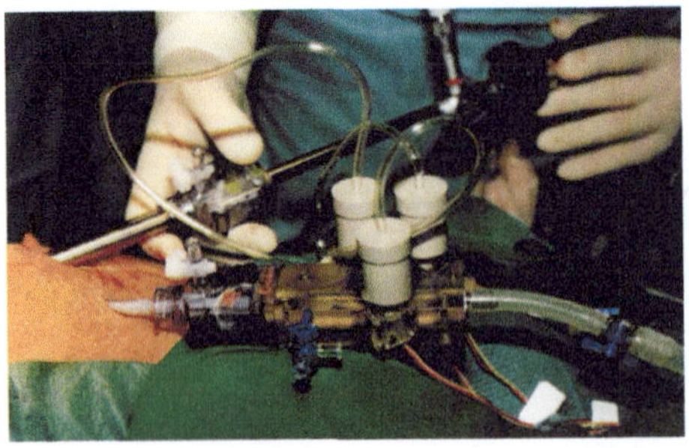

Fig. 7.2. First prototype of a micropump for PIPAC application. The device is built directly into a commercially available 5 mm trocar (Endopath, Ethicon Endosurgery, Norderstedt, Germany).

closed-loop control system. The control system allows for weighted-factor drug delivery according to the patient's condition and the level of intervention (EPO application 95908180.3). It is therefore possible to know precisely at each moment of the operation the amount of therapeutic substance that has been administrated to the patient (Figure 7.2).

7.2 Results

7.2.1 In vitro trial

The aim of the in vitro trials was to work out the kind of solutions that can be aerosolized by the micropump, the influence of viscosity, the maximal flow, and the optimal droplet size.

Kinds of solutions

We have shown that the micropump is able to aerosolize liquids such as water, ethanol, and various solutions including:

- taurolidine (Taurolin®, Geistlich, Wolhusen, Switzerland)
- 5-FU (Wyeth-Lederle, Wolfrathshausen, Germany)
- mitoxanthronhydrochlorid (Novantron®, Wyeth-Lederle, Wolfrathshausen, Germany)
- betadine (Betaisodona®, Mundipharma, Limburg, Germany), with some limitations due to PVP adhesive characteristics.

These solutions have pH values between 6.0 and 9.0.

Influence of viscosity

Since all the aforementioned solutions have low viscosity coefficients (< 300 centipoises), we were not able to observe any negative influence of viscosity.

Maximal flow

Gas and drug flow calculations were based on measurements using input and output pressure sensors for determination of the differential pressure. Flows between 6 and 20 ml/s were achieved with one spraying unit (Figure 7.3).

Because of a redundancy of spray devices (e.g. three in the current prototype), a continuous reliable operation of the drug delivery system and an enhanced peak flow were obtained in vitro.

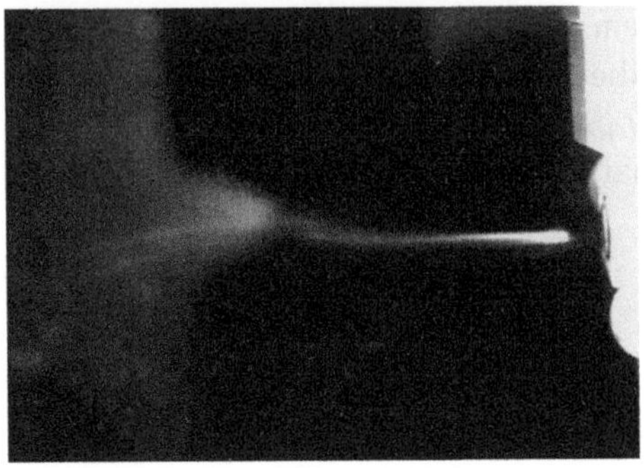

Fig. 7.3. Diffusion of the aerosol (polarized light) in the engineering laboratory.

Droplet size

A microdroplet size smaller than 10 μm was selected to allow maximal diffusion. It was observed that droplet size is inversely proportional to the excitation frequency of the monodispersive spray unit.

7.2.2 In vivo trial

The decision to use taurolidin in the current animal trial was based on a study of Jacobi et al. [12] showing that the application of taurolidin in the rat model significantly reduced the incidence of port-site recurrences. Furthermore, the toxicity of taurolidin in the pig model is known to be low (data on file, Geistlich, Wolhusen, Switzerland).

Surgical procedure

After official permissions were obtained, two German landrace pigs (weight, 21.3 and 20.4 kg, respectively) were anesthetized using routine protocols. Pneumoperitoneum of 12 mm Hg was established using a Veres needle. At the beginning of the procedure, a further 5 mm commercially available trocar (Endopath) was inserted into the left upper quadrant, and the introducer was replaced by the micropump. A laparoscopically-assisted resection of the sigmoid colon with transanal double stapling was performed in both animals, using a four-trocar technique. Operating times were 90 and 97 minutes, respectively. The CO_2 volumes were 156 and 195 liters. (An artificial leak was created by opening a valve on the right lower trocar.) During the operation, a solution of taurolidin 2% was aerosolized into the abdominal cavity.

Drug distribution

The distribution of the active principle within the abdominal cavity was assessed by aerosolizing 3 ml of a 50% methylene blue solution into a pig cadaver after installation of a pneumoperitoneum of 12 mm Hg for 30 min. This assay showed a dispersion of the microdroplets within the entire abdominal cavity, including the anterior abdominal wall where trocar sites had been placed. It is important that nonexposed surfaces such as the bursa omentalis and the inferior liver aspect were not stained. The trocars were not moved during this experiment. As expected, the distribution was not homogeneous, and staining was enhanced in the vicinity and axis of the trocar where the micropump had been introduced.

Unexpected problems

Both surgical procedures, performed by two experienced laparoscopic surgeons, showed no technical difficulties. In particular, vision was not impaired. Cardiorespiratory instability was observed in both animals by the anesthesiologist, which could be explained by the hypotonic nature of the 2% taurolidine solution that should have been corrected with saline. As soon as the relative humidity in the intraperitoneal cavity approached 100%, the micropump was not able to aerosolize any longer. For this reason, we had to create a continuous artificial gas leak through a trocar tap and a usual gas line. This allowed the micropump to function throughout the procedure, but modified the standard laparoscopic procedure, in which the gas flow is usually interrupted in the absence of any gas leak.

7.3 Discussion

We propose the novel concept of "therapeutic capnoperitoneum," defined as the association of a carrier gas such as CO_2 with an aerosolized therapeutic substance. Results show that it is possible to create a therapeutic capnoperitoneum with the drug delivery device used in the current study. It was possible to simultaneously perform resections of the sigmoid colon with no special surgical difficulty. This study was a feasibility test in a large animal model. Positive or negative target effects of drugs were not assessed at this stage of development. Therefore, this study provides no proof of the interest that therapeutic capnoperitoneum may have in clinical practice. Nevertheless, therapeutic capnoperitoneum has several interesting properties related to intraperitoneal pharmacokinetics.

The pharmacokinetic problems in peritoneal drug administration were reviewed recently by Dedrick and Flessner [13]. Both theory and clinical studies demonstrate that drug concentrations in the peritoneal cavity can greatly exceed concentrations in the plasma after intraperitoneal administration. This regional advantage has been associated with clinical activity [14]. Two pharmacokinetic problems appear to limit the effectiveness of intraperitoneal therapy: poor tumor penetration by the drug and incomplete irrigation of serosal surfaces by the drug-containing solution. In both respects, the current invention might have major advantages over conventional irrigation.

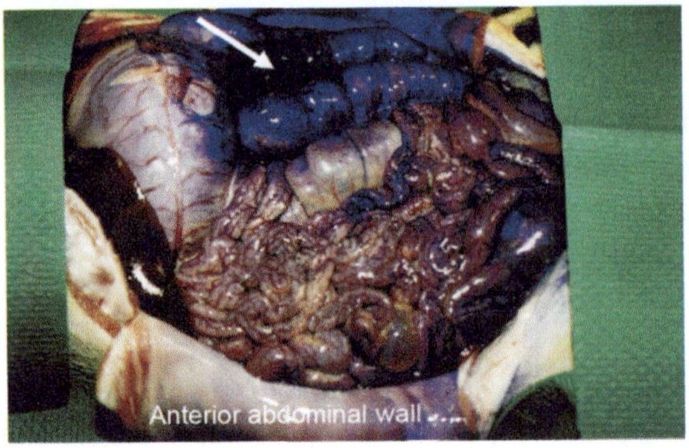

Fig. 7.4. Staining of the abdominal cavity of a German landrace pig with the first generation micropump. All exposed surfaces are stained, but there is a staining gradient from the main stream direction (arrow indicates trocar direction) towards the periphery.

7.3.1 Increasing exposure of the peritoneal surface

Various observations in experimental animals suggest limited exposure of the peritoneal surface under conditions of peritoneal dialysis. In general, definitive studies have not been conducted on the potential peritoneal surface area of human subjects. The likelihood exists that much of the residual tumor burden after surgery is untreated or undertreated by conventional intraperitoneal irrigation. If the peritoneal surfaces are not exposed to drug-containing solutions or if they are inadequately exposed, then the rationale for regional administration is compromised [13]. Theoretical considerations suggest that the therapeutic capnoperitoneum should be capable of carrying microdroplets of active substances to all exposed peritonteal surfaces. These considerations were confirmed by the current pilot study conducted in two animals, in which all exposed peritoneal surfaces were stained by methylene blue, suggesting that the active principle is distributed throughout the abdomen (Figure 7.4).

7.3.2 Increasing hydrostatic intraabdominal pressure

The mechanical model described by Dedrick and Flessner [13] implies that obtaining large increases in the tissue penetration of lowmolecular-weight drugs may be difficult. As shown in their equation (see Chapter 5), the penetration distance is equal to the square root of the ratio of the intratissue diffusivity and the rate constant for drug removal from the tissue $(D/k)^{1/2}$. Increasing the penetration distance requires an increase in D and/or a decrease in k. Because of the square-root relationship, the ratio D/k would have to be quadrupled to produce a doubling of penetration. The tissue diffusivity is a function of the tissue structure and the drug properties; it is equal to the diffusivity in the interstitial space of the tissue (which incorporates the tortuous path that a molecule must traverse) and the volume fraction of tissue interstitial space.

Introducing dialysis solution into the peritoneal cavity of rats and raising the intraperitoneal pressure from 0 to 4 cm H_2O caused the extracellular space of the anterior abdominal wall to double (Flessner MF: unpublished observations). This expansion of the interstitium likely increases the effective diffusivity. In the meantime, further data support the potential benefit of increasing intraperitoneal hydrostatic drugs. When the intraabdominal pressure was raised, an increased intratumoral accumulation [15] and antitumor effect of i.-p. doxorubicin and cisplatin was observed in the animal model [16, 17]. Clinical applications of hyperpressure have been limited to palliating malignant ascites with laparoscopic HIPEC at 10–15 mm Hg [18].

Against this framework, therapeutic capnoperitoneum has theoretical advantages over intraperitoneal irrigation, by applying a hydrostatic intraperitoneal pressure of 12 to 15 mm Hg (16 to 20 cm H_2O).

7.3.3 Applications of therapeutic capnoperitoneum

Therapeutic pneumoperitoneum has numerous potential applications, particularly in the following fields.

Prevention of local recurrence after cancer surgery

The main causes of local recurrence are intraoperative tumor cell implantation and inadequate excision of the primary tumor or the lymphatic drainage. Because they are breaking the natural barrier formed by the mesothelium and hyaluronic acid [20], peritoneal wounds [21] such as those of trocar sites [22] or anastomoses are major causes of recurrence.

The presence of growth factors and other cytokines in surgical wounds after cancer resections might stimulate growth of minimal residual disease. Avoidance of unnecessary surgical trauma by gentle techniques, control of spilled cells by intraoperative locoregional cytostatic drug delivery, and treatment of peritoneal wounds by aerosolizing coating agents therefore could reduce the local recurrence rate.

Prevention of port-site recurrences

Jacobi et al. [12] have shown that intraperitoneal lavage with taurolidine in cancer laparoscopy was able to reduce markedly the incidence of port-site recurrences in the rat model. At this point, the micropump has been shown to aerosolize a 2% taurolidine solution, and because the therapeutic substance reaches the anterior and lateral abdominal walls in the current animal model, it can be hypothesized that a preventive effect will be achieved. Therapeutic capnoperitoneum also might be used in thoracoscopy. Because port-site recurrences also have been described during such procedures [23], aerosolization of taurolidine or other hyaluoronates might be indicated as well.

Intraperitoneal and intrapleural chemotherapy

The response of established carcinoma or sarcoma implants to intraperitoneal and intrapleural chemotherapy is multifactorial. Two of the factors that influence the pharmacokinetics of intraperitoneal drugs are pressure and hyperthermia. The application of an intraperitoneal hyperpressure such as capnoperitoneum in laparoscopy and heated CO_2 might be a promising approach to increase the drug diffusion into the tumor and to enhance the efficiency of intraperitoneal chemotherapy. These points deserve further research because in the case of colorectal adenocarcinoma there are insufficient data on which to base a clear-cut conclusion concerning real benefits [25].

Modulation of tumor immunogeneity

In the animal model, stress factors such as butyrate (associated or not with heat) in peritoneal carcinosis of colorectal origin have been shown to enhance tumor immunogenicity. In the rat model, immunomodulation followed by passive immunotherapy using intraperitoneal interleukin-2 (IL-2) application achieved some complete tumor responses in established peritoneal carcinosis [26].

Benign disease: infections and adhesions

Other possible applications of therapeutic pneumoperitoneum concern benign disease such as intraabdominal or intrapleural infections and prevention of postoperative adhesions.

Perioperative analgesia

Since it has been shown that intraoperative bupivacain irrigation reduces both frequency and intensity of shoulder pain after laparoscopic procedures [27], therapeutic capnoperitoneum also might be used for postoperative or even intraoperative analgesia.

Remaining challenges

It is important to note, however, that technical challenges remain. To aerosolize drug solutions into the gas stream, it was necessary to maintain a gas flow throughout the procedure, so that large volumes of CO_2 were used. Technically, this was possible by opening a trocar tap and diverting the therapeutic pneumoperitoneum over a usual line into a special waste recipient. Alternatively, the gas might be diverted into an active coal filter. This might have caused some degree of hypothermia in the patient. Despite the laminar air flow in modern operating rooms to prevent exposure of the surgical team to potentially hazardous drugs, no therapeutic pneumoperitoneum should be allowed to escape into the environment during the procedure. Such gas leaks should be prevented during laparoscopic cancer surgery because they appear to promote implantation and growth of free intraperitoneal tumor cells at port sites [28] and might be toxic when tissue has been cauterized [29]. In the particular case of intraperitoneal chemotherapy using cytostatic drugs, it might be necessary for the operating team to leave the room during the application of the drug (e.g. at the end of the procedure).

Using monopolar cautery in the presence of an aqueous taurolidine solution was possible with no limitation. Nevertheless, further study using flammable solvents such as ethanol is necessary to identify potential hazards.

In summary, we introduce the novel concept of "therapeutic capnoperitoneum" in laparoscopic and thoracoscopic surgery to prevent some side effects of CO_2 pneumoperitoneum without increasing the difficulty of the surgical procedures nor the risks to the patient. Expected and unexpected effects of various drugs now need to be assessed in appropriate studies. These might be exciting fields of research for engineers, pharmaceutical companies, oncologists, and laparoscopic surgeons.

Bibliography

[1] Semm K. Die Automatisierung des Pneumoperitoneums für die endoskopische Abdominalchirurgie. Arch Gyn 232 (1980) 738.

[2] Jones DB, Guo LW, Reinhard MK, Soper NJ, Philpott GW, Connet J, Fleshman JW. Impact of pneumoperitoneum on trocar-site implantation of colon cancer in hamster model. Dis Colon Rectum 38 (1995) 1182–1188.

[3] Bloechle C, Emmermann A, State T, Scheurlen UJ, Schneider C, Achilles E, Wolf M, Mack D, Zornig C, Broelsch CE. Laparoscopic vs. open repair of gastric perforation and abdominal lavage of associated peritonitis in pigs. Surg Endosc 12 (1998) 212–218.

[4] Bouvy ND, Marquet RL, Jeekel H, Bonjer HJ. Impact of gas(less) laparoscopy and laparotomy on peritoneal tumor growth and abdominal wall metastases. Surg Endosc 10 (1996) 1618 [abstract].

[5] Paolucci V, Gutt CN, Schaeff B, Encke A. Gasless laparoscopy in abdominal surgery. Surg Endosc 9 (1995) 497–500.

[6] Watson DI, Mathew G, Ellis T, Baigrie CF, Rofe AM, Jamieson GG. Gasless laparoscopy may reduce the risk of port-site metastases following laparoscopic tumor surgery. Arch Surg 132 (1997) 166–168.

[7] Dorrance HR, Oein K, O'Dwyer PJ. Laparoscopy promotes tumor growth in an animal model. Surg Endosc 10 (1996) 559 [abstract].

[8] Jacobi CA, Sabat R, Ordemann J, Muller JM. Influence of different gases on the tumor cell growth in laparoscopic surgery: preliminary results of an experimental study in a rat model. Langenbecks Arch Chir 381 (1996) (Suppl 1): 127–130.

[9] Bongard FS, Pianim N, Liu SY, Lippmann M, Davis I, Klein S. Using helium for insufflation during laparoscopy. JAMA 266 (1991) 3131 [letter].

[10] Southern DA, Mapleson WW. Which insufflation gas for laparoscopy. BMJ 307 (1993) 1424 [letter].

[11] Reymond MA, Hu B, Garcia A, Reck T, Köckerling F, Hess J, Morel P. Feasibility of therapeutic pneumoperitoneum in a large animal model using a microvaporisator. Surg Endosc. 14, 1 (Jan 2000) 51–55.

[12] Jacobi CA, Ordemann J, Bohm M, Zieren HU, Sabat R, Muller JM. Inhibition of peritoneal tumor cell growth and implantation in laparoscopic surgery in a rat model. Am J Surg 174 (1997) 359–363.

[13] Dedrick RL, Flessner MF. Pharmacokinetic problems in peritoneal drug administration: tissue penetration and surface exposure. J Natl Cancer Inst 89 (1997) 480–487.

[14] Alberts DS, Liu PY, Hannigan EV, O'Toole R, Williams SD, Young JA. Intraperitoneal cisplatin plus intravenous cyclophosphamide versus intravenous cisplatin plus intravenous cyclophosphamide for stage III ovarian cancer. N Engl J Med 335 (1996) 1950–1955.

[15] Los G, Mutsaers PH, Lenglet WJ, Baldew GS, McVie JG. Platinum distribution in intraperitoneal tumors after intraperitoneal cisplatin treatment. Cancer Chemother Pharmacol 25 (1990) 389–394.

[16] Esquis P, Consolo D, Magnin G, Pointaire P, Moretto P, Ynsa MD, Beltramo JL, Drogoul C, Simonet M, Benoit L, Rat P, Chauffert B. High intra-abdominal pressure enhances the penetration and antitumor effect of intraperitoneal cisplatin on experimental peritoneal carcinomatosis. Ann Surg 24, 4 (2006) 106–112.

[17] Jacquet P, Stuart OA, Chang D, Sugarbaker PH. Effects of intra-abdominal pressure on pharmacokinetics and tissue distribution of doxorubicin after intraperitoneal administration. Anticancer Drugs 7 (1996) 596–603.

[18] Garofalo A, Valle M, Garcia J, Sugarbaker PH. Laparoscopic hyperthermic chemotherapy for palliation of debilitating malignant ascites. Eur J Surg Oncol 32 (2006) 682–685.

[19] Abulafi AM, Williams NS. Local recurrence of colorectal cancer: the problem, mechanisms, management, and adjuvant therapy. Br J Surg 81 (1994) 7–19.

[20] Jones LM, Gardner MJ, Catterall JB, Turner GA. Hyaluronic acid secreted by mesothelial cells: a natural barrier to ovarian cancer cell adhesion. Clin Exp Metastasis 13 (1995) 373–380.

[21] van den Tol PM, van Rossen EE, van Eijck CH, Bonthuis F, Marquet RL, Jeekel H. Reduction of peritoneal trauma by using nonsurgical gauze leads to less implantation metastasis of spilled tumor cells. Ann Surg 227 (1998) 242–248.

[22] Schneider C, Jung A, Reymond MA, Tannapfel A, Balli J, Franklin ME, Hohenberger W, Köckerling F. Efficacy of surgical measures in preventing port-site recurrences in a porcine model. Surg Endosc. 15, 2 (Feb 2001) 121–125.

[23] Downey RJ, McCormack P, LoCicero III J, and the Video-Assisted Thoracic Surgery Study Group Dissemination of malignancies following video-assisted thoracic surgery. J Cardiovasc Thor Surg 111 (1996) 954–960.

[24] Sugarbaker PH. Intraperitoneal chemotherapy and cytoreductive surgery for the prevention and treatment of peritoneal carcinomatosis and sarcomatosis. Semin Surg Oncol 14 (1998) 254–261.

[25] Penna C, Nordinger B. Locoregional therapy for adjuvant treatment of colorectal adenocarcinoma. Eur J Cancer 32 (1996) 1117–1122.

[26] Perrin P, Burg C, Vavasseur F, Galmiche JP, Bornet F, Meflah K. Treatment with butyrate/Il-2 combination in peritoneal carcinomatosis of colonic origin. C R Acad Sci III 316 (1993) 611–614.

[27] Cunniffe MG, McAnena OJ, Dar MA, Calleary J, Flynn N. A prospective randomized trial of intraoperative bupivacaine irrigation for management of shoulder tip pain following laparoscopy. Surg Endosc 176 (1998) 258–261.

[28] Tseng LNL, Berends FJ, Wittich P, Bouvy ND, Marquet RL, Kazemier G, Bonjer HJ. Port-site metastases: impact of local tissue trauma and gas leakage. Surg Endosc 12 (1998) 1377–1380.

[29] Hensman C, Baty D, Willis RG, Cuschieri A. Chemical composition of smoke produced by high-frequency electrosurgery in a closed gaseous environment. Surg Endosc 12 (1998) 1017–1019.

W. Solass, A. Hetzel, T. Schwarz, G. Nadiradze, E. Sagynaliev, and M. A. Reymond

8 PIPAC Technology

In 1999, we proposed the concept of "therapeutic capnoperitoneum" in order to take advantage of the physical properties of gas and pressure by applying drug into the peritoneal cavity as a pressurized aerosol [1]. In the last ten years, only few papers about laparoscopic nebulizers and their experimental or clinical applications were published. Alkhamesi et al. showed that nebulized heparin and hyaluronic acid attenuates peritoneal tumor growth after laparoscopic surgery in a rodent model [2]. Sharon et al. examined the effect of continuous intraabdominal nebulization of lidocaine during gynecological laparoscopic procedures in a limited number of patients [3]. A prospective randomized trial showed efficacy of aerosolization of anesthetics in laparoscopic surgery [4]. This result was confirmed in obesity surgery [5]. Druckrey-Fiskaaen et al. examined laparoscopic spray application of fibrin sealant effects on hemodynamics and spray efficiency at various application pressures and distances [6]. Recently, Greib et al. compared various gas humidifying devices as a means of intraperitoneal local anesthetic administration, and only one of them was able to generate a therapeutic aerosol [7]. However, the opportunities offered by a therapeutic capnoperitoneum were recognized as a potential "revolution in laparoscopic surgery" [8].

The advantages of aerosol routes for the delivery of specific drugs have become well recognised in pulmonary medicine. The drugs often begin to act very rapidly, and, as a smaller dose can be used than with oral or intravenous delivery, there is generally a reduction in the incidence of systemic side effects [9]. Moreover, these aerosols avoid the first pass effect in the liver and gastrointestinal tract toxicities. In some cases, lower drug dosages can be used which has the additional benefit of minimizing adverse reactions. Using these routes also provides a viable alternative for administration of drugs that exhibit erratic pharmacokinetics after oral or parenteral administration. Thus, it appears logical to expand the domains of application of aerosol medicine to other body parts such as the peritoneal or the pleural cavity. Moreover, combining aerosol delivery with artificial hydrostatic pressure creates further synergies in taking advantage of physical laws.

8.1 Aerosol

An aerosol is a suspension of particles (in our example of liquid droplets) in a gas (in our case carbon dioxide, CO_2). Hundred of aerosols products are on the market, including medical devices, in particular in pulmonary medicine. Usually, an inert gaseous

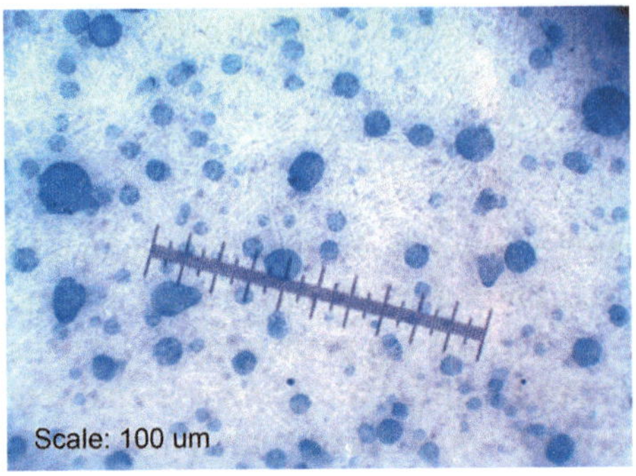

Fig. 8.1. The micropump generates aerosol droplets with a mean diameter of 11 µm. However, droplet size is heterogeneous ranging from 3–15 µm after sedimentation. Magnification: 80×.

compound under pressure serves as a propellant. The propellant serves several purposes:

- pushing the product out of the can
- vaporizing after leaving the container, producing a spray or foam
- acting as a solvent for the product (in most cases)

PIPAC technology differs from usual aerosol can technology. No propellant gas is needed, but during PIPAC a liquid solution is aerosolized into a gaseous (CO_2) environment, using a specific nozzle. Energy is provided by applying an upstream mechanical force gradient for a given period of time.

The size of the particles has a major influence on their behavioural properties, and the aerosol particle radius or diameter is a key property used to characterize aerosols. During PIPAC, the micropump does not generate a monodisperse aerosol (i.e. all particle have the same size) but a polydisperse aerosol. Thus, it is necessary to describe the sizes of the aerosol particles with a size distribution; a distribution that gives the concentration of particles having a certain size (or diameter, Figure 8.1).

Current PIPAC technology allows aerosolizing solutions with higher viscosity, including polymers, glucoses and lipids. Moreover, it has been shown to work in environments highly saturated with humidity; in other words it can generate fog in fog. This is a significant progress compared to the first generation micropump prototype (see Chapter 4) where severe dysfunctions were observed in such demanding environments. In particular, surface tension caused microperforations on the silicium chips to be immediately sealed by liquid films as soon as the vaporization process was interrupted. Moreover, these microperforations were also sealed by sticky solutions such as heparin-like substances (e.g. taurolidine) or glucose-based solutions.

When applying therapeutic aerosols, it is useful to remember that they are subject to physical laws. These general laws, including size distribution, terminal velocity, aerodynamic diameter, dynamics and dynamics regime, partitioning, activation and coagulation, are relatively complex and are described in detail elsewhere [10].

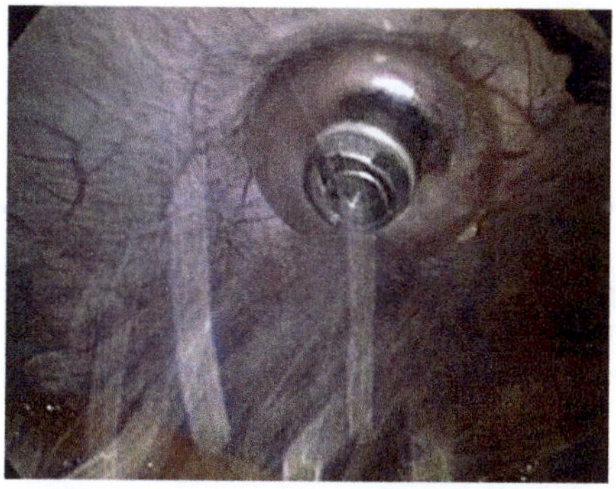

Fig. 8.2. Intraoperative picture of the micropump (MIP®, Reger Medizintechnik, Rottweil) showing aerosol movement 30 minutes after application.

Aerosols used in medicine provide an airborne mist and produce particles that are usually less than 50 µm in size. This small size ensures that the dispersed droplets or particles will remain airborne for a prolonged period of time. A one second burst from a typical space spray will produce 120 million particles in which a substantial number will remain airborne for about an hour. Microdroplets produced during PIPAC measure around 11 µm in size and, at the end of a typical PIPAC application time (30 minutes), videoendoscopy confirms that microdroplets are still moving in the gaseous environment (Figure 8.2).

Therapeutic aerosols have been best investigated in pulmonary medicine, and there is little knowledge about intraperitoneal aerosols. However, intraabdominal or intrapleural administration appears easier and more reproducible than pulmonary applications, for following reasons:

- Physical laws governing aerosol deposition are concerned principally with inertial impaction and gravitational sedimentation. Inertial impaction occurs chiefly in pulmonary medicine with larger particles whenever the transporting airstream is fast, changing direction, or turbulent (for example in the oropharynx or at bifurcations between successive airway generations). Inertial deposition is therefore influencing aerosol delivery by capturing a significant part of the therapeutic substance in the upper airways. This problem does not exist within the peritoneal cavity, where deposition mainly follows gravitational sedimentation.
- One of the most critical manoeuvres during pulmonary administration is to coordinate the actuation of the aerosol with the patient's inspiration. This problem does not exist during intraperitoneal administration.
- Gas molecules travel in random paths and collide with one another and the organ walls. These collisions exert a pressure per unit area and also cause the gases to occupy a volume. Both the pressure and volume are affected by temperature. The interrelationships between these three variables were formulated by Boyle, Charles, and Gay-Lussac [11], and can be applied to pharmaceutical aerosols. PIPAC allows modification of the intraabdominal or intrapleural temperature by applying cooled or heated CO_2, which is barely possible in pulmonary medicine (Figure 8.3).

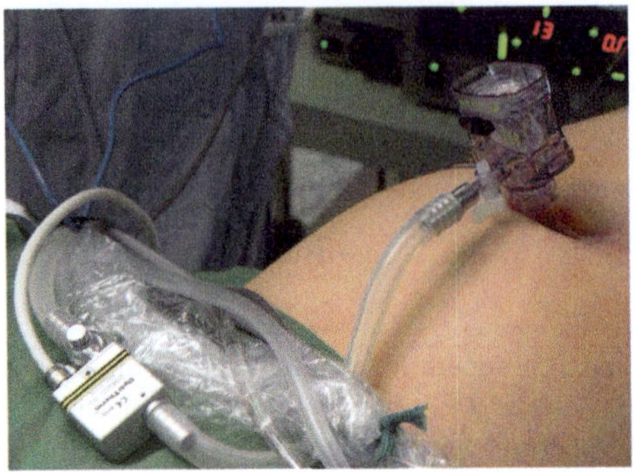

Fig. 8.3. Example of a CO_2 heating device (OptiTherm, Karl Storz, Germany) used during laparoscopy. Alternatively, some CO_2 insufflators (e.g. Thermoflator, Karl Storz, Germany) generate heated CO_2.

8.2 Pressure

Intraabdominal pressure increases intratumoral drug concentration. Dedrick et al. postulated that the penetration distance is equal to the square root of the ratio of the tissue diffusivity and the rate constant for drug removal from the tissue (D/k)1/2 [12]. Animal experiments [13], [14] confirmed the increased intratumoral accumulation and antitumor effect of intraperitoneal doxorubicin and cisplatin when the intraabdominal pressure was raised. Increased intraabdominal pressure is thought to generate a convective flux that forces the drug from the peritoneal cavity into the subperitoneal tissue. At the same time, intraabdominal pressure might counteract the hydraulic capillary pressure and slow the outflow of the drug to the body compartment. Measurement of local cisplatin concentrations along the radii of peritoneal tumor nodules showed platinum penetration far greater than 1 mm [15]. The clinical limit of usable intraabdominal pressure enhancement is dictated by respiratory and hemodynamic tolerance. Clinical applications of HIPEC in intraabdominal pressure settings has so far been limited to palliating debilitating malignant ascites with laparoscopic HIPEC at 10–15 mm Hg [16].

8.3 Micropump

We have developed a device allowing effective aerosolization of drugs into the peritoneal cavity, under normal laparoscopy conditions. This device has been optimized for clinical use and received CE certification as a class 2 medical device. Two patent applications have been filed, and the technology transfer process was supported by a grant of the German BMWI to Reger Medizintechnik in Rottweil, Germany (Figure 8.4).

The micropump (MIP®) has a diameter of 9 mm and consists of three parts: a connecting port, a shaft and a nozzle.

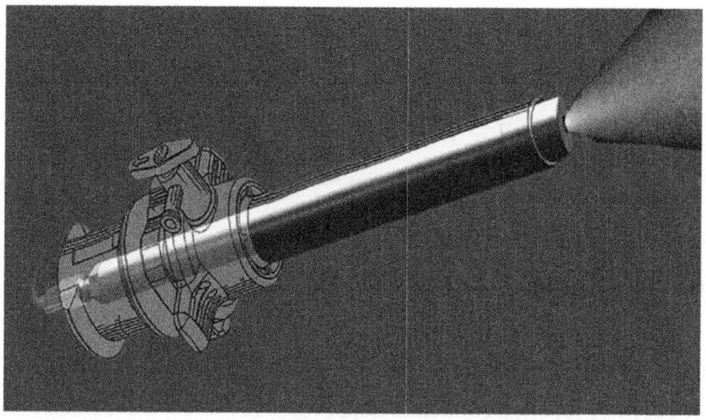

Fig. 8.4. Technical drawing of the micropump (MIP®, Reger Medizintechnik, Rottweil, Germany), inserted into an industry-standard trocar.

General recommendations and guidelines for dealing with drugs, for example with cytotoxic drugs, are to be implemented. The application of drugs occurs solely under the responsibility of the physician.

The MIP® can only be operated by a trained physician or by trained qualified personnel under the supervision of a physician. The MIP® should only be used in a closed abdomen or thorax. The MIP® is inserted through a 10–12 mm balloon trocar into the abdomen or chest and its correct position is checked by videoendoscopy. The tightness of the abdomen must be examined before use; in case of doubt a protective adhesive film must be applied over the entire abdomen. Only trocars ensuring the tightness of the abdomen should be used. All unused trocar valves must be closed by a safety cap.

The MIP® may only be operated within an operating room with laminar air flow with a complete air change in maximum every four minutes. The MIP® may only be activated with a remote control system from outside the operating room. It is assumed that the ventilation system in all operating rooms meet in terms of size and maintenance the requirements of norms DIN 1946 Part 2 "Air-conditioning – Health Technical Requirements" and DIN 4799 "Test air management systems for operating theatres". Occupational health workplace measurements according to TGRS 40 are recommended during the first use of the MIP® and should be repeated at regular intervals. Should a physician or an assistant enter the operating room during the procedure, this shall be kept as short as possible.

The use of specific safety checklists is highly recommended.

8.4 High-pressure injector

A high-pressure injector is connected to the micropump via a high-pressure line in order to deliver the therapeutic solution under adequate upstream pressure (20 bar) to the micropump.

High-pressure injectors are medical devices and their use can be potentially hazardous to the patient or to other persons, including the medical team. These potential hazards include:
- air embolism
- contamination of the environment
- cross-contamination (between syringes)
- delay in the administration of the solution.

According to the documentation of the manufacturers, these hazards could lead to severe injuries or even death. Therefore, high-pressure injectors have to be operated according to the instructions of the manufacturers in order to ensure the safety of the patient and of the operating team.

High-pressure injectors were developed for delivering contrast enhancement agents and rinsing solutions for CT-angiographies or for endovascular surgery in human patients. Thus, in most cases, the producer excludes any liability for any use outside the certified field of applications. Administration of chemotherapy might even be explicitly excluded from the application field.

According to the operating instructions of the high-pressure injectors manufacturers, any accessories have to be certified according to the norm EN 60601-1/IEC 60601-1 in order to be connected with the high-pressure injector. Furthermore, these accessories have to fulfil all configurations of the norm system EN 60601-1-1/IEC 60601-1-1. All individuals connecting an accessory with the input- or output-interface of a high-pressure injector are configuring a medical system and are liable, that this configuration fulfil the norm EN 60601-1-1/IEC 60601-1-1 (Figure 8.5).

The micropump (Reger Medizintechnik, Rottweil, Germany) is CE-certified (CE 0483). The question of the compatibility of the micropump with industry-standard high-pressure injectors has been addressed in detail within the framework of the CE-certification of the micropump and of the risk assessment protocols. In particular, the micropump was part of a conformity assessment process according to the German MedizinProdukteGesetz (MPG), that concluded that the micropump can be used together with any CT- or angiography- high pressure injector up to a pressure of 20 bar. Each micropump is tested individually before delivery at a pressure of 40 bar. The manufacturer of the micropump (Reger Medizintechnik, Rottweil, Germany) has delivered a certificate of conformity that can be requested on demand. In practice, the micropump can be connected to any CE-certified, industry-standard high-pressure injector, up to an upstream pressure of 20 bar. Of course, only high-pressure lines certified for such use can be used for connecting the micropump with the injector.

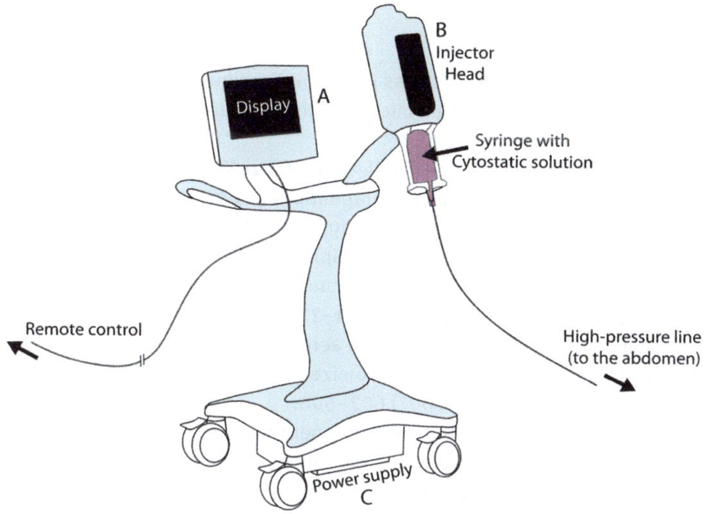

Fig. 8.5. Example of a high-pressure injector developed for vascular surgery (Mark 7 Arterion®-injection system, Medrad, Germany) that we are using in our institution for PIPAC application. A: display steering unit. B: injector head. C: power unit.

8.5 Training and documentation

European and German regulations require that any user of medical product devices has to receive a specific instruction and this instruction has to be documented. Such training is provided by representatives of the manufacturer of the MIP®. Contact data can be downloaded from http://www.reger-med.de. According to European law, such training has to be documented, and only physicians having received this training are allowed to use the MIP® in clinical practice.

8.6 Limited sales

PIPAC technology is only sold to physicians or hospitals. A training certificate is required to gain access to the technology. Moreover, in the present stage of technology development, where emphasis on clinical studies and scientific validation is needed, customers are required to contribute to a prospective registry with pseudoanonymized patient data, including follow up.

Bibliography

[1] Reymond MA, Hu B, Garcia A, Reck T, Köckerling F, Hess J, Morel P. Feasibility of therapeutic pneumoperitoneum in a large animal model using a microvaporisator. Surg Endosc. 14, 1 (Jan 2000) 51–55.

[2] Alkhamesi NA, Ridgway PF, Ramwell A, McCullough PW, Peck DH, Darzi AW. Peritoneal nebulizer: a novel technique for delivering intraperitoneal therapeutics in laparoscopic surgery to prevent locoregional recurrence. Surg Endosc. 19, 8 (Aug 2005) 1142–1146.

[3] Sharon A, Hirsh I, Kaufman Y, Ostrovski L, Brandes-Klein O, Spiegel D, Shenderey A, Lissak A. The effect of continuous intraabdominal nebulization of lidocaine during gynecological laparoscopic procedures – a pilot study. Gynecol Surg 5 (2008) 221–225.

[4] Alkhamesi NA, Peck DH, Lomax D, Darzi AW. Intraperitoneal aerosolization of bupivacaine reduces postoperative pain in laparoscopic surgery: a randomized prospective controlled double-blinded clinical trial. Surg Endosc. 21, 4 (Apr 2007) 602–606.

[5] Alkhamesi NA, Kane JM, Guske PJ, Wallace JW, Rantis PC. Intraperitoneal aerosolization of bupivacaine is a safe and effective method in controlling postoperative pain in laparoscopic Roux-en-Y gastric bypass. J Pain Res. 1 (Dec 1 2008) 9–13.

[6] Druckrey-Fiskaaen KT, Janssen MW, Omidi L, Polze N, Kaisers U, Nur I, Goldberg E, Bokel G, Hauss J, Schön MR. Laparoscopic spray application of fibrin sealant effects on hemodynamics and spray efficiency at various application pressures and distances. Surg Endosc 21 (2007) 1750–1759.

[7] Greib N, Schlotterbeck H, Dow WA, Joshi GP, Geny B, Diemunsch PA. An evaluation of gas humidifying devices as a means of intraperitoneal local anesthetic administration for laparoscopic surgery. Anesth Analg 107 (2008) 549–551.

[8] Canis M, Matsuzaki S, Bourdel N, Jardon K, Cotte B, Botchorishvili R, Rabischong B, Mage G. [Peritoneum and laparoscopic environment]. Bull Cancer 94 (2007) 1043–1051. Review.

[9] Newman SP, Clarke SW. Therapeutic aerosols 1-Physical and practical considerations. Thorax 38 (1983) 881–886.

[10] Hinds WC. Aerosol Technology (2nd edn.). Wiley – Interscience, 1999.

[11] USC Eshelman School of Pharmacy, http://pharmlabs.unc.edu/labs/aerosols/physical_laws.htm, consulted on 27.4.2014.

[12] Dedrick RL, Flessner MF. Pharmacokinetic problems in peritoneal drug administration: tissue penetration and surface exposure. J Natl Cancer Inst. 89, 7 (Apr 2 1997) 480–487. Review.

[13] Esquis P, Consolo D, Magnin G, Pointaire P, Moretto P, Ynsa MD, Beltramo JL, Drogoul C, Simonet M, Benoit L, Rat P, Chauffert B. High intra-abdominal pressure enhances the penetration and antitumor effect of intraperitoneal cisplatin on experimental peritoneal carcinomatosis. Ann Surg 244 (2006) 106–112.

[14] Jacquet P, Stuart OA, Chang D, Sugarbaker PH. Effects of intra-abdominal pressure on pharmacokinetics and tissue distribution of doxorubicin after intraperitoneal administration. Anticancer Drugs 7 (1996) 596–603.

[15] Los G, Mutsaers PH, Lenglet WJ, Baldew GS, McVie JG. Platinum distribution in intraperitoneal tumors after intraperitoneal cisplatin treatment. Cancer Chemother Pharmacol 25 (1990) 389–394.

[16] Garofalo A, Valle M, Garcia J, Sugarbaker PH. Laparoscopic hyperthermic chemotherapy for palliation of debilitating malignant ascites. Eur J Surg Oncol 32 (2006) 682–685.

M. A. Reymond, A. Tannapfel, C. Schneider, H. Scheidbach,
S. Köver, A. Jung, T. Reck, H. Lippert, and F. Köckerling

9 Preclinical experiments

First we developed an intraperitoneal tumor xenograft model in the large animal, being able to grow human HeLa cells in port-site wounds of German landrace pigs. Before the first in-human use, we have shown that therapeutic capnoperitoneum improves both distribution and penetration of an active substance into the peritoneum. Moreover, we were able to show an increased biological activity in human peritoneal carcinomatosis ex vivo (nuclear toxicity using Dbait). This was the first proof of concept in human tissue showing genotoxiciy induced by jamming DNA repair pathways. These preclinical experiments are detailed below.

9.1 Xenograft intraperitoneal model in the pig

M. A. Reymond, A. Tannapfel, C. Schneider, H. Scheidbach, S. Köver, A. Jung, T. Reck, H. Lippert, and F. Köckerling

Experimental animal studies are necessary if the results of minimally-invasive oncological surgery are to be improved. Since small animals such as rodents are inappropriate for such laparoscopic surgical studies, there is a requirement for a large animal tumor model. For years, farm and miniature pigs have been widely used in laboratory medicine [1]. Since the introduction of surgical laparoscopy, the pig model has been increasingly used not only in experimental studies, but also for the training of laparoscopic surgeons. Various aspects of laparoscopy such as venous blood flow [2], peritonitis [3], formation of adherences [4], and so on, have been investigated using the pig model.

Over the last few years, the problem of tumor cell spillage during cancer laparoscopy has been extensively studied. Various measures have been proposed to reduce the incidence of port-site recurrence [5, 7]. To assess the efficacy of such measures, a large animal model permitting survival experiments is necessary. In a series of publications [8, 9], Allardyce et al. reported on a clinically relevant model of laparoscopic colectomy in the pig, using suspended 51Cr-labeled, fixed HeLa cells injected intraperitoneally. The authors suggested that this model might be useful for evaluating surgical factors impacting on the contamination of port wounds with tumor cells. While alternative animal models are also available for use in oncological laparoscopy, for example the hamster [10] or the rat [11], many surgeons believe them to be inappropriate for assessing the effect of technical measures on oncological outcome due to the limited applicability of usual surgical techniques and instruments in small animals. The model described by Allardyce et al. [12] has not been tested in survival studies. In particular, it was not clear whether cultured HeLa cells would survive labeling with 51Cr – a toxic isotope. The present study aimed to find an answer to this question and develop a porcine model for testing current laparoscopic surgical practice and the effectiveness of protective measures in survival studies.

9.1.1 Material and methods

The trial was approved by the Committee on Animal Research in Thüringen, Germany. Nine randomly selected nonsyngeneic German farm pigs aged 6 to 8 weeks at operation and weighing a mean of 31 ± 6.6 kg were employed in the trial.

9.1.2 Anesthesia

After premedication with intramuscular azaperone 1–2 mg/kg and atropine 0.05 mg/kg, a canula was inserted into the ear vein, and orotracheal intubation performed. Anesthesia was achieved with N_2O, analgesia with intravenous fentanyl and droperidol, and muscle relaxation with pancuronium in accordance with usual protocols (Table 9.1).

Table 9.1. Anesthesia protocol.

Indication	Drug
Premedication	Azeparone 1–2 mg/kg im Atropine 0.05 mg/kg im
Sedation for intubation	Methomidate 4–8 mg/kg iv
Muscle relaxation	Succinylcholine, followed by pancuronium organon 0.1 mg/kg iv
Inhalation anesthesia	O2/NO2 mixture
Analgesia	Fentanyl 0.005 mg/kg iv Droperidol 0.2 mg/kg iv
Muscle relaxation	Pancuronium organon 0.1 mg/kg iv

9.1.3 Operative procedure: sigmoid colectomy

After induction of anesthesia, a water enema (2 liters) was given to prepare the bowel. The extremities of the animal were tied to the operation table with the pelvis slightly elevated, using a triangular support to facilitate transanal double stapling.

The abdominal wall was disinfected with 10% povidone-iodine solution. After insufflating the abdomen with CO_2 via a Veress needle, the first 12 mm trocar (Ethicon, Norderstedt, Germany) was inserted above the umbilicus and a pneumoperitoneum of 12 mm Hg created. Next, 10^7 freshly prepared HeLa cells were injected into the abdominal cavity through the umbilical trocar. Three further 12 mm trocars were inserted into the right upper and the right and left lower quadrants, the latter being positioned at the proximal end of a 40 mm line marking the position of the minilaparotomy. A classical laparoscopic, short sigmoid resection was then performed, an extraperitoneal purse string suture placed, a 25 mm stapler head (Ethicon Endosurgery, Norderstedt, Germany) inserted and an intracorporeal anastomosis done by transanal double stapling. Sterile gloves were used, and instruments were sterilized between the procedures. Disposable trocars and Veress-cannulas were used.

9.1.4 Postoperative care

In the immediate postoperative period, the animals were kept in boxes warmed with infrared light, and monitored. When awake, they were allowed to drink milk. Beginning on postoperative day one, all pigs were allowed free access to normal food and water.

9.1.5 Cell line

HeLa cells were grown in EMEM (supplemented with 1 x non essential aminoacids, 2 mM L-glutamine, 250 g/ml penicillin/streptomycin, 50 mM 2-mercaptoethanol [Life-Technologies, Eggenstein, Germany]) in a 5% CO_2 incubator at 37 °C until 80–90% confluence was reached. The cells were washed twice in PBS, detached by incubating for four minutes in trypsine-versene solution (Life-Technologies, Eggenstein, Germany) at 37 °C, spun down (400 xg, 10 minutes, room temperature) and split threefold. For injection into the pigs, the cells were harvested at 60–70% confluence, counted and resuspended at a density of 1×10^7 cells/ml in EMEM for transport.

9.1.6 Labeling of HeLa cells

To investigate the effects of chromium (CrO_4^{2-}) on the long term viability of HeLa cells we adopted the protocol used by Allardyce et al. [12]. Since these authors did not specify the activity used we followed standard protocols for chromium release experiments [13]. HeLa cells were incubated overnight (for at least 14 hours) in EMEM in the presence of 150 µM, 340 µM or 430 µM Na_2CrO_4 (SIGMA, Münich, Germany). The next day the chromium-containing medium was removed and the cells were washed three times in 37 °C warm PBS. Fresh medium was added and the viability of the cells monitored after 6, 12 and 24 hours.

9.1.7 Immunohistochemistry

Tissue samples free of necrosis or hemorrhage were obtained from all animals. The material was routinely fixed in 4% formaldehyde solution and embedded in paraffin. After slicing into 4 μm thick sections, the preparations were dewaxed in xylene and then rehydrated. Endogenous peroxidase activity was blocked by 3% hydrogen peroxide in methanol for 30 minutes. After brief rinsing in phosphate buffered saline, sections were preincubated with avidin-biotin (Camon SP 2001) for 15 minutes to reduce nonspecific background staining. The slides were incubated overnight with a 1 : 50 dilution of primary antibody (mouse, monoclonal; pan cytokeratin, Clone MNF 116, Dako Diagnostik, Hamburg, Germany) at room temperature. After incubation with biotinylated goat antibody to mouse immunoglobulin (DakoDiagnostik, Hamburg, Germany), the slides were covered with streptavidin-biotin-peroxidase complex. The peroxidase reaction proceeded for eight minutes, with 3-amino-9-ethylcarabazole solution as substrate in phosphate-buffered saline with hydrogen peroxide. Slides were counterstained with haematoxylin and finally mounted. Sections known to stain positively were included in each run; negative controls were also performed by replacing the primary antibody with mouse or goat ascites fluid (Sigma-Aldrich Biochemicals, St. Louis, MO).

9.1.8 In vitro study of chromate toxicity

After 14 hours incubation with 150, 340 and 430 μM Na_2CrO_4 and subsequent washing, no cells survived following 24 hours culture in EME (Figure 3). In comparison, the number of cells of the control (without Na_2CrO_4) had doubled.

9.1.9 Intraoperative complications

No intraoperative complications were observed. In one case, a primary anastomotic leak was laparoscopically oversewn. In no cases did conversion become necessary.

9.1.10 Port site recurrence

In all animals nodules were observed macroscopically at at least one port site (Figure 9.1). Peritoneal carcinosis was not present in any of the animals.

Local necrosis was usually present, sometimes associated with pus, rendering macroscopic differentiation between inflammation and tumor difficult (Figure 9.2). In the opinion of the senior pathologist (A. T.), tumor diagnosis using conventional histological analysis alone was not reliable enough.

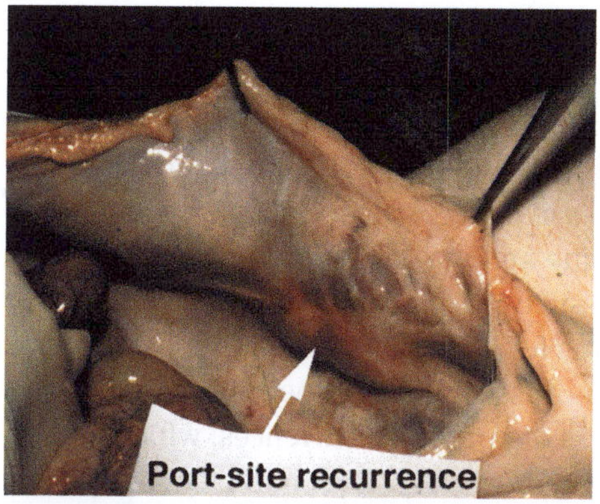

Fig. 9.1. Macroscopic appearance of a port-site recurrence in the left paraumbilical trocar position. Notice the position of the four trocars and of the 4 cm long minilaparotomy in the left lower quadrant (reproduced from [6]).

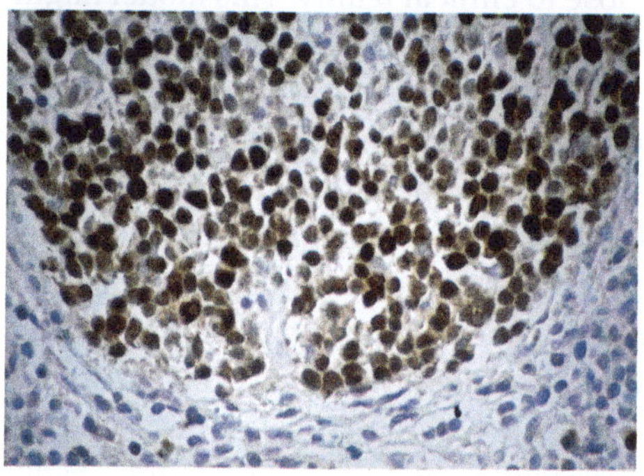

Fig. 9.2. Immunohistochemistry of a port site metastasis, showing xenografting of the HeLa cell line in the surgical wound in an nonimmunodeficient German landrace pig (reproduced from [6]).

Table 9.2. Histopathological analysis of port sites after autopsy; number of port-site recurrences.

	Port site recurrences (n = 9 animals)
Trocar 1 (RLQ)	7
Trocar 2 (RUQ)	6
Trocar 3 (LLQ)	5
Minilaparotomy (LUQ)	5
Total	**23**

Analysis after immunohistological staining confirmed the presence of a tumor at 23 out of 36 (63.8%) port sites and minilaparotomies, and infirmed clearly the presence of tumor in all other samples (Table 9.2).

9.1.11 Postoperative course

All the animals survived the surgical procedure, and no postoperative anastomotic leakage was observed. One case of postoperative pneumonia was observed and treated with intramuscular antibiotics. Mean weight gain was 9.1 ± 4.7 (from 31.0 ± 6.6 to 40.2 ± 7.9) kg.

9.1.12 Discussion

Our results show that it is possible to establish an intraperitoneal xenograft tumor in the pig, using a human cell line. In other words, the model first described by Allardyce et al. [8, 9] can be adapted for survival studies in cancer surgery. This is an important point, since the influence of surgical technique and the effect of protective measures on tumor recurrence can best be assessed in such survival studies.

In the present trial, tumor recurrence was found only within peritoneal wounds such as port sites and anastomoses, and was not associated with peritoneal carcinosis. This is in accord with the clinical presentation of port site recurrences, which by definition, are not associated with peritoneal carcinosis [14]. The characteristics of this xenogeneic tumor model are therefore very close to clinical reality. This model might be used for studies not only on port site recurrences in laparoscopy, but also on anastomotic recurrences following open or laparoscopic surgery.

Na_2CrO_4 labeled, fixed HeLa cells are not suitable for survival studies in vivo, as is documented by cellular death in vitro in the presence of chromate. Since such tumors are difficult to identify macroscopically or with conventional histology alone, another method of identification had to be found. This proved possible with immunohistochemistry. After staining the nodules with a pancytokeratin mouse anti-human MNF-116 monoclonal antibody, tumor cells were identified with a high degree of reliability.

Abandoning radiolabeling did not prevent accurate identification of tumor cells. Moreover, the abandonment of isotopes facilitated the experiment, since compliance with state regulations was easier. In a survival trial using radiolabeled cells, the animals, their urine and stools would have been considered radioactive and in need of appropriate handling and isolation. Our experimental farm had no authorization for handling radioactive isotopes, and our radioisotope laboratory was not licensed to keep large animals.

Numerous recent studies investigating mechanisms of tumor recurrence after surgery have been published in recent years. Obviously, such trials cannot be conducted in humans, and all the studies employed animal models. Nevertheless, using animals for xenogeneic tumor trials is no trivial matter, and adequate consideration must be given to the stress inflicted on the animals. Following Swiss Federal regulations, the present animal model can be classified in accordance with the following points.

- Type of surgical procedure.
  A bowel resection is considered a severe stress for the animal (degree 3), but no difference is made in the Swiss regulations between open and laparoscopic approaches. In the present trial, the animals quickly recovered from the surgical procedure, and were able to take normal food and water after 12 hours. The senior veterinarian observed no distress behavior, and the animals gained weight normally throughout the postoperative period. Because the bowel resection was

performed laparoscopically, we would tend to classify the surgical procedure as degree 2 (moderate), considering that the stress is slight but lasts a relatively long period of time.

- Xenogeneic tumor.
  The recurrent tumor was always small (under 3 cm) at sacrifice after four weeks, and caused no detectable symptoms. The tumor trial should be classified as degree 2 (moderate) because the experiment was terminated before any abdominal or digestive dysfunction occurred [15].

The present model permits the investigation of the influence of surgical technique and the effect of protective measures on tumor recurrence following laparoscopy or other surgical procedures. It is doubtful that the same information could be obtained using a small animal model. Some limitations of small animal models are related to the surgical instruments. For example, transanal stapling is impossible in the rat, the mouse or the hamster. Further limitations are related to the surgeon; the amplitude and number of movements do not reflect clinical reality. In our opinion, small animal models are therefore less suitable for assessing the quality of the laparoscopic technique. Small animal models do, however have other advantages: they are relatively inexpensive and involve the use of extensively studied animals. These factors have facilitated the investigation of many physiological or physiopathological effects of minimal access surgery [11, 16].

In summary, we present a human xenogeneic tumor model in the pig that enables survival studies to be performed. The stress imposed on the animals is moderate. The effects of surgical technique and of various protective measures that might be used perioperatively to prevent tumor recurrence can be tested using this model.

Bibliography

[1] Mount LE, Ingram DL. The pig as a laboratory animal. London: Academic Press, 1–175, 1971.
[2] Tagaki S. Hepatic and portal vein blood flow during carbon dioxide pneumoperitoneum for laparoscopic hepatectomy. Surg Endosc 12 (1998) 427–431.
[3] Greif WM, Forse RA. Hemodynamic effects of the laparoscopic pneumoperitoneum during sepsis in a porcine endotoxic shock model. Ann Surg 227 (1998) 474–480.
[4] Chen MD, Teigen CA, Reynolds HT, Johnson PR, Fowler JM. Laparoscopy vs. laparotomy: an evaluation of adhesion formation after pelvic and paraaortic lymphadenectomy in a porcine model. Am J Obstet Gynecol 178 (1998) 499–503.
[5] Jacobi CA, Ordemann J, Bohm M, Zieren HU, Sabat R, Muller JM. Inhibition of peritoneal tumor cell growth and implantation in laparoscopic surgery in a rat model. Am J Surg 174 (1997) 359–363.
[6] Reymond MA et al. Description of an intraperitoneal tumor xenograft survival model in the pig. Eur J Surg Oncol. 2, 6 (2000) 393–397
[7] Reymond MA, Kastl S, Schneider C, Hohenberger W, Köckerling F. Techniques for the prevention of port-site metastases. Surg Endosc 11 (1997) 533. (Abstract)

[8] Franklin ME, Rosenthal D, Abrego-Medina D et al. Techniques on tumor implantation following laparoscopy, Prospective Comparison of Open vs. Laparoscopic Colon Surgery for Carcinoma. Dis Colon Rectum 39 (1996) S35–S46.
[9] Allardyce RA, Morreau P, Bagshaw PF. Operative factors affecting tumor cell distribution following laparoscopic colectomy in a porcine model. Dis Colon Rectum 40 (1997) 939–945.
[10] Allardyce RA, Morreau PN, Frizelle FA, Bagshaw PF. Tumor cell wound distribution after colectomy in a porcine model. Aust NZ J Surg 68 (1998) 363–366.
[11] Jones DB, Guo LW, Reinhard MK et al. Impact of Pneumoperitoneum on Trocar Site Implantation of Colon Cancer in Hamster Model. Dis Colon Rectum 38 (1995) 1182–1188.
[12] Berguer R, Gutt CN. Laparoscopic colon surgery in a rat model. A preliminary report. Surg Endosc 8 (1994) 1195–1197.
[13] Allardyce R, Morreau P, Bagshaw P. Tumor Cell Distribution Following Laparoscopic Colectomy in a Porcine Model. Dis Colon Rectum 39 (1996) S47–S52.
[14] Wunderlich J, Shearer G. In: Coligan JE, Kruisbeek AM, Margulies DH, Shevach EM, Strober W (eds). Current Protocols in Immunology. New York: Wiley & Sons Inc, 1994:
[15] Reymond MA, Schneider C, Hohenberger W, Köckerling F. The pathogenesis of port-site recurrences. J Gastrointest Surg 1 (1997) (In Press)
[16] Protection des animaux. Berne: Swiss Federal Veterinary Office, 1994.
[17] Berguer R, Gutt C, Stiegmann GV. Laparoscopic surgery in the rat. Description of a new technique. Surg Endosc 7 (1993) 345–347.

9.2 Staining experiments with aerosolized methylene blue in the pig

W. Solass, A. Hetzel, G. Nadiradze, E. Sagynaliev, and M. A. Reymond

9.2.1 Introduction

The present experimental study presents the first results obtained with the PIPAC technology in the large animal model. Our general aim was to examine what happens within the abdominal cavity during nebulization of a vital stain (methylene blue). Our specific aims were to examine if better stain distribution throughout the peritoneal cavity and better direct penetration of the stain into the peritoneum can be achieved compared to conventional peritoneal lavage under similar conditions.

9.2.2 Material and Methods

Study design

This is an experimental in vivo study in the large animal model, comparing the effect of therapeutic capnoperitoneum (four animals) with the effect of conventional lavage (one control animal).

Nebulizer

The nebulizer consists of several components including an injector, a line and a nozzle. The nozzle had a diameter of 0.2 mm and a pressure of about 8 bar was delivered upfront of the nozzle. The nebulizer was inserted through a 5 mm trocar and generated an aerosol within the abdominal cavity. The gaseous phase consisted of CO_2; the liquid phase of microparticles of methylene blue.

Animal model

After obtaining the authorization of the animal experiment review board of the State of Thüringen, we operated on five German female landrace pigs, weighing between 45–60 kg, under anesthesia using routine protocols. Pneumoperitoneum of 12 mm Hg was established using a Veres needle. In the first step, a transvaginal cholecystectomy was performed in a three-trocar technique. In the second step, a peritoneal lavage or the application of therapeutic capnoperitoneum was performed according to the protocols below. The animals were euthanatized at the end of the procedure and immediately autopsied.

Experimental protocol

Similar protocols were applied for the control and test animals.

- Control animal ($n = 1$) with conventional peritoneal lavage. Twenty milileters of methylene blue (1% Methylenblau VITIS®, Neopharma, Aschau i. Chiemgau, Germany) were diluted into six liters of isotonic saline solution (0.9% NaCl). One inflow line and two outflow lines were placed into the abdomen and the abdomen was filled with two liter solution. A continuous peritoneal lavage was maintained for 30 minutes with an inflow of 1 L/min over a rolling pump.
- Test animals ($n = 4$) with therapeutic capnoperitoneum. Methylene blue (5 ml) was diluted into 10 ml isotonic saline solution (0.9% NaCl). The nebulizer was inserted into a 5 mm trocar. The solution was nebulized by hand pressure at room temperature (20 °C) over a few seconds into the abdominal cavity and an intraabdominal pressure of 12 mm Hg maintained for 30 minutes. The aerosol was eliminated using a pressure-limited waste system including valve and filter (Figure 9.3).

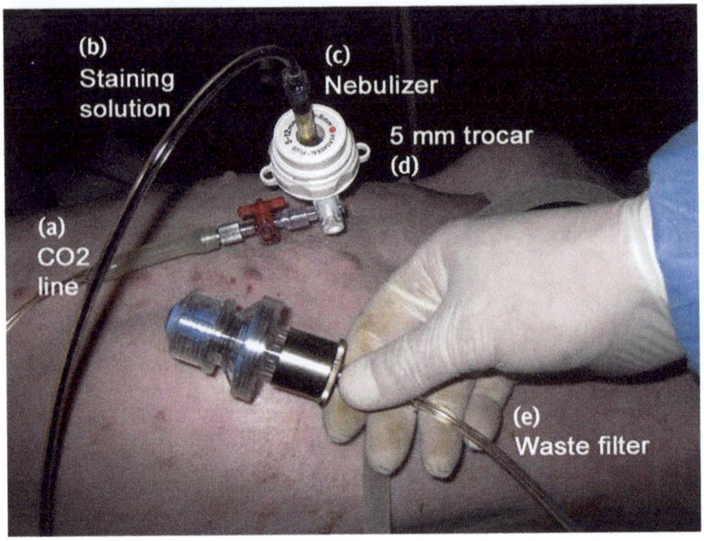

Fig. 9.3. The CO_2 line (a) is connected as usual with a 5 mm trocar (d). The liquid solution (methylene blue) is transported through a conventional IV line (b) to the nebulizer (c). An overpressure in the abdominal cavity is prevented by a valve connected to a filter (e) (reproduced from [1]).

9.2.3 Results

Procedures could be performed as planned both in the test group (four animals with nebulization) and in the control animal (conventional peritoneal lavage) and delivered the expected results.

The nozzle allowed rapid and effective nebulization of the methylene blue solution into the abdomen. Videoscopic control showed an immediate (within five seconds) staining of the complete abdominal cavity, including bowel loops, liver, anterior abdominal wall and diaphragmatic peritoneum (Figure 9.4).

No droplet formation was observed and the surgeon's view was not blurred. No hyperpressure developed in the abdominal cavity, as checked by the CO_2 insufflator The pressure-controlled valve of the waste filter did not open. No adverse cardiovascular nor pulmonary effect was registered. No gas leak was detected during the experiment. At the end of the procedure, the aerosol could be completely collected into the waste filter.

Adequacy of stain distribution throughout the entire peritoneal cavity was clearly superior in the nebulization group, as compared to the control (Figure 9.5).

Immediate autopsy confirmed that staining of the serosal surfaces was better distributed after nebulization than after peritoneal lavage. In particular, hidden surfaces were stained in the nebulization group, but not in the control animal. This was the case for anatomical structures located in the anterior, upper part of the abdomen (such as the abdominal wall).

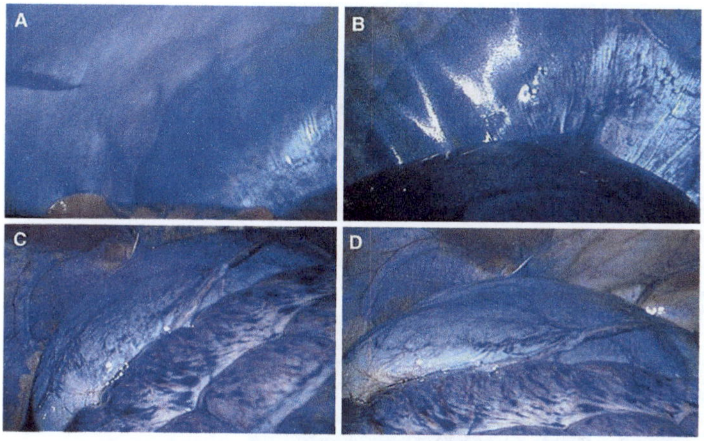

Fig. 9.4. Real-time endoscopic monitoring of nebulization showed immediate staining of the complete abdominal cavity, including the anterior abdominal wall and diaphragmatic peritoneum (a, b), liver (b), bowel loops and visceral peritoneum (c, d) (reproduced from [1]).

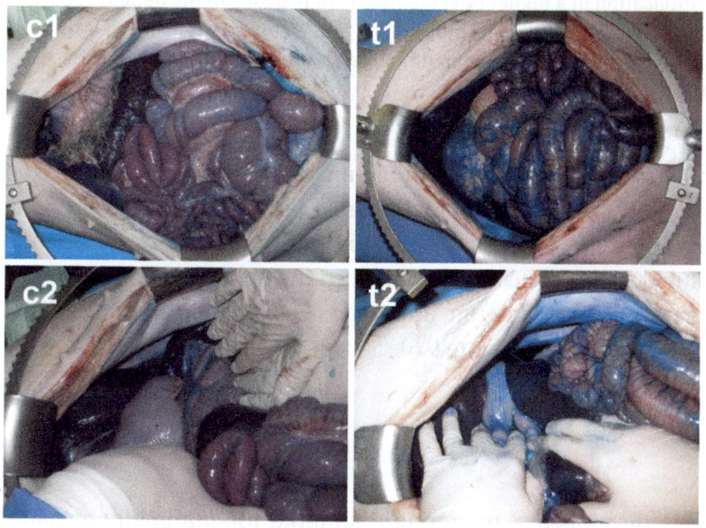

Fig. 9.5. Adequacy of stain distribution. Autopsy findings in the control (c1, c2) and test (t1, t2) animals. Staining of the serosal surfaces is better distributed after nebulization than after peritoneal lavage. Importantly, the hidden, anterior aspect of the stomach (*) is stained only in the nebulization group, as is the anterior abdominal wall (+) (reproduced from [1]).

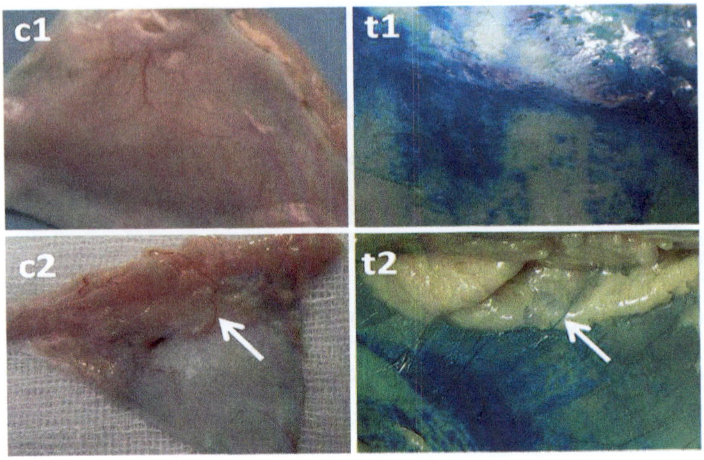

Fig. 9.6. Direct penetration of stain into the peritoneum. Autopsy findings in the control (c) and test (t) animals. c1 and t1 show the front side of the peritoneum (towards the abdomen), c2 and t2 show the backside of the peritoneum. Almost no staining of the peritoneum is observed in the control group, despite the application of a higher (4 ×) methylene blue dosis. In the nebulization group, staining has a patchy aspect (t1). Methylene blue staining has reached capilllary vessels in the retroperitoneal fat tissue in the nebulization group (t2, arrow) but not in the control animal (c2, arrow) (reproduced from [1]).

Direct penetration of the stain into the peritoneum was enhanced by nebulization (with the application of a pressure of 12 mm Hg) as compared to the conventional lavage. Importantly, this difference was obtained in spite of the application of a higher (4 ×) total methylene blue dosis in the control animal. In the nebulization group, the stain reached the backside of the peritoneum, as demonstrated by the staining of isolated retroperitoneal capillary vessels (Figure 9.6).

9.2.4 Discussion

About ten years ago, we developed a micropump suitable for minimally-invasive surgery procedures that allowed microdroplets of therapeutic substances to be distributed into the pneumoperitoneum (CO_2), creating the so-called "therapeutic pneumoperitoneum", or better said, the "therapeutic capnoperitoneum" [10]. The aerosol was produced by piezoelectric crystals stimulating three microperforated silicium chips. A feedback system was regulating the amount of drug delivery depending on the effective gas flow. In vitro, the micropump was shown to be able to aerosolize various aqueous and ethanol solutions, including cytostatic and bacteriostatic drugs and adhesion modulating agents. However, the function of the micropump was limited in vivo because of water condensation on the surface of the chips so that further development was abandoned.

In the last ten years, only few papers about laparoscopic nebulizers and their experimental or clinical applications were published. Alkhamesi et al. showed that nebulized heparin and hyaluronic acid attenuates peritoneal tumor growth after laparoscopic surgery in a rodent model [11]. Sharon et al. examined the effect of continuous intraabdominal nebulization of lidocaine during gynecological laparoscopic procedures in a limited number of patients [12]. Druckrey-Fiskaaen et al. examined laparoscopic spray application of fibrin sealant effects on hemodynamics and spray efficiency at various application pressures and distances [13]. Recently, Greib et al. compared various gas humidifying devices as a means of intraperitoneal local anesthetic administration, and only one of them was able to generate a therapeutic aerosol [14]. However, the opportunities offered by a therapeutic capnoperitoneum were recognized as a potential "revolution in laparoscopic surgery" [15].

To our knowledge, no nebulizer has so far obtained EC or FDA certification so that it could be used for intraperitoneal drug application in the clinical setting. Moreover, no pharmacokinetics studies are available proving that therapeutic capnoperitoneum improves drug distribution throughout peritoneal cavity or drug penetration into the tissues, as compared to peritoneal lavage.

This experimental study was aimed at examining in the effect of nebulization of a vital stain into the abdominal cavity during laparoscopy. In particular, we wanted to determine distribution of methylene blue within the abdominal cavity, and penetration of the stain into the peritoneal layers. The current standard of care (peritoneal lavage) was used as a control.

Experimental data obtained in the animal model suggest limited exposure of the peritoneal surface during conventional peritoneal lavage. When peritoneal dialysis was carried out in rodents with a solution containing methylene blue and bovine serum albumin, autopsy findings showed that large parts of the visceral and parietal peritoneum displayed no stain or very little stain [16]. In particular, the hidden aspects of the caecum and stomach as well as large portions of the small and large intestines and of the diaphragm remained unstained. Our results confirm this finding, namely that distribution of methylene blue within the peritoneal cavity is poor after peritonal lavage.

Our results are encouraging, since they confirm that peritoneal nebulization allows a better distribution of a substance throughout the abdominal cavity, as compared with conventional lavage. Immediate distribution of the stain all over the peritoneum was an impressive feature of the videoendoscopic monitoring during the procedure. It appears legitimate to extrapolate from our qualitative observations in a large animal model to the human setting. Unfortunately, quantitative data on the fraction of the peritoneum exposed to the lavage solution are not available in human patients. Moreover, functional peritoneal surfaces appear highly variable depending on the conditions [17]. To our knowledge, application of a therapeutic capnoperitoneum is one of the first concepts to increase exposure of the serosal surface and peritoneal tumor nodules. Such a therapeutic concept addresses an important medical need because much of the residual tumor burden is probably untreated or undertreated by conventional techniques such as HIPEC.

Our data also show an advantage in direct penetration of the stain into the normal peritoneum. The peritoneum is a single-layer cellular, mesothelial membrane that is supported by connective tissue. It offers protection against infection and tumor invasion [18]. However, in advanced cancer stages, tumor cells spread onto the peritoneal surface and into surgical wounds and they develop macroscopic nodules up to several centimeters diameter. Experimental data show very limited penetration of drugs into the peritoneum and peritoneal nodules. Los et al. [19] measured platinum concentrations in CC531 colon adenocarcinoma growing intraperitoneally in the rat by proton-induced x-ray emission following intraperitoneal and intravenous administration of cisplatin. Tumor concentration was significantly elevated at 1 mm from the periphery but not at 1.5 mm. The same authors obtained similar results in tumor-bearing rats, in which the drug concentration was significantly elevated at a depth of 1 mm in the tumor nodules 24 hours (single dose) or 48 hours (three injections) after intraperitoneal administration [20]. Thus, the current principle is to treat the macroscopic (visible) malignant peritoneal disease with CRS and, immediately after, to treat the remaining microscopic (nonvisible) malignant peritoneal disease with HIPEC. However, the efficacy of HIPEC remains hampered by the pharmacokinetics aspects defined above.

Dedrick has shown that limited direct penetration of drugs into tumor tissue remains an important practical and theoretical concern for regional drug therapy in the peritoneal cavity [9]. The present experiment has shown that, after nebulization, methylene blue reaches the backside of the peritoneum and the capillary vessels located in the retroperitoneum. This is an exciting experimental finding, showing that nebulization of a substance into the abdominal cavity might be significant progress towards mastering this penetration problem, and in turn could help to improve clinical results of intraperitoneal drug therapy by allowing therapy of larger tumor nodules. However, an enhanced local drug delivery might be associated with specific locoregional toxic effects like abdominal pain, bowel perforation, anastomotic leakage, infection, or postoperative ileus that need to be carefully evaluated.

Unfortunately, this finding is also generating concerns about potential systemic toxicity. Drug uptake by capillary flow into the general circulation might increase systemic side effects, and paradoxically decrease the delivery of drug to the tumor. The fundamental goal of intraperitoneal chemotherapy is to increase exposure of the contents of the peritoneal cavity while reducing systemic toxic effects. On the one side, poor drug penetration is limiting cytotoxicity and tumor response. On the other side, it may protect sensitive normal cells, for example the mucosa of the gastrointestinal tract. Thus, an increased drug distribution and tissue penetration (e.g. through nebulization) could result in an increased regional advantage but a higher systemic toxicity, since the gradient between peritoneal and plasma concentrations will narrow.

Up to now, there is a single experimental study assessing the pharmacokinetics of intraperitoneal ropivacaine, a local anesthetic, administered by instillation or nebulization in five pigs [21]. The pharmacokinetic profile of ropivacaine nebulization was found to be similar to direct intraperitoneal instillation, but with a lower absorption rate. This is an interesting result that is supporting further development of our concept of therapeutic capnoperitoneum.

Safety aspects of manipulating a toxic aerosol are significant and will be object of further studies. Our preliminary research has shown that appropriate technical solutions are available, which are routinely used in other applications, in particular in the automobile and chemical industry. These technical solutions will now be adapted for protecting both the patient and the medical team from possible side effects.

Careful and detailed pharmacokinetics and toxicity studies are also necessary to define the optimal framework for applying this novel, promising therapeutic approach in the human patient.

Bibliography

[1] Solass W et al. Description of a novel approach for intraperitoneal drug delivery and the related device. Surg Endosc. 26, 7 (Jul 2012) 1849–1855.
[2] Markman M. Intracavitary chemotherapy. Crit Rev Oncol Hematol. 3 (1985) 205–233. Review.
[3] Sugarbaker PH, Gianola FJ, Speyer JL, Wesley R, Barofsky I, Myers CE. Prospective randomized trial of intravenous v. intraperitoneal 5-FU in patients with advanced primary colon or rectal cancer. Semin Oncol 12 (1985) 101–111.
[4] Sugarbaker PH. Peritonectomy procedures. Ann Surg 221 (1995) 29–42.
[5] Elias D, Lefevre JH, Chevalier J, Brouquet A, Marchal F, Classe JM, Ferron G, Guilloit JM, Meeus P, Goéré D, Bonastre J. Complete cytoreductive surgery plus intraperitoneal chemohyperthermia with oxaliplatin for peritoneal carcinomatosis of colorectal origin. J Clin Oncol 27 (2009) 681–685.
[6] Alberts DS, Liu PY, Hannigan EV, O'Toole R, Williams SD, Young JA, Franklin EW, Clarke-Pearson DL, Malviya VK, DuBeshter B. Intraperitoneal cisplatin plus intravenous cyclophosphamide versus intravenous cisplatin plus intravenous cyclophosphamide for stage III ovarian cancer. N Engl J Med 335 (1996) 1950–1955.
[7] Maggiori L, Elias D. Curative treatment of colorectal peritoneal carcinomatosis: current status and future trends. Eur J Surg Oncol 36 (2010) 599–603. Review.
[8] Markman M. Intraperitoneal antineoplastic drug delivery: rationale and results. Lancet Oncol 4 (2003) 277–283.
[9] Dedrick RL, Flessner MF. Pharmacokinetic Problems in Peritoneal Drug Administration: Tissue Penetration and Surface Exposure. J Natl Cancer Inst 89 (1997) 480–487.
[10] Reymond MA, Hu B, Garcia A, Reck T, Kockerling F, Hess J, Morel P. Feasibility of therapeutic pneumoperitoneum in a large animal model using a microvaporisator. Surg Endosc 14 (2000) 51–55.
[11] Alkhamesi NA, Ridgway PF, Ramwell A, McCullough PW, Peck DH, Darzi AW. Peritoneal nebulizer. A novel technique for delivering intraperitoneal therapeutics in laparoscopic surgery to prevent locoregional recurrence. Surg Endosc 19 (2009) 1142–1146.

[12] Sharon A, Hirsh I, Kaufman Y, Ostrovski L, Brandes-Klein O, Spiegel D, Shenderey A, Lissak A. The effect of continuous intraabdominal nebulization of lidocaine during gynecological laparoscopic procedures- a pilot study. Gynecol Surg 5 (2008) 221–225.
[13] Druckrey-Fiskaaen KT, Janssen MW, Omidi L, Polze N, Kaisers U, Nur I, Goldberg E, Bokel G, Hauss J, Schön MR. Laparoscopic spray application of fibrin sealant effects on hemodynamics and spray efficiency at various application pressures and distances. Surg Endosc. 21 (2007) 1750–1759.
[14] Greib N, Schlotterbeck H, Dow WA, Joshi GP, Geny B, Diemunsch PA. An evaluation of gas humidifying devices as a means of intraperitoneal local anesthetic administration for laparoscopic surgery. Anesth Analg 107 (2008) 549–551.
[15] Canis M, Matsuzaki S, Bourdel N, Jardon K, Cotte B, Botchorishvili R, Rabischong B, Mage G. [Peritoneum and laparoscopic environment]. Bull Cancer 94 (2007) 1043–1051. Review.
[16] Flessner MF. Small-solute transport across specific peritoneal tissue surfaces in the rat. J Am Soc Nephrol 7 (1996) 225–233.
[17] Steller MA, Egorin MJ, Trimble EL, Bartlett DL, Zuhowski EG, Alexander HR, Dedrick RL. A pilot phase I trial of continuous hyperthermic peritoneal perfusion with high-dose carboplatinum as primary treatment of patients with small-volume residual ovarian cancer. Cancer Chemother Pharmacol 43 (1999) 106–114.
[18] Elias D, Goéré D. [Treat the peritoneum with respect! It's our first-line of defense against carcinomatosis]. J Chir (Paris) 144 (2007) 275–276.
[19] Los G, Mutsaers PH, van der Vijgh WJ, Baldew GS, de Graaf PW, McVie JG. Direct diffusion of cis-diamminedichloroplatinum(II) in intraperitoneal rat tumors after intraperitoneal chemotherapy: a comparison with systemic chemotherapy. Cancer Res 49 (1989) 3380–3384.
[20] Los G, Mutsaers PH, Lenglet WJ, Baldew GS, McVie JG. Platinum distribution in intraperitoneal tumors after intraperitoneal cisplatin treatment. Cancer Chemother Pharmacol 25 (1990) 389–394.
[21] Betton D, Greib N, Schlotterbeck H, Joshi GP, Ubeaud-Sequier G, Diemunsch P. The pharmacokinetics of ropivacaine after intraperitoneal administration: instillation versus nebulization. Anesth Analg 111 (2010) 1140–1145.

9.3 Ex vivo experiments with Dbait on diseased peritoneum

W. Solass, A. Herbette, T. Schwarz, A. Hetzel, J. S. Sun, M. Dutreix, and M. A. Reymond

Current therapy of peritoneal carcinomatosis, when possible, includes cytoreductive surgery associated or not with hyperthermic intraperitoneal chemotherapy [1]. However, this therapy is linked to significant morbidity and mortality, and results are still limited [2]. Thus, there is a need for novel therapeutic approaches, including preventive strategies during initial surgery [3].

The ability of cancer cells to recognize damage and initiate DNA repair is an important mechanism of resistance to treatment. Pharmacological inhibition of DNA repair for a short period during treatment has the potential to make cancer cells more vulnerable to the damaging effects of therapy, therefore increasing the response to treatment [4]. Dbait acts by baiting and hijacking the enzyme complexes that repair DNA double strand breaks (DSB), diverting them away from their primary objective, the DSB on chromosomes [5]. Such DSB are currently caused by treatment, such as radiotherapy (RT) and DNA-damaging chemotherapy. Dbait increases the sensitivity of HNCC, melanoma and glioblastoma to irradiation [6], and the sensitivity of colorectal cancer to chemotherapy [7]. However, a limitation of this approach is tumor access and penetration into tumor nodes, so that it can only be applied to superficially spreading tumors.

Laparoscopy offers a unique opportunity to control and to steer the operating environment during surgery, by loading carbon dioxide with a therapeutic substance and creating the so-called therapeutic capnoperitoneum [8]. Recently, we have shown that therapeutic peritoneum allows homogeneous distribution of a therapeutic substance within the peritoneal cavity and an improved penetration depth into normal and diseased tissue compared with conventional peritoneal lavage [9]. However, working with toxic therapeutic aerosols is only possible under strongly regulated conditions. Interestingly, preclinical studies with Dbait in the primate have shown no toxicity of the molecule on healthy tissues (data on file). Thus, there is a rationale for combining Dbait with therapeutic capnoperitoneum to obtain a synergy. In particular, a local increase in chemosensitivity could improve efficacy of both intraperitoneal and systemic chemotherapy on peritoneal carcinomatosis.

The general purpose of the present ex vivo experiment was to test possible advantages of combining both technologies for treating a human peritoneal carcinomatosis tumor nodule, in particular concerning tumor access (distribution and penetration). A second specific goal was to examine whether genotoxicity can be demonstrated in a tumor nodule of human peritoneal carcinomatosis after loading capnoperitoneum with Dbait.

9.3.1 Material and methods

The current study was designed to investigate the biodistribution of Dbait in a peritoneal carcinomatosis nodule ex vivo, immediately after surgical resection. For this purpose, a tumor nodule was exposed to Dbait aerosol using the micropump (MIP®) spraying device under 12 mm Hg of CO_2 pressure in a closed box modelling the peritoneal cavity. An electrical gradient was generated to focus drug distribution onto the peritoneal surface and to enhance tissue penetration. As controls, two further experiments were conducted: (1) the experiment as above without Dbait, and (2) lavage of a peritoneal carcinomatosis nodule with Dbait in a glucose solution. The following parameters have been measured:

(a) surface homogeneity of Dbait distribution within the simulated peritoneal cavity;
(b) Dbait diffusion into the peritoneal nodule, and;
(c) Dbait bioactivity in cancer cells under oxidative stress.

9.3.2 Study design

This ex vivo study involved tumor tissue from a single human patient suffering peritoneal carcinomatosis from endometrial origin. Because patient therapy was not influenced by the experiment, no authorization from an ethical committee was required. Ex vivo research on human tissue is allowed at our institution by a valid authorization of the common ethics committee of the Westfalian University – Medical Chamber of Westfalia-Lippe (AeKWL, Figure 9.7).

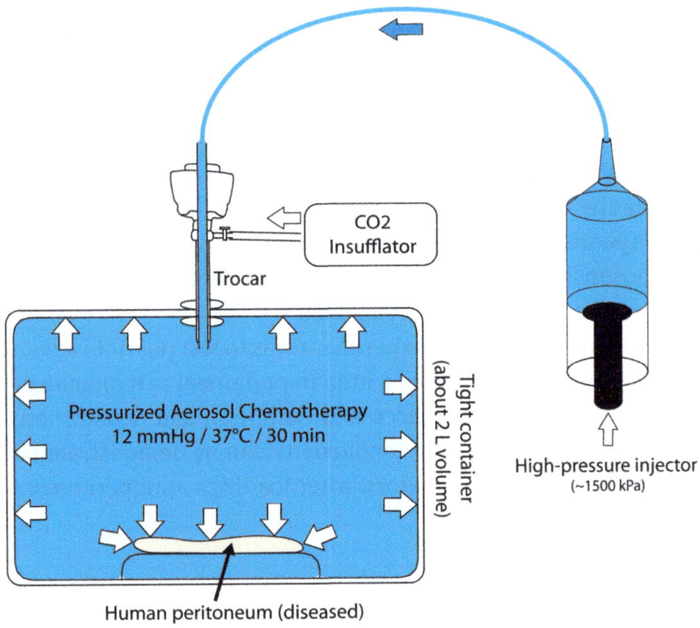

Fig. 9.7. Laparoscopy-like ex vivo experiment on fresh operation specimen of diseased human peritoneum (peritoneal carcinomatosis from endometrial origin). Therapeutic capnoperitoneum (12 mm Hg) was established in a plastic box. An electrostatic gradient of 60 V was generated between the MIP® and the biological tissue, placed on a neutral electrode. MIP® micropump (reproduced from [10]).

9.3.3 Nebulizer

The nebulizer has been described elsewhere [9] and consists of several components, including an injector, a line, and a nozzle. The nozzle had a diameter of 0.2 mm, and a pressure of approximately 8 bars was delivered upfront of the nozzle. The nebulizer was inserted through a 10 mm trocar and generated an aerosol within the plastic box mimicking the abdominal cavity. The gaseous phase consisted of CO_2; the liquid phase of microparticles of Dbait (100 lg/ml).

9.3.4 Patient characteristics, cytoreduction, and intraperitoneal hyperthermic chemotherapy

A female patient suffering peritoneal carcinomatosis from endometrial cancer was selected for the experiment and gave her written, informed consent. Chloroquine 100 mg qd was administered for one week before the operation. First, a complete cytoreduction was achieved (CRS). In a second step, intraperitoneal hyperthermic chemotherapy was applied with cisplatin 75 mg/m^2 body surface and doxorubicin 15 mg/m^2 body surface, according to usual protocols.

9.3.5 Tumor characteristics

Immediately after surgical cytoreduction, a peritoneal fragment of approximately 10 × 9 × 10 cm, showing macroscopic peritoneal nodules, was selected for experimental purpose. The remaining surgical specimen was sent to the pathologist for diagnostic purposes. Microscopic analysis showed a poorly differentiated (G3) clear cell adenocarcinoma with few small necrosis foci.

9.3.6 Experimental protocol

The three surgical samples were treated as follows.

a) The first peritoneal nodule was inserted into the experimental box, placed on the electrode, and exposed to CO_2 capnoperitoneum at room temperature for 30 minutes. After dilution into 90 ml of glucose 5%, 9 mg of Cy5-labelled Dbait (1 : 1 dilution with non fluorescent Dbait) was aerosolized into the box.
b) A second peritoneal nodule was exposed to "peritoneal lavage" using 0.1 mg/ml Dbait-Cy5 diluted into 10 ml of glucose 5%.
c) A third peritoneal nodule was exposed to identical conditions as (a) without Dbait (negative control).

Immediately after the experiment, all three samples were split into two halves. The first half was fixed in formalin solution and sent to the pathologist, the second half was immediately frozen at −80 °C for further biological analysis.

9.3.7 Microscopic analysis

For analysis, formalin-fixed specimens were stained with H&E according to usual protocols. For microscopic fluorescence analysis, samples were fixed with PFA 4% for 20 minutes at room temperature (RT), followed by exposure to Triton 0.5% for 10 minutes at room temperature. Then, samples were washed out in SVF diluted in PBS solution for one hour at room temperature, followed by incubation with c-H2AX mouse antibody (Millipore, Billerica, MA, USA) diluted 1/200 (SVF in PBS) for two hours at room temperature. After washing, samples were incubated with secondary anti-mouse FITC (Sigma-Aldrich Chimie Sarl., Lyon, France) diluted 1/100 for 45 minutes at room temperature. Nuclei were counterstained with Dapi 0.5 lg/ml for five minutes at room temperature. Analysis was performed with an inverted microscope.

9.3.8 Results

The experiment was performed according to the schedule. No technical difficulty was encountered. In particular, MIP® generated the Dbait aerosol without any difficulty. Remote control of the injection device was possible without direct intervention in the operating room. All six sides of the experimental box were stained; however, an intensity gradient was observed from the bottom to the top of the box (not shown).

Microscopic analysis revealed homogeneous peritoneal distribution of Dbait-Cy5 in the therapeutic capnoperitoneum sample (arrows), only minimal uptake in the lavage sample, and no staining (or only marginal staining) in the control sample (Figure 9.8).

Fluorescence was detected within the tumor up to 1 mm depth in the therapeutic capnoperitoneum sample but not in the lavage sample. Thus, aerosolization of the molecule allowed significantly better tumor access and better bioavailability of Dbait than conventional lavage (Figure 9.9).

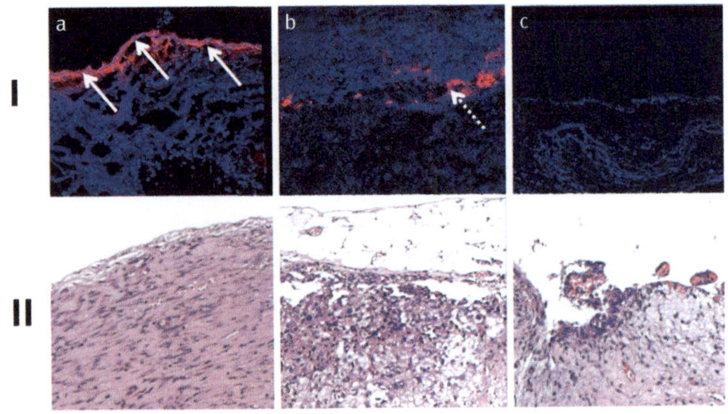

Fig. 9.8. Diffusion of therapeutic substance onto the peritoneum. I: Cryosection of human peritoneum, red: Dbait-Cy5 staining, blue: Dapi (nucleus). (a): After nebulization of Dbait, (b): after lavage with Dbait, (c): after nebulization without Dbait. Staining reveals homogeneous peritoneal fluorescence in the therapeutic capnoperitoneum sample (arrows), only minimal uptake in the lavage sample, and no staining in the control sample. II: H&E staining (reproduced from [10]).

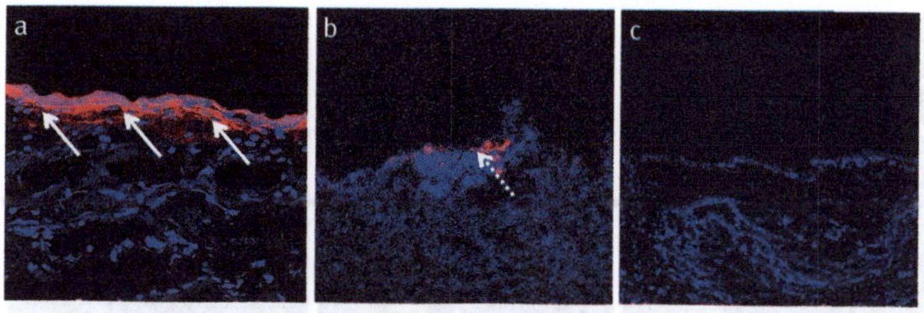

Fig. 9.9. Penetration of therapeutic substance into the peritoneum. Cryosection of human peritoneum, red: Dbait-Cy5 staining, blue dapi (nucleus). (a): After nebulization of Dbait, (b): after lavage with Dbait, (c): after nebulization without Dbait. Staining reveals fluorescence up to seven cellular layers in the therapeutic capnoperitoneum sample (a), no tissue uptake in the lavage sample (b) and no staining in the control sample (c) (reproduced from [10]).

Biological results showed intranuclear phosphorylation of H2AX in the nebulized sample and almost no activity in the lavage sample (Figure 9.10).

The low activity detected in the lavage sample is due to the presence of spontaneous chromosomal damage in peritoneal carcinomatosis cells. Detection of histone gamma-H2AX (phosphorylated H2AX) reveals the nuclear activation of DNA-dependent protein kinase (DNA-PK) by Dbait. Dbait was taken up by cancer cells, and a biological activity was detected up to 1 mm depth. Importantly, tumor nodules showed more activity at the tumor invasion front (Figure 9.11).

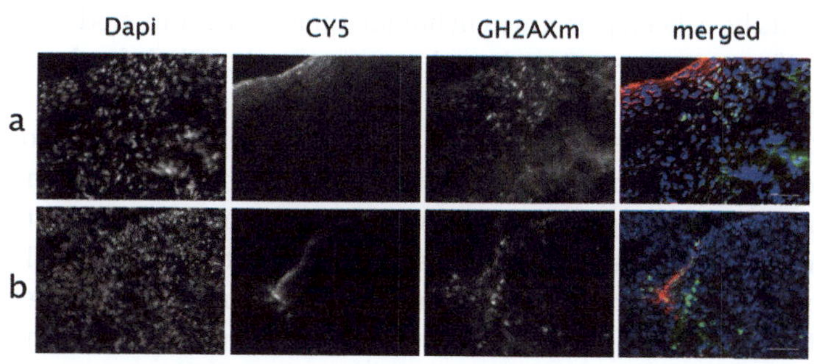

Fig. 9.10. Biological activity. Cryosection of human peritoneum. Detection of early Dbait activity marker: Phosphorylated H2AX. Red: Dbait-Cy5 staining, blue: Dapi staining (nucleus), green: c-H2AX. (a): After nebulization of Dbait, (b): after lavage with Dbait. Intranuclear phosphorylation of H2AX is observed the nebulized sample and only artifactual staining (no nuclear staining) in the lavage sample. Detection of histone c-H2AX (phosphorylated H2AX) reveals activation of DNA-Phosphokinase by Dbait, which has been shown to be the key step for sensibilization to genotoxic therapy (reproduced from [10]).

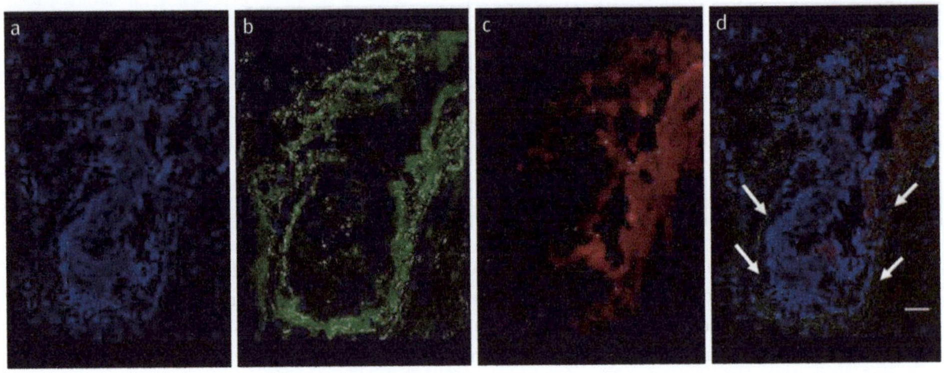

Fig. 9.11. Tumor specificity. Detection of early Dbait activity marker: cryosection of human peritoneum; A blue: Dapi staining (nucleus); B green: c-H2AX after nebulization of Dbait, C red: Dbait-Cy5 staining, D merged: H2AX activation is maximal at the tumor invasion front (arrow) (reproduced from [10]).

9.3.9 Discussion

This ex vivo experiment was designed to examine possible advantages of combining Dbait with therapeutic capnoperitoneum for treating a human tumor nodule of peritoneal carcinomatosis ex vivo, in particular concerning tumor access (distribution and penetration). A second specific goal was to examine whether bioactivity of Dbait could be demonstrated.

This is the first time that the biological activity of Dbait is proved in human patient tissue. So far, experiments have been performed in human tumor xenograft models in the animal. This is significant progress toward regulatory approval of Dbait for therapeutic use in patients.

The above-mentioned results are encouraging, because they evidence a homogeneous distribution of Dbait onto the peritoneum and a better penetration into the peritoneum than after conventional peritoneal lavage. This excellent bioavailability of Dbait in human peritoneal tissue ex vivo confirms the results obtained previously in the large animal model showing a better vital staining of the abdominal cavity after aerosolization than after lavage with methylene blue [9]. Another important finding was intranuclear phosphorylation of H2AX in the nebulized sample, proving Dbait uptake up to 1 mm depth, and showing biological activity. Detection of histone gamma-H2AX (phosphorylated H2AX) reveals nuclear activation of DNA-PK by Dbait, a significant result because this activation has been shown to be the key step for chemosensibilization to genotoxic therapy [5, 6]. Moreover, this result has been obtained under oxidative stress conditions (warm ischemia) in human tumoral tissue, and not in an animal model. Importantly, tumor nodules showed more activity than the neighbor, normal peritoneum, in particular at the tumor invasion front. Thus, the present experiment delivers the proof of principle for combining Dbait with systemic or intraperitoneal chemotherapy to produce significant synergy. Of course, this proof of principle ex vivo should now be confirmed by corresponding in vivo studies.

Current intraperitoneal hyperthermic chemotherapy guidelines recommend the application of an intraperitoneal temperature of 41–43°C [11]. Recently, we observed that numerous Heat Shock proteins were phosphorylated in cells treated by Dbait. Moreover, in vitro, Dbait sensitizes cells to temperature shifts (unpublished data). Thus, it will be interesting to perform these efficacy studies under hyperthermic conditions to increase the biological effect of Dbait. In this experiment, biological response was observed already after less than one hour. This was a surprise because preclinical data obtained in the animal model showed maximal biological response after three hours. This can be explained by the application of an electrostatic gradient of 60 V, which is similar to the condition of cellular electroporation. This was obviously helpful for uptake of very large amounts of Dbait molecules. Preoperative therapy with chloroquine also might have contributed to this improved cellular drug uptake: chloroquine is known to fragilize the membranes of the endosomes, so that the release of Dbait molecules into the cytoplasm is facilitated [12]. The biological effect was achieved with a low Dbait dose, only 9 mg for a volume corresponding to the entire abdominal cavity. Dbait effect is strictly dose-dependent, as demonstrated in several tumor systems [6]. In the preclinical model, a dose of 4 mg was considered adequate for treating small tumor xenografts (data submitted). Thus, an excellent intracellular uptake of Dbait was achieved under experimental conditions.

Another, major point of interest is that Dbait has shown no toxicity in preclinical studies in the primate (data on file). Thus, aerosolization of Dbait might be possible in clinical practice without particular safety measures for protecting both patient and surgical team. This favourable safety profile might speed up implementation of therapeutic capnoperitoneum in cancer surgery.

In summary, combining Dbait with therapeutic capnoperitoneum appears to have several practical advantages. Peritoneal carcinomatosis is a superficial and diffuse tumor that is accessible to Dbait. Pressure enhances Dbait penetration into tumor tissue. CO_2 as a carrier ensures excellent drug distribution onto the peritoneum. Application of an electrostatic gradient optimizes both drug distribution and drug uptake, probably by inducing cellular electroporation. Dbait has no toxicity demonstrated in the primate so that its clinical use appears easily possible. Finally, intraperitoneal hyperthermia might enhance the efficacy of Dbait by creating cellular stress, but this has not been investigated in the present proof-of-principle experiment. The development of procedures easily applicable to the clinical setting that might improve outcome in peritoneal carcinomatosis should be given high priority. This proof-of-principle experiment opens a new avenue for treating peritoneal carcinomatosis that should now be followed by adequate clinical studies, a precondition for regulatory approval of this new, challenging therapeutic approach.

Bibliography

[1] Roviello F, Caruso S, Marrelli D, Pedrazzani C, Neri A, De Stefano A, Pinto E. Treatment of peritoneal carcinomatosis with cytoreductive surgery and hyperthermic intraperitoneal chemotherapy: state of the art and future developments. Surg Oncol 20, 1 (2011) e38–e54.

[2] Baratti D, Kusamura S, Laterza B, Balestra MR, Deraco M. Early and long-term postoperative management following cytoreductive surgery and hyperthermic intraperitoneal chemotherapy. World J Gastrointest Oncol 2, 1 (2010) 36–43.

[3] Kusamura S, Baratti D, Zaffaroni N, Villa R, Laterza B, Balestra MR, Deraco M. Pathophysiology and biology of peritoneal carcinomatosis. World J Gastrointest Oncol 2, 1 (2010) 12–18.

[4] Helleday T, Petermann E, Lundin C, Hodgson B, Sharma RA. DNA repair pathways as targets for cancer therapy. Nat Rev Cancer 8 (2008) 193–204.

[5] Quanz M, Chassoux D, Berthault N, Agrario C, Sun JS, Dutreix M. Hyperactivation of DNA-PK by double-strand break mimicking molecules disorganizes DNA damage response. PLoS One 4, 7 (2009) e6298.

[6] Quanz M, Berthault N, Roulin C, Roy M, Herbette A, Agrario C, Alberti C, Josserand V, Coll JL, Sastre-Garau X, Cosset JM, Larue L, Sun JS, Dutreix M. Small-molecule drugs mimicking DNA damage: a new strategy for sensitizing tumors to radiotherapy. Clin Cancer Res 15, 4 (2009) 1308–1316.

[7] Devun F et al. Assessing chemotherapy efficacy enhancement by inhibition of DSBs repair by Dbait32Hc in colorectal cancers developed in genetically engineered mouse models. J Gastroenterol, in press.

[8] Reymond MA, Hu B, Garcia A, Reck T, Kockerling F, Hess J, Morel P. Feasibility of therapeutic pneumoperitoneum in a large animal model using a microvaporisator. Surg Endosc 14, 1 (2000) 51–55.

[9] Solass W, Hetzel A, Nadiradze G, Sagynaliev E, Reymond MA. Description of a novel approach for intraperitoneal drug delivery and the related device. Surg Endosc, in press.

[10] Solass W et al. Therapeutic approach of human peritoneal carcinomatosis with Dbait in combination with capnoperitoneum: proof of concept. Surg Endosc. 26, 3 (Mar 2012) 847–852.

[11] Piso P. Basisprotokoll für ein multimodales chirurgisches therapiekonzept zur behandlung von Patienten mit Peritonealcarcinose mittels Peritonektomie/multiviszeralresektion und hyperthermer intraperitonealer chemotherapie. Deutsche Gesellschaft für Allgemein-und Viszeralchirurgie, Berlin, 2007.

[12] Guy J, Drabek D, Antoniou M. Delivery of DNA into mammalian cells by receptor-mediated endocytosis and gene therapy. Mol Biotechnol 3, 3 (1995) 237–248.

W. Solass, R. Kerb, T. Mürdter, U. Giger-Pabst, D. Strumberg, C. Tempfer, J. Zieren, M. Schwab, and M. A. Reymond

10 First PIPAC in-human application

10.1 Introduction

Life expectancy in peritoneal carcinomatosis (PC) is limited due to advanced tumor stage and poor therapeutic response. Resistance of peritoneal carcinomatosis to systemic chemotherapy (SC) is explained by molecular mechanisms [1] and by limited drug distribution [2]. This is the rationale for locoregional therapy combining cytoreductive surgery (CRS) with intraperitoneal chemotherapy [3]. However, this approach is debated [4]: intraperitoneal chemotherapy is hampered by limited drug distribution within the abdominal cavity and poor penetration into peritoneal carcinomatosis nodules [5]. Thus, the benefit of combined CRS and intraperitoneal chemotherapy over CRS alone might be marginal [6].

We have proposed applying chemotherapy as a pressurized aerosol within the abdominal cavity [7], in order to take advantage of following physical properties: applying an aerosol allows a homogeneous repartition of the substance within a closed space; and generating an artificial pressure gradient counterbalances tumoral interstitial fluid pressure, an obstacle in cancer therapy [8]. In the large animal model, a pressurized aerosol improved both distribution of a vital stain within the abdominal cavity, and depth of penetration into the peritoneum, as compared to peritoneal lavage with a liquid solution [9]. When treating human peritoneal carcinomatosis ex vivo, we achieved a superior distribution onto the peritoneum and a better penetration into peritoneal carcinomatosis nodules than intraperitoneal chemotherapy [10]. This was the rationale for the first application in the human patient.

10.2 Methods

10.2.1 Patients

PIPAC was offered as a treatment option to three patients suffering from a fatal disease for which no satisfactory alternative therapy was available, pursuant to the individual compassionate use of medicinal products according to the German Medical Act (AMG) and with documented favorable opinion by the Ethics Committees of the University of Münster, Germany. Patients were evaluated by our multidisciplinary team before onset of treatment and provided written informed consent. Clinical and histological confirmation of peritoneal carcinomatosis including small bowel involvement was required. No patient had parenchymatous metastases. Patient histories are summarized in Table 10.1. PIPACs were performed between November 2011 and March 2013.

10.2.2 Surgical procedures

After insufflation of a 12 mm Hg capnoperitoneum at 37 °C, two balloon trocars (Applied Medical, Düsseldorf) were placed. Explorative laparoscopy was performed as usual and Peritoneal Carcinomatosis Index [11] determined. Parietal biopsies were taken and ascites removed. A nebulizer (MIP®, Reger Medizintechnik, Rottweil) was connected to a high-pressure injector (Injektron 82M, MedTron, Saarbruecken) and inserted into the abdomen through a trocar. A pressurized aerosol containing cisplatin (Hexal, Barleben) at a dose of 7.5 mg/m^2 body surface in 150 ml NaCl 0.9% was applied immediately followed by doxorubicin (Hexal, Barleben) 1.5 mg/m^2 in 50 ml NaCl 0,9%. Then, the system was kept in steady-state for 30 minutes (application time). Toxic aerosol was exhausted over a closed system. Trocars were retracted. PIPAC was repeated two to five times at various time intervals (Figure 10.1). Occupational health safety aspects are described elsewhere [12].

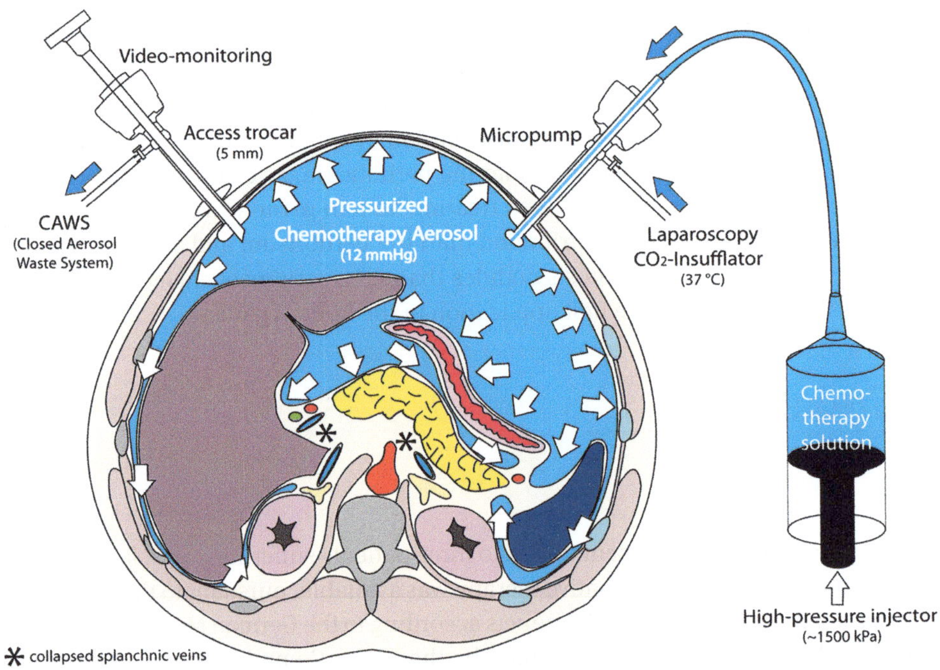

Fig. 10.1. Technique of Pressurized IntraPeritoneal Aerosol Chemotherapy (PIPAC). A capnoperitoneum of 12 mm Hg is established as usual during laparoscopy. A chemotherapy aerosol is generated at the tip of a mechanical micropump introduced through a balloon trocar, and maintained for 30 min at 37 °C. Then, the toxic aerosol is exsufflated over a secure system (CAWS: Closed Aerosol Waste System) into the outside environment (reproduced from [13]).

10.2.3 Safety and Efficacy assessments

Assessments for patient safety and tolerability were performed from days one to five after treatment, and included medical examination and routine laboratory measures. Adverse effects were graded according to the NCI Criteria for Adverse Events (CTCAE) [14]. Tumor response was assessed by laparoscopy with macroscopic assessment, histology and immunohistochemistry, as part of the next PIPAC cycle. Patients were followed up for analysis until June 20th, 2013 or until death.

10.2.4 Histology and immunohistochemistry

Multiple biopsies were analyzed for possible tumor response by conventional HE microscopy.

10.2.5 Clinical Pharmacology

Analysis is based on eight PIPAC in three patients. Blood samples were drawn before, during and up to 12 hours after the start of PIPAC. At the end of PIPAC biopsies from peritoneal tissue and tumor nodules were snap frozen. Doxorubicin plasma levels were determined by UHPLC-MS/MS using [13C2H3]-doxorubicin as internal standard. Pharmacokinetics parameters were derived by noncompartmental analysis (WinNonLin 6.3, Pharsight, Cary, NC). The area under the plasma concentration-time curve (AUC) was calculated by the linear trapezoidal rule.

10.3 Results

10.3.1 Patient 1

A 45-year-old male patient was operated on because of acute bowel obstruction due to peritoneal carcinomatosis from signet-ring appendiceal cancer. Postoperative high-dose chemotherapy (5-FU) was interrupted due to acute heart failure. After recovery, Karnovsky Index was 40%. First PIPAC was performed, showing a PCI of 16 (Figure 10.2 panels a1 and b1). Four weeks later, second PIPAC showed stable disease. Four weeks later, third PIPAC showed hard, glassy nodules (a2), histology showed regres-

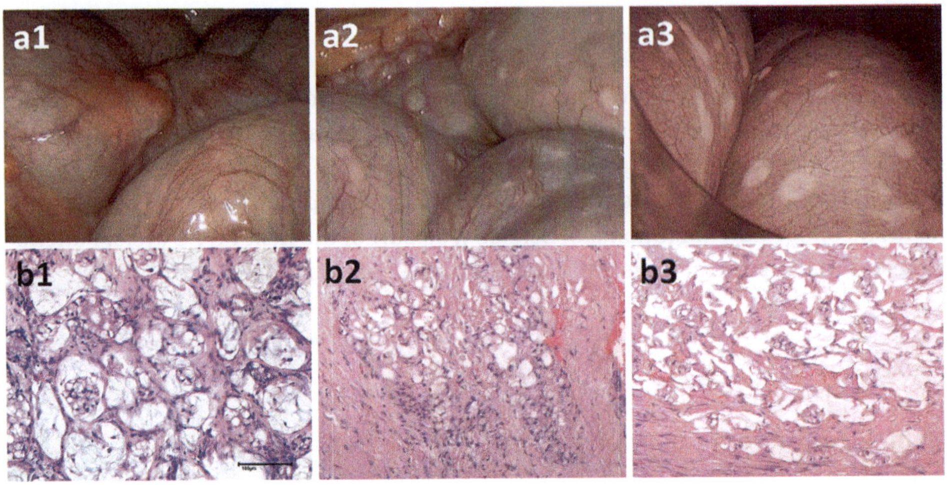

Fig. 10.2. Macroscopical and histological response after PIPAC. Forty-five-year-old male patient with diffuse peritoneal carcinomatosis (PCI = 16) from a signet-ring cells appendiceal cancer with inaugural small bowel obstruction. Macroscopy before (a1), after first (a2) and after third PIPAC (a3) showing regression of small bowel peritoneal carcinomatosis nodules. Histology shows vital tumor before PIPAC (b1), inflammatory reaction with nodular sclerosis after first PIPAC (b2) and large areas of devitalized tumor after third PIPAC (b3). Scale bar 100 lm (reproduced from [13]).

sive changes with nodular sclerosis (b2). Six weeks later, small bowel nodules were regressive (a3), histology showed regressive changes with 60% vital cells and large devitalized areas (b3, Figure 10.2).

Complete CRS was performed, and fourth PIPAC administered. A postoperative bowel perforation required surgical revision. After recovery, the patient developed bowel obstruction and tumor progression was confirmed by laparotomy. He died 187 days after first PIPAC.

10.3.2 Patient 2

A 38-year-old male patient with a two year history of signet-ring gastric cancer, gastrectomy and two chemotherapy lines presented with tumor progression and end-stage disease requiring parenteral nutrition. Karnovsky index was 40%. A PCI of 6 was documented at first PIPAC (Figure 10.3, panel a1). Four weeks later, during the second PIPAC, macroscopy showed complete remission (a2), multiple biopsies confirmed absence of tumor cells (b2). Eight weeks later the patient developed liver and bone metastases, and died 109 days after the first PIPAC. Two weeks before death abdomen CT showed no evidence of peritoneal carcinomatosis (Figure 10.3).

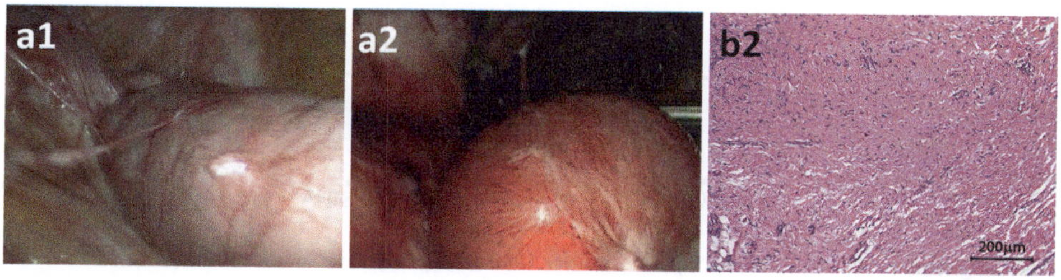

Fig. 10.3. Thirty-eight-year-old patient with signet-ring gastric cancer and peritoneal carcinomatosis. Laparoscopy 6 weeks after first PIPAC, including small bowel resection (blind-loop at the Roux-Y oesophago-jejunal anastomosis). Mascroscopy: tumor nodes scarring. Histology: All biopsies negative. Complete intraperitoneal remission (CR). Patient developed liver metastases four weeks later and died after 109 days without evidence of intraabdominal recurrence on the CT scan (reproduced from [13]).

10.3.3 Patient 3

A 73-year-old female patient with a ten year history of ovarian cancer, surgery and multiple chemotherapy regimen presented with tumor progression and hemorrhagic ascites. Karnovsky index was 40%. At first PIPAC, a PCI of 14 was documented and 2.5 L ascites removed (Figure 10.4, panels a1 and b1). At second PIPAC after four weeks, peritoneal carcinomatosis nodules were hard and glassy, ascites volume dropped to one liter. Histology showed no regression (not shown). Six weeks later at the third PIPAC,

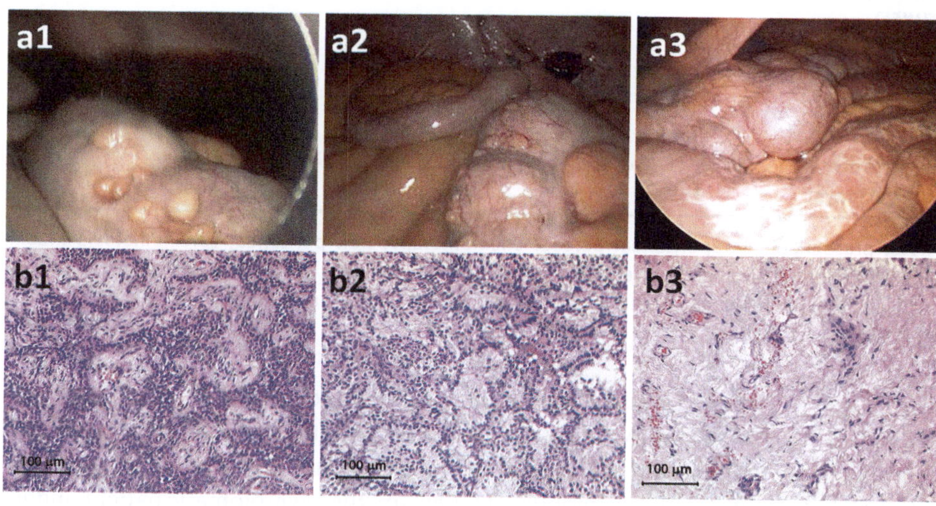

Fig. 10.4. Seventy-three-year-old patient (patient 3) with therapy-resistant peritoneal carcinomatosis and malignant ascites of ovarian origin. Shown is the macroscopic (upper fig) and histological (HE staining, lower fig) appearance before (left column), after PIPAC (middle column) and at later stages of follow up (right column). (a), (b) show partial and then complete macroscopic and microscopic tumor remission after repeated PIPAC. Scale bar 100 lm (reproduced from [13]).

Table 10.1. Patient characteristics and therapy summary.

Patient	1	2	3
Sex	M	M	F
Age at first PIPAC	38	45	73
Diagnosis	Gastric Ca, signet ring	Appendix Ca, signet ring	Ovarian Ca
First diagnosis	2009 (2 y.)	9.2011 (6 w.)	2001 (10 y.)
Previous surgery	Gastrectomy, LAD D2	Ileo-caecal resection	Hysterectomy, Adnexectomy, LAD
Previous Chemotherapy Regimen	ECF, paclitaxel	5-FU	Multiple regimens
Karnovsky before PIPAC therapy	40%	40%	40%
PCI before PIPAC therapy	6	16	14
PIPAC application (n)	2	4	4
Secondary CRS	No	Yes	No
Adverse effects (Grade CTAEC)	Fever [2], Vomiting [2], Pain [2]	Bowel perforation* [4]	Fatigue [1]
Intraperitoneal tumor remission: macroscopy	CR	PR	CR
Intraperitoneal tumor remission: histology	CR	PR	CR
Tumor Apoptosis (TUNEL)	N/A#	Yes	Yes
Tumor ascitis control	N/A	N/A	Yes
Max. Karnovsky after therapy	40%	70%	90%
Status	Dead	Dead	Alive
Cause of death	Metastasis, cachexia	Bowel obstruction	N/A
Survival (days)	109	187	400

PIPAC: pressurized intraperitoneal aerosol chemotherapy; PCI: peritoneal carcinomatosis index; CRS: cytoreductive surgery. * bowel perforation after CRS combined with PIPAC; # not enough material archived; N/A: not relevant; LAD: lymphadenectomy; PR: partial (intraperitoneal) remission; CR: complete (intraperitoneal) remission.

ascites was < 500 ml (a2), histology showed partial tumor response with fibrotic reaction (b2). Karnovsky index was 90%. Eight months after first PIPAC, fourth PIPAC showed complete remission (a3), multiple biopsies showed apoptotic inflammatory cells (b3) but no tumor. After 15 months of follow up, the asymptomatic patient underwent control laparoscopy, tumor was documented in two out of five peritoneal biopsies, so that fifth PIPAC was applied. Six weeks later, a single, 6 cm large tumor node was resected, all other biopsies were negative; sixth PIPAC was applied (Figure 10.4). After 567 days, the patient is alive with an excellent quality of life.

10.4 Safety

All eleven PIPAC procedures were technically easy to perform. For PIPAC alone, mean operating time was 93 ± 13 min. No intraoperative complication was noted. PIPAC alone was very well tolerated, no adverse effect > 2 CTCAE was noted (Table 10.1).

After PIPAC alone, patients were discharged from hospital two to five days after treatment. In two instances, PIPAC was combined with another operation (small bowel resection, complete cytoreductive surgery): in the latter case a postoperative bowel perforation (see Patient 1 above) required surgical revision.

10.5 Clinical Pharmacology

The plasma concentration-time curve fitted best to a two-compartment model with first order absorption. Peak doxorubicin plasma concentrations were low (4.0–6.2 ng/ml) and were reached with the end of nebulization. Doxorubicin was eliminated from the body with a clearance (Cl/F) of 2.6–6.0 ml/min. Half-lives and AUCs ranged from 86 to 468 min and 415 to 915 ng/ml×min, respectively (Figure 10.5).

In tumor nodules, local tissue concentration of doxorubicin was high (mean 1.70 µg/g) and variable (SD ± 1.45 µg/g). Fluorescence microscopy showed nuclear presence of doxorubicin up to 500 µm depth (Figure 10.6).

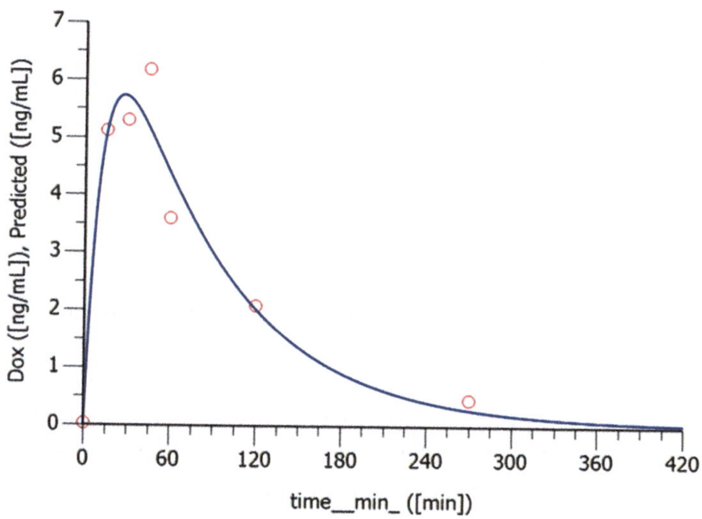

Fig. 10.5. Systemic doxorubicin exposure during PIPAC, showing a typical pharmacokinetic profile in peripheral venous blood after PIPAC with doxorubicin 1.5 mg/m^2 body surface for 30 minutes at an intraabdominal pressure of 12 mm Hg. Peak doxorubicin plasma concentrations were low (4.0–6.2 ng/ml). Line predicted profile. Dots experimental values (reproduced from [13]).

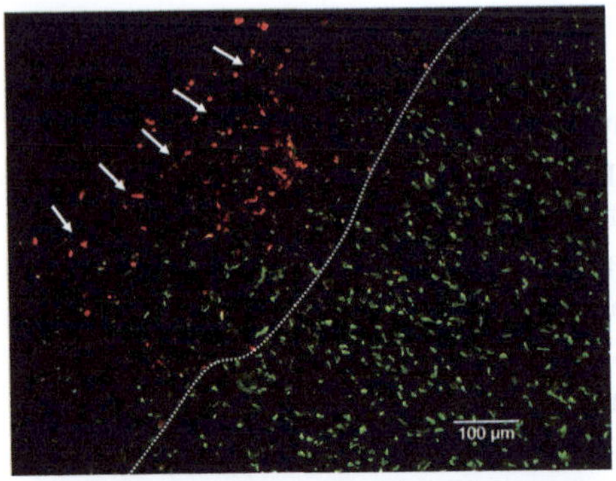

Fig. 10.6. Local doxorubicin exposure in peritoneal tumor nodes immediately after PIPAC. Local disposition is high with 1.70 ± 1.45 lg/g. In a fluorescence microscopy shows a nuclear presence of doxorubicin up to 500 lm depth. Red doxorubicin. Green picogreen nuclear counterstaining. Scale bar 100 lm (reproduced from [13]).

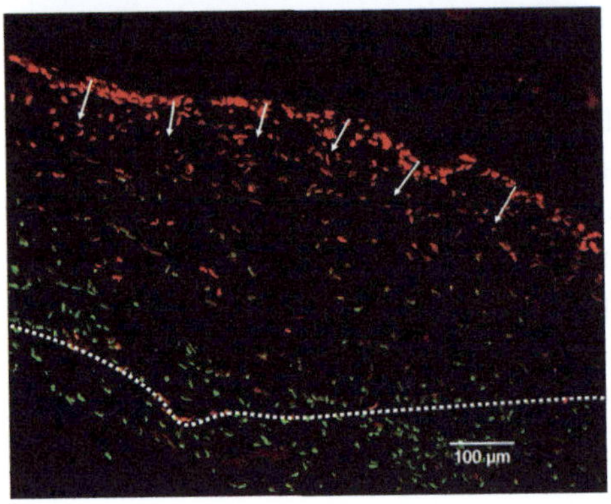

Fig. 10.7. Local doxorubicin exposure in normal peritoneum immediately after PIPAC. Fluorescence microscopy shows a nuclear presence of doxorubicin up throughout the whole peritoneal layer into the properitoneal fatty tissue (> 600 µm depth). Red doxorubicin. Green picogreen nuclear counterstaining. Scale bar 100 lm (reproduced from [13]).

In adjacent, normal peritoneum, fluorescence microscopy showed staining throughout the whole peritoneal layer into the properitoneal fatty tissue (> 600 µm). Highest concentration was achieved within 100 to 200 µm from the surface (Figure 10.7).

10.6 Discussion

To our knowledge, this is the first report of successful application of chemotherapy as a pressurized aerosol within the abdomen of human patients.

It has been predicted that innovative concepts overcoming pharmacologic limitations of intraperitoneal chemotherapy could improve, perhaps dramatically, its efficacy [5]. A superior dose-response ratio after PIPAC could be expected from preclinical data. In the human patient, plasma concentration-time profile analysis now confirms such a superior ratio between dose, systemic and local drug concentration: PIPAC required only a tenth of the doxorubicin dose to achieve higher tumor concentrations (0.03–4.1 µmol/g) as reported for HIPEC (0.02 µmol/g) [16]. In contrast, systemic availability of doxorubicin after PIPAC and HIPEC was equal as indicated by the approximately ten times lower maximal plasma concentration after PIPAC.

We [9, 10] as well as others [16, 17] reported that increasing intraperitoneal pressure enhanced particularly the uptake of drugs into the tumor, resulting in a higher local disposition. After PIPAC, doxorubicin was not only detected in significant concentrations in peritoneal carcinomatosis nodules, but nuclear staining was demonstrated throughout the peritoneum, up to deeply into the retroperitoneal fatty tissue. Another explanation for superior local disposition could be the high drug concentration in the aerosol. Although only a a tenth of the total dose was used, doxorubicin concentration in the aerosol (52 μM) is three times higher as in the intraperitoneal fluid usually used in HIPEC (18 μM) [16] without impairing tolerability as it was reported after applying higher concentrations of intraperitoneal chemotherapy [18].

Tumor response was observed in all three cases after PIPAC, as a consequence of the well-documented antitumor activity of doxorubicin and cisplatin and the superior local disposition. However, we were surprised by the extent of macroscopic and microscopic response in these multidrug-resistant tumors. We documented a complete remission of peritoneal carcinomatosis in two patients, which was indeed unexpected.

At this stage, it would be clearly premature to claim that combined PIPAC with cisplatin and doxorubicin improves survival in advanced peritoneal carcinomatosis. However, in our three patients with multiresistant tumors, low performance index and very limited life expectancy, we observe a mean survival over 288 days. Remarkably, 567 days after her first PIPAC patient 3 is still alive.

In sharp contrast to HIPEC, PIPAC was very well tolerated and the only severe adverse effect observed was a bowel perforation after CRS (Table 10.1). Otherwise, postoperative courses were uneventful, with early hospital discharge.

PIPAC might create synergies with systemic chemotherapy (SC). Liver and renal tests showed neither acute nor cumulative toxicity after PIPAC [20], which appears reasonable bearing in mind the 90% dose reduction as compared to conventional systemic chemotherapy. Moreover, PIPAC permits repeated cycles of intraperitoneal chemotherapy, and therefore might allow effective regimen combining systemic chemotherapy and PIPAC. Importantly, repeated laparoscopy enables objective staging, assessment of therapeutic response and adaptation of further therapy accordingly, which was barely possible until now. Finally, considering that all three patients were in poor physical condition with a low performance index, PIPAC might allow therapy in polymorbid patients, when SC is contraindicated.

We observed tumor regression even in platinum-resistant tumors, after application of cisplatin and doxorubicin. This is not surprising since drug effect is usually dose-dependent. PIPAC might become an alternative therapy for platinum-resistant tumors, in particular in women with ovarian cancer where tumor progression is diagnosed after first-line therapy with carboplatinum-taxol.

Repeated intraoperative analysis of the environmental air showed that PIPAC is safe for staff and meets the requirements of the German working safety regulations [12].

In conclusion, these early data appear promising. PIPAC can induce remission in end-stage, therapy-resistant peritoneal carcinomatosis, and first safety data are encouraging. PIPAC is well tolerated, a decisive feature in patients with limited life expectancy. By requiring only 10% of the dose of conventional intraperitoneal chemotherapy, PIPAC shows an excellent local distribution with low systemic exposure. Furthermore, PIPAC permits repeated cycles of intraperitoneal chemotherapy as well as objective tumor staging and response assessment. PIPAC is easy to use. PIPAC is complying with EC occupational safety regulations. The potential of this generic technology for a variety of indications and drugs has now to be determined in adequate studies.

Bibliography

[1] Griffiths RW, Zee YK, Evans S, Mitchell CL, Kumaran GC, Welch RS, Jayson GC, Clamp AR, Hasan J. Outcomes after multiple lines of chemotherapy for platinum-resistant epithelial cancers of the ovary, peritoneum, and fallopian tube. Int J Gynecol Cancer. 21, 1 (Jan 2011) 58–65.

[2] Minchinton AI, Tannock IF. Drug penetration in solid tumors. Nat Rev Cancer. 6, 8 (Aug 2006) 583–592. Review.

[3] Macrì A, Fortugno A, Saladino E. Rationale and techniques of CRS and peritoneal chemohyperthermia. World J Gastrointest Oncol. 3, 12 (Dec 15 2011) 169–174.

[4] Sugarbaker PH, Ryan DP. Cytoreductive surgery plus hyperthermic perioperative chemotherapy to treat peritoneal metastases from colorectal cancer: standard of care or an experimental approach? Lancet Oncol. 13, 8 (Aug 2012) e362–369.

[5] Dedrick RL, Flessner MF. Pharmacokinetic Problems in Peritoneal Drug Administration: Tissue Penetration and Surface Exposure. J Natl Cancer Inst 89 (1997) 480–487.

[6] Elias D, Gilly F, Boutitie F, Quenet F, Bereder JM, Mansvelt B, Lorimier G, Dubè P, Glehen O. Peritoneal colorectal carcinomatosis treated with surgery and perioperative intraperitoneal chemotherapy: retrospective analysis of 523 patients from a multicentric French study. J Clin Oncol. 28, 1 (Jan 1 2010) 63–68.

[7] Reymond MA, Hu B, Garcia A et al. Feasibility of therapeutic pneumoperitoneum in a large animal model using a microvaporisator. Surg Endosc 14 (2000) 51–55.

[8] Heldin CH, Rubin K, Pietras K, Ostman A. High interstitial fluid pressure – an obstacle in cancer therapy. Nat Rev Cancer. 4, 10 (Oct 2004) 806–813. Review.

[9] Solass W, Hetzel A, Nadiradze G, Sagynaliev E, Reymond MA. Description of a novel approach for intraperitoneal drug delivery and the related device. Surg Endosc. 26, 7 (Jul 2012) 1849–1855.

[10] Solass W, Herbette A, Schwarz T, Hetzel A, Sun JS, Dutreix M, Reymond MA. Therapeutic approach of human peritoneal carcinomatosis with Dbait in combination capnoperitoneum: proof of concept. Surg Endosc. 26, 3 (Mar 2012) 847–852.

[11] Elias D, Souadka A, Fayard F, Mauguen A, Dumont F, Honore C, Goere D. Variation in the peritoneal cancer index scores between surgeons and according to when they are determined (before or after cytoreductive surgery). Eur J Surg Oncol. 38, 6 (Jun 2012) 503–508.

[12] Solass W, Giger U, Borgstedt U, Zieren J, Reymond MA. Pressurized IntraPeritoneal Aerosol Chemotherapy (PIPAC): occupational health and safety aspects. Ann Surg Oncol 2013 Jun 14. [Epub ahead of print].

[13] Solass W et al. Intraperitoneal chemotherapy of peritoneal carcinomatosis using pressurized aerosol as an alternative to liquid solution: first evidence for efficacy. Ann Surg Oncol. 21, 2 (Feb 2014) 553–559.

[14] http://ctep.cancer.gov/protocolDevelopment/electronic_applications/ctc.htm, downloaded on Dec 31st, 2012.

[15] Sugarbaker PH, Van der Speeten K, Anthony Stuart O, Chang D. Impact of surgical and clinical factors on the pharmacology of intraperitoneal doxorubicin in 145 patients with peritoneal carcinomatosis. Eur J Surg Oncol. 37, 8 (Aug 2011) 719–726.

[16] Jacquet P, Stuart OA, Chang D, Sugarbaker PH. Effects of intra-abdominal pressure on pharmacokinetics and tissue distribution of doxorubicin after intraperitoneal administration. Anticancer Drugs. 7, 5 (Jul 1996) 596–603.

[17] Esquis P, Consolo D, Magnin G, Pointaire P, Moretto P, Ynsa MD, Beltramo JL, Drogoul C, Simonet M, Benoit L, Rat P, Chauffert B. High intra-abdominal pressure enhances the penetration and antitumor effect of intraperitoneal cisplatin on experimental peritoneal carcinomatosis. Ann Surg. 244, 1 (Jul 2006) 106–112.

[18] Ozols RF, Young RC, Speyer JL, Sugarbaker PH, Greene R, Jenkins J, Myers CE. Phase I and pharmacological studies of adriamycin administered intraperitoneally to patients with ovarian cancer. Cancer Res. 42, 10 (Oct 1982) 4265–4269.

[19] Markman M. Intraperitoneal antineoplastic drug delivery: rationale and results. Lancet Oncol 4 (2003) 277–283.

[20] Blanco A, Giger U, Solass W, Cruciger O, Zieren J, Reymond MA. Renal and hepatic toxicities after Pressurized IntraPeritoneal Aerosol Chemotherapy (PIPAC). Ann Surg Oncol 20, 7 (Jul 2013) 2311–2316.

A. Blanco, U. Giger-Pabst, W. Solass, J. Zieren, and M. A. Reymond

11 Renal and liver toxicities

In spite of significant progress in chemotherapy regimen, peritoneal carcinomatosis (PC) still has poor prognosis and remains an unmet medical need. Systemic chemotherapy is the standard therapy in this palliative situation, but survival benefit is limited, with for example median survival of 22 months in recurrent ovarian cancer and 16 months in colorectal cancer [1–3]. The limited results of chemotherapy are explained in part by the mechanisms of chemoresistance in these advanced tumors but also by poor penetration of the therapeutic substance into tumor tissue [4, 5]. Over the last decade, locoregional delivery of chemotherapy into the abdominal cavity has been increasingly applied for treating peritoneal carcinomatosis, with the aim of increasing the drug concentration ratio between tumor cells and plasma compartment. This approach has been validated by pharmacological studies, and more recently by clinical studies, for example, in ovarian cancer and colorectal cancer [4, 6–8]. However, the efficacy of intraperitoneal chemotherapy is impaired by two main pharmacological limitations, namely poor penetration into tumor nodules and limited distribution within the abdomen [6]. Therefore, prior complete surgical cytoreduction is required for effective intraperitoneal chemotherapy [9]. Pressurized intraperitoneal aerosol chemotherapy (PIPAC) is an innovative technique, applying chemotherapeutic drugs as a pressurized aerosol into the abdomen during laparoscopy [10]. In an animal model and in ex vivo surgical specimens, PIPAC has been shown to improve the local bioavailability of drug and staining substances, as compared with conventional peritoneal lavage [11, 12]. Recently, this excellent bioavailability in the nodules of peritoneal carcinomatosis has been confirmed in human patients, and pharmacokinetic analysis showed a low drug concentration in peripheral venous blood [13].

While these results are encouraging, it remains unclear whether PIPAC causes significant hepatic or renal toxicity. In theory, local drug delivery into the abdomen combined with the artificial intraabdominal pressure might increase the risk for first-pass hepatic toxicity and direct toxic renal parenchymal injury. Herein we report data on liver and renal toxicity from a pilot study of patients subjected to PIPAC.

11.1 Patients and methods

11.1.1 Study Design

This is a prospective data collection (phase 0 study) within the framework of off-label use of an approved drug as defined by Arzneimittelgesetz (German Drug Act). The procedures were performed at the Evangelisches Krankenhaus Bielefeld and at Marien Hospital Herne, Ruhr-University Bochum, Germany.

11.1.2 Ethics

The protocol was approved by the Institutional Review Board (Ethikkommission der WW-Universität Müster and Medical Chamber of Westfalia-Lippe). The patients were extensively informed about the procedure and included in the study if they gave their written consent. The procedures were performed according to the Declaration of Helsinki and EC and German laws and regulations. In particular, occupational health and safety risks were evaluated by two independent audits (data on file).

11.1.3 Patients

Eight PIPAC procedures were performed in three patients at 4–6-week intervals, between November 2011 and February 2012. Patient and disease characteristics are summarized in Table 11.1.

Table 11.1. Patients characteristics.

	Pat. 1	Pat. 2	Pat. 3
Sex	M	M	F
Age (years)	38	45	74
Cancer localisation	Gastric	Appendiceal	Ovarian
First diagnosis	2 years	2 months	9 years
Previous surgery	Gastrectomy, lymphadenectomy	Ileo-caecal resection, lymphadenectomy	ovarectomy, hysterectomy, omentectomy, lymphadenectomy
Previous systemic chemotherapy	2 lines + experimental	1 line	2 lines + experimental
Reason for therapy interruption	MDR	Severe toxicity	MDR
PIPAC sessions (*n*)	2	3	3

M: male. F: female. PIPAC: Pressurized IntraPeritoneal Aerosol Chemotherapy. MDR: multidrug resistance.

11.1.4 Therapy

After insufflation of 12 mm Hg capnoperitoneum, two balloon trocars (12 mm and 5 mm; Applied Medical, Düsseldorf, Germany) were inserted into the abdominal wall. Diagnostic laparoscopy was performed, and the possibility of cytoreductive surgery excluded. Extent of peritoneal disease was documented by video recordings in all quadrants, and parietal biopsies were taken for anatomopathology, genomics studies, and functional research. Ascites was removed, and the volume documented. Then, a 9 mm micropump (MIP®, Reger Medizintechnik, Rottweil, Germany) was connected to a high pressure injector (Injektron 82 M; MedTron, Saarbruecken, Germany) and inserted into the abdomen. A pressurized aerosol containing cisplatin at a dose of 7.5 mg/m^2 body surface and doxorubicin 1.5 mg/m^2 body surface was then applied via the high-pressure injector and nebulizer. Therapeutic capnoperitoneum (TC) was maintained for 30 minutes at body temperature (37 °C). Then, TC was exhausted using a closed system including a particle filter into the waste air system of the hospital. Finally, trocars were retracted and laparoscopy ended. No drainage of the abdomen was applied. All surgical procedures were performed by the same surgeon (M. A. R.).

11.1.5 Sampling

Peripheral venous blood was collected preoperatively and then daily until the fifth postoperative day. Blinded analysis was performed in the clinical chemistry laboratory of our hospital according to routine protocols.

11.2 Statistical Analysis

Statistics were performed using SPSS version 14.0 software. Descriptive statistics included mean, median, percentiles, and confidence interval. Data are presented as box plots. Comparative statistics over time were performed by one-way repeated analysis of variance (ANOVA).

11.3 Results

Discrete signs of liver toxicity were observed after PIPAC with cisplatin 7.5 mg/m^2 body surface and doxorubicin 1.5 mg/m^2 body surface (Figure 11.1). First, we observed a doubling of serum gamma-GT levels with a peak on the fourth postoperative day (POD), followed by a decrease on POD 5 (one-way ANOVA, $p = 0.22$). Discrete liver cytolysis was detected, with maximal GPT (ALAT) serum level of 135 ± 177 U/l on POD 4 versus a preoperative value of 35 ± 31 U/l ($p = 0.57$). We also observed an increase of GOT (ASAT) serum levels, with a peak of 76 ± 33 U/l on POD 3 versus a preoperative value of 35 ± 8 U/l ($p = 0.68$).

Liver synthesis was also discretely impaired after PIPAC application. Quick-test dropped from 103 ± 8% (preoperatively) to 84 ± 2% on POD 4. However, the mean values remained within the normal range (70–100%) (Figure 11.1). Total bilirubin serum levels remained within the normal range, increasing slightly on POD 1 and then returning to the preoperative value within four days (Figure 11.1).

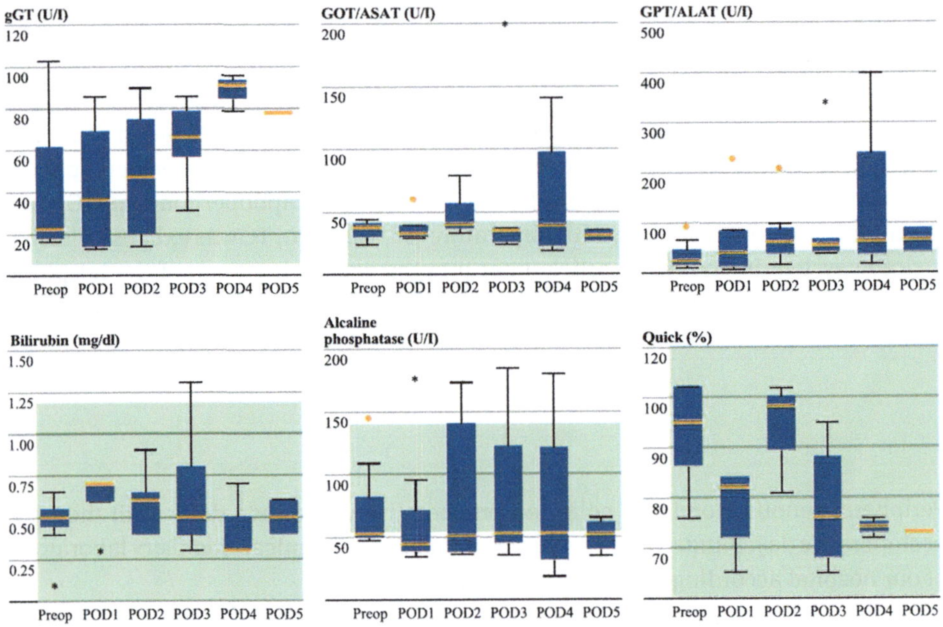

Fig. 11.1. Liver toxicity: discrete liver toxicity was observed after PIPAC, with increase of serum gamma-GT levels (ANOVA, $P < 0.05$). No liver cytolysis was detected, with GOT (ASAT) and GPT (ALAT) remaining within the normal range. ANOVA: repeated analysis of variance. Normal values: gamma-GT 9–36 U/l; GOT (ASAT) 5–31 U/l; GPT (ALAT) 0–34 U/l. Liver function: Liver metabolism was not significantly impaired after PIPAC application. Liver synthesis function, as monitored by quick-test, remained within the normal range. ANOVA: repeated analysis of variance. Normal values: alkaline phosphatase 40–150 U/l; total bilirubin\1.2 mg/dl; Quick 70–120%. Green shaded areas: normal range of measured parameters (reproduced from [16]).

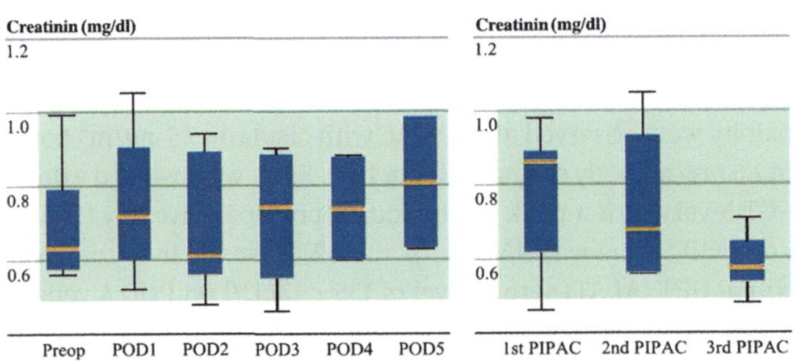

Fig. 11.2. Renal function: serum creatinine levels did not increase significantly (ANOVA) after PIPAC application and remained within the normal range. ANOVA: repeated analysis of variance. Normal value: 0.5–0.9 mg/dl. Cumulative renal toxicity of repeated PIPAC with cisplatin 7.5 mg/m2 body surface and doxorubicin 1.5 mg/m^2 body surface over 2–3 months of observation time. Preoperative serum creatinine value before first PIPAC (three patients), second (three patients), and third PIPAC (two patients). Creatinine levels remain within the normal range. Normal value: 0.5–0.9 mg/dl. Green shaded areas: normal range of measured parameters (reproduced from [16]).

Renal function was not impaired. Serum creatinine levels remained within the normal range (Figure 11.2), with a peak of 0.75 ± 0.19 mmol/l on POD 1 versus a preoperative mean value of 0.70 ± 0.17 mmol/l. No cumulative toxicity was observed after repeated PIPAC application at four-week intervals. All three patients received PIPAC two or three times. The preoperative mean serum creatinine level was not increased, as compared with the reference value before the first application, so that cumulative renal injury could be reasonably excluded (Figure 11.2). A similar pattern was observed for liver toxicity. Serum GOT, GPT, and bilirubin as well as quick-test did not increase significantly with repeated PIPAC application (data not shown).

11.4 Discussion

These pilot data obtained in the first patients treated with PIPAC worldwide show that, with the drugs above and with the dose range tested, PIPAC did not induce significant renal or hepatic toxicity. This is remarkable since application of chemotherapy was repeated twice or three times at four-week intervals.

For hyperthermic intraperitoneal chemotherapy (HIPEC), a combination of cisplatin and doxorubicin appears to be one of the most effective available regimens with tolerable locoregional toxicity. Currently, all patients with peritoneal carcinomatosis managed at our institution with cytoreductive surgery (CRS) and HIPEC are given doxorubicin and cisplatin. Pharmacological aspects of intraperitoneal administration of these drugs are well known: Doxorubicin shows a much more advantageous plasma:peritoneal area under the curve (AUC) ratio than cisplatin (162 ± 113 and 20 ± 6, respectively). On the other hand, very high intraperitoneal concentrations of cisplatin can be achieved without inflicting significant systemic toxicity. Penetration of the tumor mass is greater for cisplatin than doxorubicin, as reviewed previously [14]. After parenteral administration, cisplatin is present as an unreactive, noncharged dichloride complex in the extracellular space. This lack of electrical charge facilitates transport across the vascular wall and the cellular membrane. Within the cell, the chloride concentration is low (4 mmol/l) and the chloride ions of the complex are exchanged by OH-groups and free water molecules so that highly reactive water-hydroxide-chloride complexes are formed. These complexes have a toxic alkylating effect and cannot leave the cell anymore because of their electric charge, eventually causing cellular death. Cisplatin is mainly eliminated via the kidney, so that hepatic side effects of cisplatin are minimal. In the kidney, the various metabolites of cisplatin reach high local concentration, and the drug has dose-dependent renal toxicity, as reviewed previously [15]. In clinical practice and with a standard systemic cisplatin regimen (75–100 mg/m^2 body surface), tubular function is impaired in about 30% of patients, resulting in some cases in nonreversible tubular necrosis and chronic renal failure [17]. We have observed in our patients comparable side effects after HIPEC with cisplatin doses over 75 mg/m^2 body surface (unpublished data). Parent platinum-based chemotherapeutics such as carboplatin or oxaliplatin have the same mechanism of action, but with a lower incidence of side effects, as reviewed previously [18].

Doxorubicin belongs to the family of anthracyclines and induces radical reactions (covalent binding to various molecules) as well as formation of superoxide radical anions (O_2^-) and hydrogen peroxide (H_2O_2). In the process of inactivation of these molecules, highly reactive and toxic hydroxide radicals (OH–) are generated, which in turn cause single- and double-strand DNA breaks, as reviewed previously [15]. Cellular death after doxorubicin therapy does not only occur by apoptosis, but is a sort of "dirty death" with release of toxic metabolites into the surrounding tissue, initiating a local chain reaction involving neighboring cells. This explains why extravasation of doxorubicin during intravenous delivery provokes extensive local tissue necrosis. After parenteral application, tissue uptake of doxorubicin is rapid, and elimination occurs mainly via biliary excretion after hepatic metabolism. Interestingly, doxorubicin has only moderate liver toxicity [19]. During PIPAC, only about 10% of a usual systemic drug dose is applied into the abdomen. Moreover, systemic drug concentration is minimal, about 1% of a systemic dose or 5% of a HIPEC dose.

However, the discussion should not be limited to the dose applied but should also consider particular aspects of PIPAC such as delivery in the immediate vicinity of target organs, pressure application, and hemodynamic effects, with the risk of inducing direct local toxicity. The drug dose for our first experimental PIPAC protocol was determined based on the dosage used for intravenous delivery, with the assumption that systemic toxicity could not be more pronounced than after intravenous delivery, since systemic uptake cannot exceed 100%. However, we were concerned about possible local side effects within the abdomen such as bowel necrosis, and decided to use the same concentration in the chemotherapy solution as during HIPEC. Since the maximal volume that can be nebulized during PIPAC is about 200 ml, the total dose to be applied has to be limited to about 10% of a standard HIPEC dose. In light of our first observations in human patients, it appears that this cautious protocol design was probably life saving since the local bioavailability in PIPAC appears much higher than after HIPEC. During PIPAC, chemotherapy is nebulized into the peritoneal cavity under pressure of 12 mm Hg. The rationale for increasing the intraperitoneal pressure was to create a gradient counteracting interstitial fluid pressure within tumors. Since interstitial pressure is responsible for poor penetration of chemotherapeutic drugs into tumors, bioavailability is expected to be enhanced when the intraabdominal pressure is artificially raised [5]. This hypothesis has been confirmed in small animal experiments, in a large animal model, as well as ex vivo on a human specimen of peritoneal carcinomatosis [6, 11, 12]. Our results in vivo provide further proof that bioavailability in tumor nodules is excellent after PIPAC, exceeding what can be achieved with HIPEC (unpublished data).

A third topic of interest is that increasing the intraperitoneal pressure impairs both portal and renal blood flow. As a consequence, renal function is decreased during capnoperitoneum, depending on the level of hydration, intraabdominal pressure, patient positioning, and procedure duration [20]. An increase of the intraabdominal pressure by 5 mm Hg (from 10 to 15 mm Hg) resulted in a blood flow decrease by 39% to the liver (portal venous flow) and by 60% to the peritoneum. Splanchnic blood flow decreased along with operative time, in spite of constant intraarterial pressure [21]. On the basis of these data and our own observations, it appears reasonable to propose that PIPAC is advantageous over other delivery routes, because of limited blood inflow into the intraabdominal organs during the uptake phase. This results in limited outflow from the splanchnic circulation to the systemic compartment, which leads to high tissue bioavailability and low systemic plasma concentration. The pharmacological data collected in the first patients confirm that the systemic AUC of doxorubicin after PIPAC is only about 1% of that of systemic administration and 5% of that of HIPEC administration (see page 121).

Finally, we did not observe any cumulative toxicity. PIPAC can be applied several times without any difficulties, since no therapy-related adhesions developed. This is indeed an important feature for developing effective locoregional chemotherapy regimens including several cycles and is a clear advantage over HIPEC, for which repeated application is exceptional. However, repeated administration of anthracyclines is known to induce cumulative organ toxicity. For example, application of doxorubicin is followed by severe fibrosis induction, and cardiotoxic effects are known to develop with a delay of up to six months, being irreversible and eventually lethal. Thus, the maximal total dose of doxorubicin applicable is limited to 550 mg/m^2 [15]. In our first patients, no signs of cumulative renal or hepatic toxicity were observed after the second or third PIPAC administration. Moreover, no clinical symptoms of cardiac toxicity were detected, in spite of the fact that one of the patients had previously developed a life-threatening cardiac failure after systemic administration of 5-fluorouracil (5-FU).

In conclusion, the first toxicity data obtained after PIPAC are promising. No clinically relevant liver cytolysis was observed, and neither metabolic nor synthetic hepatic functions were significantly impaired. Renal function remained within the normal range. PIPAC could be repeated without inducing cumulative toxicity. Thus, it appears reasonable to propose that PIPAC causes less hepatic and renal toxicity than other chemotherapy delivery routes, due to lower therapeutic doses and favorable kinetics. While promising, the data presented here have to be considered as preliminary and need to be confirmed in future studies including appropriate dose-finding and safety studies in various cancer types and with different chemotherapeutic drugs.

Bibliography

[1] Van Lierde S, Denys H, Peeters M. Systemic chemotherapy in patients with peritoneal carcinomatosis from non colorectal origin. Cancer Treat Res. 134 (2007) 441–448.

[2] Bristow RE, Puri I, Chi DS. Cytoreductive surgery for recurrent ovarian cancer: a meta-analysis. Gynecol Oncol. 112, 1 (Jan 2009) 265–274.

[3] Zani S, Papalezova K, Stinnett S et al. Modest advances in survival for patients with colorectal-associated peritoneal carcinomatosis in the era of modern chemotherapy. J Surg Oncol. 18 (2012) Jul. Epub ahead of print.

[4] Markman M. Intraperitoneal antineoplastic drug delivery: rationale and results. Lancet Oncol 4 (2003) 277–283.

[5] Minchinton AI, Tannock IF. Drug penetration in solid tumors. Nat Rev Cancer. 6, 8 (Aug 2006) 583–592.

[6] Dedrick RL, Flessner MF. Pharmacokinetic problems in peritoneal drug administration: tissue penetration and surface exposure. J Natl Cancer Inst 89 (1997) 480–487.

[7] Jaaback K, Johnson N, Lawrie TA. Intraperitoneal chemotherapy for the initial management of primary epithelial ovarian cancer. Cochrane Database Syst Rev. 9, 11 (Nov 2011) CD005340. Review.

[8] Elias D, Lefevre JH, Chevalier J et al. Complete cytoreductive surgery plus intraperitoneal chemohyperthermia with oxaliplatin for peritoneal carcinomatosis of colorectal origin. J Clin Oncol. 27 (2009) 681–685.

[9] Macrì, A, Fortugno A, Saladino E. Rationale and techniques of cytoreductive surgery and peritoneal chemohyperthermia. World J Gastrointest Oncol. 3, 12 (Dec 2011) 169–174.

[10] Reymond MA, Hu B, Garcia A et al. Feasibility of therapeutic pneumoperitoneum in a large animal model using a microvaporisator. Surg Endosc 14 (2000) 51–55.

[11] Solass W, Hetzel A, Nadiradze G et al. Intraoperative intraperitonal drug delivery using a nebulizer: rationale and pharmacokinetic results. Surg Endosc. 26, 7 (Jul 2012) 1849–1855.

[12] Solass W, Herbette A, Schwarz T et al. Therapeutic approach of human peritoneal carcinomatosis with Dbait in combination with capnoperitoneum: proof of concept. Surg Endosc. 26, 3 (Mar 2012) 847–852.

[13] Reymond M. Therapeutic aerosolized chemotherapy for peritoneal carcinomatosis. In: Eurocancer 2012. John Libbey Eurotext, Paris 2012, 55–56.

[14] Rossi CR, Mocellin S, Pilati P et al. Pharmacokinetics of intraperitoneal cisplatin and doxorubicin. Surg Oncol Clin North Am. 12, 3 (Jul 2003) 781–794. Review.

[15] Estler CE, Schmidt H (eds). Pharmakologie und Toxikologie (6th edn.) Schattauer, Stuttgart; 2007.

[16] Blanco A et al. Renal and hepatic toxicities after pressurized intraperitoneal aerosol chemotherapy (PIPAC). Ann Surg Oncol. 20, 7 (Jul 2013) 2311–2316.

[17] Dos Santos NA, Carvalho Rodrigues MA, Martins NM et al. Cisplatinum-induced nephrotoxicity and targets of nephroprotection: an update. Arch Toxicol. 1 (2012) Mar. Epub ahead of print.

[18] Sakaeda T, Kadoyama K, Okuno Y. Adverse event profiles of platinum agents: data mining of the public version of the FDA adverse event reporting system, AERS, and reproducibility of clinical observations. Int J Med Sci. 8, 6 (2011) 487–491.

[19] Carvalho C, Santos RX, Cardoso S et al. Doxorubicin: the good, the bad and the ugly effect. Curr Med Chem. 16, 25 (2009) 3267–3285.

[20] Demyttenaere S, Feldman LS, Fried GM. Effect of pneumoperitoneum on renal perfusion and function: a systematic review. Surg Endosc. 21, 2 (Feb 2007) 152–160.

[21] Schilling MK, Redaelli C, Krahenbuhl L et al. Splanchnic microcirculatory changes during CO2 laparoscopy. J Am Coll Surg 184 (1997) 378–382.

C. B. Tempfer, I. Celik, W. Solass, B. Buerkle, U. Giger-Pabst, J. Zieren, D. Strumberg, and M. A. Reymond

12 PIPAC in ovarian cancer

In women with a diagnosis of ovarian cancer, disease recurrence will eventually occur in 60 to 85% of cases within five years after primary treatment [1]. Intravenous chemotherapy with platinum compounds, taxanes, anthracyclines, gemcitabine, topotecan, and trabectedin in various combinations and sequences are the mainstay of recurrence treatment with median survival rates between 4–10 months [2]. Intraperitoneal chemotherapy in the clinical setting of recurrent ovarian cancer is an experimental approach. Although proven to be effective in the adjuvant setting, intraperitoneal chemotherapy has not been demonstrated to improve survival in clinical trials in women with recurrent disease. The potential of intraperitoneal chemotherapy to improve survival, however, may be high, given its potential to prolong progression-free and overall survival of patients with minimal residual disease after initial surgery [3, 4]. At present, intraabdominal treatment strategies in recurrent ovarian cancer have been assessed in phase I and II trials predominantly in patients with malignant ascites. Agents used in these studies include chemotherapy compounds as well as antiangiogenic agents such as bevacizumab, the vascular endothelial growth factor-trap, and the trifunctional anti-EPCAM antibody catumaxomab [5]. Pharmacological limitations such as poor drug distribution within the abdominal cavity and poor penetration into peritoneal nodules have limited the success of intraperitoneal chemotherapy in women with recurrent disease and high disease burden [6]. Therefore, it has been claimed that innovative concepts overcoming these limitations should be explored in order to improve the efficacy of intraperitoneal chemotherapy [6, 7].

12.1 Off-label use

One potential way to overcome the pharmacokinetic limitations of intraperitoneal chemotherapy is to apply intraperitoneal chemotherapy as a pressurized aerosol in order to take advantage of the physical properties of gas and pressure [7]. This approach is based on the assumption that intraabdominal application of chemotherapy under pressure will enhance tumor drug uptake [8, 9]. As proof of concept, pressurized intraperitoneal aerosol chemotherapy (PIPAC) achieved a superior distribution on the peritoneum and a better penetration into peritoneal nodules compared to conventional intraperitoneal chemotherapy in an ex vivo model [10]. In addition, an in vivo experimental study using five pigs yielded a better distribution of a pressurized test dye within the abdominal cavity and a better penetration into the peritoneum compared to peritoneal lavage [11]. Specifically, the stained peritoneal surface was larger after pressurized aerosol application compared with peritoneal lavage, and staining was more intense. Hidden peritoneal surfaces as well as the anterior abdominal wall were only stained in the aerosol group and the outer aspect of the peritoneal membrane was immediately stained after pressurized spraying. Based on these data, pressurized intraperitoneal aerosol chemotherapy (PIPAC) has been tested in humans with recurrent peritoneal carcinomatosis (PC) [12]. In these preliminary applications, PIPAC induced regression of peritoneal nodules with limited hepatic and renal toxicity. Specifically, gamma-glutamyltransferase was significantly elevated in the early postoperative phase, whereas aspartate aminotransferase, alanine aminotransferase, bilirubin levels, quick-test, and serum creatinine levels were not influenced by the procedure [13]. In addition, the procedure has been shown to be safe regarding occupational health aspects such as operation theater air contamination with aerosol chemotherapy particles [14]. Here, we report on the procedures and outcomes of a preliminary series of 21 patients with recurrent, platinum-resistant ovarian cancer and peritoneal carcinomatosis treated with PIPAC in an off-label use program between December 2011 and June 2013. We aimed to test the hypothesis that PIPAC is feasible, can induce histologic tumor regression and achieve a tumor response in women with recurrent, platinum-resistant ovarian cancer and peritoneal carcinomatosis comparable to what has been observed in patients with other malignancies [12–14].

12.1.1 Patients and methods

Institutional review board approval for an off-label use program using PIPAC in women with peritoneal carcinomatosis was obtained. Between December 2011 and June 2013 21 women with recurrent ovarian cancer were treated and analysis was retrospective. All patients were presented in the interdisciplinary tumor board of our institution and indication was decided on an individual basis. All women signed an informed consent form and underwent laparoscopy during which PIPAC was applied intraabdominally.

The PIPAC procedure was performed as described before [12–14]. Briefly, after insufflation of a 12 mm Hg CO_2 pneumoperitoneum, two balloon safety trocars (5 and 12 mm, Applied Medical, Duesseldorf, Germany) were inserted into the abdominal wall in an operating room equipped with laminar airflow. Video documentation was started and the Peritoneal Carcinomatosis Index (PCI) was determined according to Sugarbaker, based on lesion size and distribution [15]. Multiple biopsies were taken for histologic confirmation of peritoneal carcinomatosis during the first procedure and all following procedures in order to ascertain tumor regression. Ascites volume was documented and ascites was removed. Then, a nebulizer (Reger Medizintechnik, Rottweil, Germany) was connected to an intravenous high-pressure injector (Injektron 82M, MedTron, Saarbruecken, Germany) and inserted into the abdomen. The tightness of the abdomen was documented via a zero-flow of CO_2. A pressurized aerosol containing cisplatin at a dose of 7.5 mg/m^2 body surface in a 150 ml NaCl 0.9% solution followed by doxorubicin at a dose of 1.5 mg/m^2 body surface in a 50 ml NaCl 0.9% solution were applied via nebulizer and injector. Injection parameters were set at a flow rate of 30 ml/min and a maximum upstream pressure of 200 psi in the high-pressure injector. The injection was remote-controlled to minimize personnel exposure. The therapeutic capnoperitoneum was maintained for 30 minutes at a temperature of 37 °C. Then, the chemotherapy aerosol was exsufflated via a closed line over two sequential microparticle filters into the airwaste system of the hospital. Finally, trocars were retracted and laparoscopy ended. No drainage of the abdomen was applied. The PIPAC procedure was repeated after 4–6 weeks until progression or limiting toxicity. In 6/21 women, PIPAC was combined with cytoreductive surgery.

Adverse events were graded according to the Common Terminology Criteria for Adverse Events (CTCAE) version 4.0 [17]. All p-values are two-tailed and a p-value < 0.05 was considered statistically significant. We performed a multivariable logistic regression model with objective tumor response (yes versus no), as dependent variable and patient age, serum CA-125 (< 1000 versus > 1000 U/mL), and presence of ascites (yes versus no) as independent variables. Survival was modelled in a Kaplan–Meier survival curve. We used the statistical software SPSS 11.0 for Windows (SPSS 11.0, SPSS Inc., Chicago, IL) for statistical analysis.

12.1.2 Results

Twenty-one women were treated. Of these, 16 women were diagnosed with ovarian cancer, four with primary peritoneal cancer, and one with primary fallopian tube cancer. The mean age was 63±13 years. Ascites and pleural effusion were present in 16 and 9 women, respectively. Patient characteristics including the number of previous chemotherapy lines are shown in Table 12.1. In 3/21 women, PIPAC was attempted, but not performed due to abdominal adhesions precluding laparoscopy. Further analyses are therefore limited to 18 women having undergone at least one PIPAC. In summary, 34 PIPAC procedures were performed. In 8/18 women, PIPAC was combined with cytoreductive surgery (CRS). In these women, PIPAC was administered immediately after CRS or within ten days thereafter.

CTCAE grade 1 to 5 toxicities were observed in 12, 0, 3, 2, and 0 women, respectively. Table 12.2 describes the observed toxicities in detail. Eleven out of the 18 patients had mild abdominal pain, fever and/or elevated acute phase proteins such as C-reactive protein (CRP). Of note, five women had CTCAE grade 3–4 events with four of them potentially related to the PIPAC procedure. Three of the four events potentially related to the PIPAC procedure occurred in women who had both CRS and PIPAC. No perioperative mortality occurred.

Ten women had one PIPAC and eight women had > 1 PIPAC. In these eight women, tumor response assessment was based on tumor regression, on histology of repeat biopsies, PCI improvement, and video-laparoscopy assessment. Six out of the eight

Table 12.1. Patient characteristics of 20 women with recurrent, platinum-resistant ovarian, fallopian tube, or primary peritoneal cancer undergoing pressurized intraperitoneal aerosol chemotherapy (PIPAC).

Patient Characteristics	Variable
Number of patients	21
Age, years (± SD)	63 (± 13)
Karnovsky Index (median, range)	70 (30–100)
No. of prior chemotherapy regimens (mean, ±SD)	4 (± 2.0)
Adjuvant radiotherapy	None
Presence of pleural effusion	9/21
Presence of ascites	16/21
PCI (mean, ± SD)	17.3 (± 6.3)
Serum CA-125 (U/mL)	1416 (± 1892)

SD = Standard Deviation; PCI = Peritoneal Cancer Index

Table 12.2. Adverse Events according to Common Terminology Criteria for Adverse Events (CTCAE) grading in 18 women undergoing Pressurized IntraPeritoneal Aerosol Chemotherapy (PIPAC).

Patient	Procedures	CTCAE Grading	Adverse Events
1	CRS, 6× PIPAC	1	Fever, elevated CRP, AP
2	1× PIPAC	1	AP
3	CRS, 2× PIPAC	1	Elevated CRP, AP
4	1× PIPAC	1	Elevated CRP, AP
5	CRS, 1× PIPAC	3	Recto-vaginal fistula* – Conservative treatment
6	CRS, 2× PIPAC	4	Postoperative small bowel perforation* – Reoperation
7	3× PIPAC	1	Elevated CRP, AP
8	CRS, 1× PIPAC	1	Elevated CRP, AP
9	1× PIPAC	4	Intraoperative colon lesion* – Immediate repair
10	1× PIPAC	1	Elevated CRP
11	2× PIPAC	1	Elevated CRP, AP
12	CRS, 1× PIPAC	3	Small bowel fistula – Conservative treatment*
13	1× PIPAC	3	Pneumonia, AP
14	CRS, 1× PIPAC	1	Elevated CRP, AP
15	2× PIPAC	1	Elevated CRP, AP
16	CRS, 1× PIPAC	1	Elevated CRP
17	3× PIPAC	1	Elevated CRP, AP, nausea
18	3× PIPAC	–	–

PIPAC = Pressurized IntraPeritoneal Aerosol Chemotherapy; CRS = CytoReductive Surgery; CTCAE = Common Terminology Criteria for Adverse Events; CRP = C-Reactive Protein; AP = Abdominal Pain; *related or potentially related to PIPAC

women had an objective tumor response. Complete remission, partial remission, and stable disease were observed in one, two, and three women, respectively (Figure 12.1, Figure 12.2).

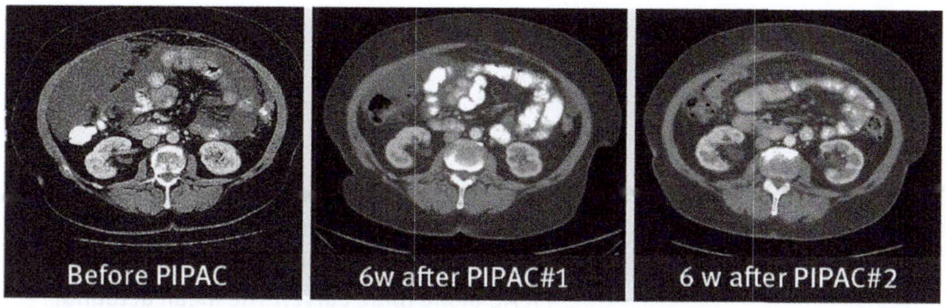

Fig. 12.1. Repeated computed tomography (CT) scans of a woman before the first PIPAC, after the first PIPAC, and after the second PIPAC demonstrating regression of ascites and peritoneal carcinomatosis (reproduced from [18]).

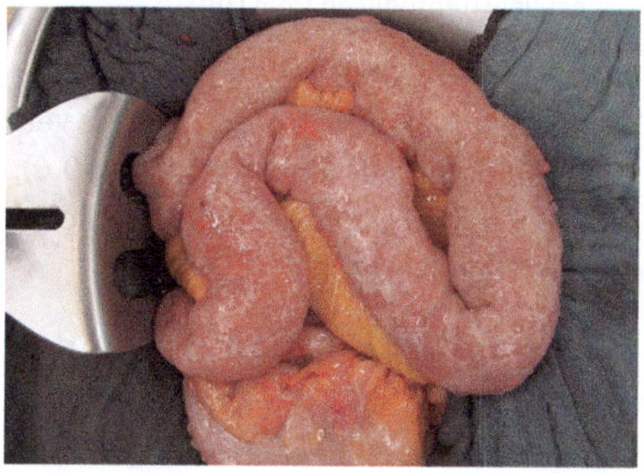

Fig. 12.2. A macroscopic image of the small bowel after four PIPACs with scarring of diffuse small bowel carcinomatosis (reproduced from [18]).

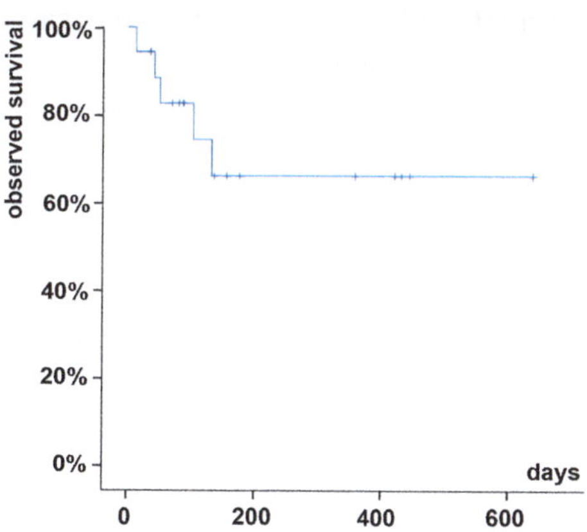

Fig. 12.3. Kaplan–Meier survival curve of 18 women who had undergone at least one PIPAC. *X*-axis: survival in days (reproduced from [18]).

Cumulative survival after 400 days was 62%. The mean actuarial survival time of all 18 women with PIPAC was 442 days. Five women died due to disease progression during follow up between 13 and 132 days after PIPAC. The median duration of follow up was 192 (minimum 13, maximum 639) days (Figure 12.3).

In a multivariable logistic regression model with objective tumor response (yes versus no) as the dependent variable and PIPAC (1 versus > 1), patient age (< 70 versus

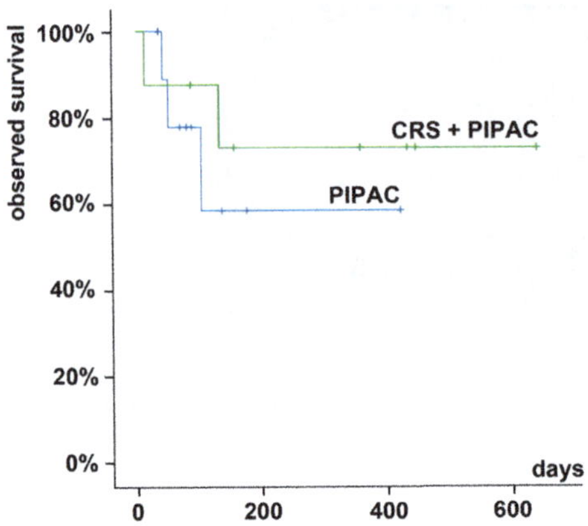

Fig. 12.4. Separate Kaplan–Meier survival curves of eight women with PIPAC combined with CRS (green curve) and ten women with PIPAC alone (blue curve). The mean actuarial survival time of patients with PIPAC combined with CRS and patients with PIPAC alone was 486 days and 268 days, respectively. Cumulative survival after 400 days was 74% and 57%, respectively (reproduced from [18]).

> 70 years), serum CA-125 (< 1000 versus > 1000 U/mL), and presence of ascites (yes versus no) as the independent variables, PIPAC ($p = 0.03$), but not patient age ($p = 0.6$), presence of ascites ($p = 0.6$), and serum CA-125 ($p = 0.5$) independently predicted objective tumor response in this patient population (Figure 12.4).

12.1.3 Discussion

In this preliminary series of 18 women with recurrent, platinum-resistant ovarian cancer, PIPAC was well tolerated and achieved an objective tumor response in 6/8 cases with > 1 PIPAC. Complete remission, partial remission, and stable disease were observed in one, two, and three women, respectively, and the cumulative survival after 400 days was 62%. This suggests that PIPAC may be a palliative treatment option for selected women with recurrent ovarian cancer, deserving further assessment in prospective clinical trials.

Our data are consistent with previous experiences with PIPAC in men and women with peritoneal carcinomatosis due to various malignancies such as gastric, colon, and appendiceal cancer [12–14]. These reports together with our data indicate that clinical benefit can be achieved in patients with recurrent cancer of various origins having spread to the peritoneum. Of note, most women in our series were heavily pretreated, indicating that PIPAC may be able to overcome platinum resistance at least in a fraction of women. This may be due to the fact that PIPAC achieves higher local chemotherapy concentrations compared to systemic chemotherapy [10, 11]. This local dose escalation may be one contributing factor explaining the therapeutic effect of PIPAC. Another factor may be a chemical peritonitis observed in most patients. Consistent with this assumption, we noted that 12/18 patients had fever and/or elevated acute phase proteins such as CRP indicating some form of local inflammatory response to PIPAC.

A potential beneficial aspect of PIPAC compared to systemic cytotoxic chemotherapy may be its side effect profile. Notorious side effects such as alopecia, peripheral neurotoxicity, nausea, and myelosuppression did not occur with PIPAC, making this treatment potentially suitable for women who had experienced severe chemotherapy-related side effects, precluding the subsequent use of another chemotherapy line. However, the observation of five WHO grade 3–4 toxicites with four of them potentially related to the PIPAC procedure is of concern. Three of these four women had both CRS and PIPAC, suggesting wound healing impairment due to high local chemotherapy concentration. Therefore, this combination should be avoided in further trials.

This preliminary report on the activity of PIPAC has a number of limitations. First, this is only a preliminary retrospective series of patients describing the technical feasibility and potential therapeutic effects in an ovarian cancer patient population. Therefore, it is only possible to state that PIPAC can be performed in recurrent ovarian cancer patients with peritoneal carcinomatosis and can achieve an objective tumor response. However, patient selection and the low number of treated patients in this small, preliminary series is a methodological limitation. In this regard, the external validity of this study is strictly limited to the women specified in the protocol. The data obtained are not applicable to the general population of women with recurrent ovarian cancer. The small number of patients in this prospective series may obscure rare adverse events and toxicities. Thus, the safety of this procedure has yet to be established.

The data reported in this retrospective series of women with ovarian cancer are in accordance with previous reports describing clinical activity of PIPAC in patients with peritoneal carcinomatosis due to colon, gastric, and appendiceal cancer [12–14]. This suggests that PIPAC may be a therapeutic option for peritoneal carcinomatosis independent of the cancer of origin. However, the clinical data available today do not allow a comparison of the efficacy or the lack thereof in different tumor entities.

In a multivariable regression analysis, presence of ascites, serum CA-125, and patient age were not suitable predictors for tumor response. This suggests that clinical parameters readily available in women with recurrent ovarian cancer are not useful as predictive markers for PIPAC. It is too early to put these preliminary results into a clinical perspective. It is clear, however, that PIPAC is easy to perform and well tolerated by most patients when applied without concomitant cytoreductive surgery. Whether or not PIPAC is a clinically meaningful therapeutic option in the setting of palliative ovarian cancer treatment, however, remains to be seen. Further clinical trials confirming the tumor response rate observed in this series as well as assessing quality of life changes during and after PIPAC are warranted.

In summary, PIPAC may be effective in women with recurrent, platinum-resistant ovarian cancer. Intraabdominal application of pressurized chemotherapy as an aerosol should be investigated in prospective clinical trials.

Bibliography

[1] Foley OW, Rauh-Hain JA, del Carmen MG. Recurrent epithelial ovarian cancer: an update on treatment.Oncology (Williston Park). 27, 4 (2013) 288–294.

[2] Hanker LC, Loibl S, Burchardi N, Pfisterer J, Meier W, Pujade-Lauraine E, Ray-Coquard I, Sehouli J, Harter P, du Bois A. AGO and GINECO study group. The impact of second to sixth line therapy on survival of relapsed ovarian cancer after primary taxane/platinum-based therapy. Ann Oncol. 23, 10 (2012) 2605–2612.

[3] Armstrong DK, Bundy B, Wenzel L, Huang HQ, Baergen R, Lele S, Copeland LJ, Walker JL, Burger RA. Gynecologic Oncology Group. Intraperitoneal cisplatin and paclitaxel in ovarian cancer. N Engl J Med. 354, 1 (2006) 34–43.

[4] Gadducci A, Conte PF. Intraperitoneal chemotherapy in the management of patients with advanced epithelial ovarian cancer: a critical review of the literature. Int J Gynecol Cancer. 18, 5 (2008) 943–953.

[5] Eskander RN, Tewari KS. Emerging treatment options for management of malignant ascites in patients with ovarian cancer. Int J Womens Health. 4 (2012) 395–404.

[6] Dedrick RL, Flessner MF. Pharmacokinetic Problems in Peritoneal Drug Administration: Tissue Penetration and Surface Exposure. J Natl Cancer Inst 89 (1997) 480–487.

[7] Reymond MA, Hu B, Garcia A et al. Feasibility of therapeutic pneumoperitoneum in a large animal model using a microvaporisator. Surg Endosc 14 (2000) 51–55.

[8] Jacquet P, Stuart OA, Chang D, Sugarbaker PH. Effects of intra-abdominal pressure on pharmacokinetics and tissue distribution of doxorubicin after intraperitoneal administration. Anticancer Drugs. 75 (1996) 596–603.

[9] Esquis P, Consolo D, Magnin G, Pointaire P, Moretto P, Ynsa MD, Beltramo JL, Drogoul C, Simonet M, Benoit L, Rat P, Chauffert B. High intra-abdominal pressure enhances the penetration and antitumor effect of intraperitoneal cisplatin on experimental peritoneal carcinomatosis. Ann Surg. 244, 1 (2006) 106–112.

[10] Solass W, Herbette A, Schwarz T, Hetzel A, Sun JS, Dutreix M, Reymond MA. Therapeutic approach of human peritoneal carcinomatosis with Dbait in combination with capnoperitoneum: proof of concept. Surg Endosc. 26, 3 (2012) 847–852.

[11] Solass W, Hetzel A, Nadiradze G, Sagynaliev E, Reymond MA. Intraoperative intraperitonal drug delivery using a nebulizer: rationale and pharmacokinetic results. Surg Endosc. 26, 7 (2012) 1849–1855.

[12] Solass W, Kerb R, Muerdter T, Giger U, Strumberg D, Tempfer C, Zieren J, Schwab M, Reymond MA. Intraperitoneal Chemotherapy of Peritoneal Carcinomatosis using Pressurized Aerosol as an Alternative to Liquid Solution: First Evidence for Efficacy. Ann Surg Oncol. 21, 2 (2014) 553–559.

[13] Blanco A, Giger-Pabst U, Solass W, Zieren J, Reymond MA. Renal and Hepatic Toxicities After Pressurized Intraperitoneal Aerosol Chemotherapy (PIPAC). Ann Surg Oncol. 20, 7 (2013) 2311–2316.

[14] Solass W, Giger-Pabst U, Zieren J, Reymond MA. Pressurized Intraperitoneal Aerosol Chemotherapy (PIPAC): Occupational Health and Safety Aspects. Ann Surg Oncol. 2013 Jun 14. 20, 11 (2013) 3504–3511.

[15] Mazzei MA, Khader L, Cirigliano A, Cioffi Squitieri N, Guerrini S, Forzoni B, Marrelli D, Roviello F, Mazzei FG, Volterrani L. Accuracy of MDCT in the preoperative definition of Peritoneal Cancer Index (PCI) in patients with advanced ovarian cancer who underwent peritonectomy and hyperthermic intraperitoneal chemotherapy (HIPEC). Abdom Imaging. 2013 Jun 7. [Epub ahead of print].

[16] Eisenhauer EA, Therasse P, Bogaerts J, Schwartz LH, Sargent D, Ford R, Dancey J, Arbuck S, Gwyther S, Mooney M, Rubinstein L, Shankar L, Dodd L, Kaplan R, Lacombe D, Verweij J. New response evaluation criteria in solid tumors: revised RECIST guideline (version 1.1). Eur J Cancer. 45, 2 (2009) 228–247.
[17] Common Terminology Criteria for Adverse Events (CTCAE) version 4.0; published: May 28, 2009 (v4.03: June 14, 2010); U.S. Department of Health and Human Services, National Institutes ofHealth, National Cancer Institute.
[18] Tempfer CB et al. Activity of Pressurized Intraperitoneal Aerosol Chemotherapy (PIPAC) with cisplatin and doxorubicin in women with recurrent, platinum-resistant ovarian cancer: preliminary clinical experience. Gynecol Oncol. 132, 2 (Feb 2014) 307–311.

12.2 PIPAC-OV1: a Phase-2 trial in the third-line palliative situation

Based on the preliminary observations made retrospectively in ovarian cancer, the first Phase-2 trial aiming to assess efficacy and safety of PIPAC was opened in March 2013 (www.clinicaltrials.gov, NCT01809379). The study title was “Feasibility, efficacy and safety of pressurized intraperitoneal aerosol chemotherapy (PIPAC) with cisplatin and doxorubicin in women with recurrent ovarian cancer: an open-label, single-arm Phase-2 clinical trial”.

12.2.1 Objectives

To evaluate the clinical benefit rate (CBR) of PIPAC in platinum-resistant ovarian cancer.

12.2.2 Study design

Single center, open-label, non-randomized, single-arm, repeated single dose study to explore the efficacy, safety, and pharmakokinetics of doxorubicin and cisplatin when given as a pressurized intraperitoneal aerosol chemotherapy (PIPAC) to ovarian cancer patients.

12.2.3 Target subject population

Female patients with recurrent ovarian cancer and disease progression with peritoneal carcinomatosis (PC) after at least two lines of previous IV chemotherapy (Table 12.3).

Table 12.3. PIPAC-OV1 study: eligibility criteria.

Ages Eligible for Study	18 Years to 80 Years
Genders Eligible for Study	Female
Accepts Healthy Volunteers	No
Inclusion criteria	At least two line previous chemotherapy
	Recurrent ovarian cancer
	Mobile patient
	Informed consent
Exclusion criteria	Ileus
	Necessity of parenteral nutrition
	Extraperitoneal metastases

12.2.4 Investigational product, dosage, and mode of administration

Doxorubicin 1.5 mg/m^2 body surface in 50 ml NaCl 0,9% and cisplatin 7.5 mg/m^2 in 50 ml NaCl 0,9% q six weeks, applied intraperitoneally as pressurized aerosol (PIPAC).

12.2.5 Duration of treatment

Three single doses in six-week intervals (18 weeks).

12.2.6 Endpoints

Primary outcome variable:
- Clinical Benefit Rate (CBR) according to RECIST criteria after 3 cycles of PIPAC with cisplatin and doxorubicin.

Secondary outcome variables:
- Duration of progression-free survival and overall survival.
- The median time to progression according to RECIST criteria after three cycles of PIPAC with cisplatin and doxorubicin.
- The Peritoneal Carcinomatosis Index (PCI) before and after therapy.
- The degree of histological regression assessed by pathological review.
- The difference in ascites volume before and after the first, second, and third PIPAC applications.
- The proportion of women with a serum CA-125 reduction of at least 50% after compared to before PIPAC applications.
- The value of initial tumor platinum sensitivity as a predictor for response to PIPAC.

12.2.7 Patient reported outcomes (PROs)

European Organization for Research and Treatment of Cancer (EORTC) quality of life questionnaires (QLQ-C30, German version).

12.2.8 Pharmacokinetics

Area under plasma concentration versus time curve (AUC), maximum plasma concentration (Cmax), time to reach Cmax (tmax), terminal half-life (t1/2), oral clearance (CL/F), oral volume of distribution (Vz/F).

12.2.9 Safety

Safety and tolerability will be assessed by collection of adverse events, according to the Common Terminology Criteria for Adverse Events (CTCAE) [1] including 12-lead ECG (electrocardiogram), echocardiography, neurological examination, blood pressure, heart rate, physical examination results and laboratory assessments (chemistry, hematology, urinalysis).

12.2.10 Statistical methods

The sample size of 50 patients was calculated on the basis of a proportion of patients with a CBR of 40% or more as proof of efficacy of PIPAC in this patient population and of less than 20% as insufficient to continue the assessment. We assumed a risk of $\alpha = 0.05$ (type I error) and $\beta = 0.10$ (type II error), and a dropout rate of 10%. Analysis will be performed using nonparametric tests since we do not assume a normal distribution of data. Safety data will be summarized at each scheduled time point by treatment using descriptive statistics.

12.2.11 Current stage

The last patient was recruited in March 2014, results are expected to be published in summer 2014.

12.3 PIPAC-OV2: a Phase-1 dose-finding study

After completion of the Phase-2 trial described above, the German federal regulatory authority (BfArm) recommended performing a dosis-finding study before applying for a comparative trial. Study title of the submitted protocol is "A Phase-1, single-arm (non-randomized), open-label, three step dose escalation study with cisplatin and doxorubicin applied as pressurized intraperitoneal aerosol chemotherapy (PIPAC) in patients with recurrent ovarian cancer and peritoneal carcinomatosis". The study protocol is currently (as of July 2014) under regulatory review.

12.4 PIPAC-OV3: a prospective Phase-2-3 randomized trial

As soon as the dosis-finding study described above is completed, we intend to submit a study protocol for a prospective, randomized trial in peritoneal carcinomatosis of platinum-resistant ovarian cancer.

Bibliography

[1] US Department of Health and Human services, National Institutes of Health, National Cancer Institute. Common Terminology Criteria for Adverse Events (CTCAE) Version 4.0, Published: May 28, 2009 (v4.03: June 14, 2010),

G. Nadiradze, W. Solass, J. Zieren, D. Strumberg, M. A. Reymond, and U. Giger-Pabst

13 PIPAC in gastric cancer

Gastric cancer is the second most common cause of death from cancer worldwide [1]. In most patients with gastric cancer, therapy is palliative and systemic chemotherapy including 5-FU/platinum combinations, with or without an anthracycline, as well as irinotecan and docetaxel-containing combinations is the current standard of care [2]. Peritoneal carcinomatosis is the most common metastatic pattern in gastric cancer and develops in more than half of patients in the course of disease [3]. Patients with gastric cancer and peritoneal carcinomatosis have a poor prognosis with a median survival of 3–5 months without treatment [4, 5]. No large-scale comparative studies document the efficacy of systemic chemotherapy in this specific situation but it appears to be modest [6].

In patients with tumors confined to the peritoneal cavity, there is established pharmacokinetic and tumor biology-related evidence that intraperitoneal drug administration is advantageous [7]. It has been suggested that intraperitoneal chemotherapy may improve survival of patients with gastric cancer and peritoneal carcinomatosis. For example, application of combined chemotherapy of intravenous and intraperitoneal paclitaxel with S-1 is active in gastric cancer patients with peritoneal carcinomatosis [8]. However, owing to the limited penetration of chemotherapy into tumor nodules, intraperitoneal chemotherapy may be best reserved for small-volume disease [9].

For treating larger lesions, it has been proposed that a complete surgical cytoreduction (CRS) is performed prior to intraperitoneal chemotherapy administration [10]. In gastric cancer, a large retrospective study suggested that combining CRS with heated intraperitoneal chemotherapy (HIPEC) might allow long-term survival in a selected group of patients with limited peritoneal carcinomatosis [11]. In the meantime, 20 prospective randomized trials with a total of 2,145 patients have been published, and two recent meta-analyses showed potential survival benefit for CRS and HIPEC in gastric cancer [12, 13], with five-year survival rates ranging from 13–28%. This multimodality treatment is currently regarded as the only therapeutic option for selected patients with peritoneal carcinomatosis of gastric origin [5]. Unfortunately, this invasive procedure is hampered by significant risks and side effects with a 30-day mortality of 5% in specialized centers [14]. Moreover, two major pharmacokinetic problems are remaining that limit the effectiveness of HIPEC: poor tumor penetration by the drug and incomplete irrigation of serosal surfaces by the drug-containing solution [15]. Thus, the benefit of combined CRS and HIPEC over CRS alone might be only marginal [16] and the role of CRS plus HIPEC in the treatment of peritoneal carcinomatosis of gastric origin remains a matter of considerable debate [17].

13.1 Off-label use

We now report our first observations after PIPAC application in patients with advanced peritoneal carcinomatosis from gastric cancer.

In fall 2011, we opened an off-label use program for treating patients diagnosed with advanced, therapy-resistant peritoneal carcinomatosis from gastric cancer with PIPAC. This program was approved by the Ethics Committees of the Wilhelms University Münster and Ruhr University Bochum, Germany, in accordance to EC regulation [25] and German law [26]. Access to this off-label use program was limited to patients who had a life-threatening disease with no satisfactory alternative therapies or could not enter a clinical trial. Therefore, only patients left without treatment options or patients whose disease did not respond or relapsed to available treatments, or for whom the treatments were contraindicated or inadequate were included.

Prior to therapy, each patient was evaluated on an individual basis by the multidisciplinary tumor board at the Marien Hospital Herne, Comprehensive Cancer Centre, Ruhr University Bochum, Germany. Specific inclusion and exclusion criteria were not defined a priori. This retrospective review concerns only patients with histologically documented peritoneal carcinomatosis of gastric origin, who had no option for complete cytoreductive surgery (CRS) and hyperthermic intraperitoneal chemotherapy (HIPEC). Most patients received prior palliative chemotherapy or were medically unfit for systemic palliative chemotherapy or had experienced severe side effects under systemic palliative chemotherapy or had refused to receive systemic chemotherapy. Patients with extraperitoneal metastatic disease were not treated (with the exception of pleural effusion), because no effect of a locoregional therapy was expected. Patients with contraindication for general anesthesia and acute infection or sepsis were not treated. Patients with reduced general condition (Karnofsky $\leq 60\%$), therapy-resistant ascites necessitating iterative drainage and partial small bowel obstruction were not excluded from therapy. All procedures were performed according to the principles of the Helsinki declaration. All patients were extensively informed and signed a consent form.

All interventions were performed under general anesthesia with a single-shot of ceftriaxone 1.5 g IV administered 30 minutes prior to surgery. A venous thromboembolism prophylaxis was given the night before surgery using certoparin 3000 IE 1× s.c. After insufflation of a 12 mm Hg CO_2 pneumoperitoneum with open access or with Veres needle, two balloon safety trocars (5 and 12 mm, Applied Medical, Düsseldorf, Germany) were inserted into the abdominal wall. Ascites were removed and the amount documented. The extent of peritoneal carcinomatosis was determined according to Sugarbaker [27] based on lesion size and distribution. Peritoneal biopsies were taken in all four quadrants for histological examination, and a local partial peritonectomy of several square centimeters was performed routinely to improve accuracy of negative findings. Then, a micropump (MIP®, Reger Medizintechnik, Rottweil, Germany) was connected to an intravenous high-pressure injector (Injektron

82M, MedTron, Saarbrücken, Germany) and inserted into the abdomen. Following safety measures were taken to exclude any exposure of the operating team [28, 29]. First, tightness of the abdomen was documented via a zero-flow of CO_2. Second, the procedure was performed in an operating room equipped with laminar air flow. Third, chemotherapy injection was remote-controlled and nobody remained in the operating room during the application. A pressurized aerosol containing doxorubicin at a dose of 1.5 mg/m^2 body surface in a 50 ml NaCl 0.9% solution followed by cisplatin at a dose of 7.5 mg/m^2 body surface in a 150 ml NaCl 0.9% solution was applied via micropump (MIP®, Reger Medizintechnik, Rottweil, Germany) and high-pressure injector. Flow rate was 30 ml/min and maximal upstream pressure was 200 psi. The therapeutic capnoperitoneum was maintained for 30 minutes at 37 °C. Then, the chemotherapy aerosol was exsufflated via a closed line over two sequential microparticle filters into the airwaste system of the hospital. Finally, trocars were retracted and laparoscopy ended. No drainage of the abdomen was applied. The PIPAC procedure was repeated after six weeks. Three PIPAC cycles were scheduled for each patient. All interventions were performed by three surgeons (M. A. R., U. G. P. and J. Z.). Survival follow up data were regularly updated by telephone calls. Patients were followed-up until Nov 21st, 2013 or until death. Clinical, laboratory and anatomopathology data were documented according to GCP rules, including electronic microfilm archiving and digital video recording of the surgical procedures. Objective tumor response was assessed by independent pathologists considering fibrosis overgrowth and proportion of vital tumor cells, as described elsewhere [30]. Adverse events were graded according to the Common Terminology Criteria for Adverse Events (CTCAE) version 4.0 [31]. Survival was modelled in a Kaplan–Meier survival curve. We used the software SPSS for Windows (SPSS 20.0, SPSS Inc., Chicago, IL, USA) for statistical analysis.

13.2 Results

Between November 2011 and June 2013, a total of 25 consecutive patients were scheduled for PIPAC. In one patient, access to the abdominal cavity was not possible due to extensive adhesions caused by prior surgery ($n = 1/25$; 4% primary nonaccess). Twenty-four patients (M : F = 12 : 12) with a mean age of 56 (± 12) years received ≥ 1 PIPAC and are objects of further analysis. Patients' characteristics and preoperative details are summarized in Table 13.1

Most tumors were classified as diffuse or signet ring cancers (18/24, 75%) and in most cases peritoneal carcinomatosis was advanced (mean PCI of 16 ± 10). Three patients had synchronous malignant pleural effusion, and liver metastasis were diagnosed at second PIPAC in a further patient, so that four patients had extraperitoneal metastasis. Five patients (21%) were in reduced general condition (Karnofsky index ≤ 60%, ECOG ≥ 2); in three patients systemic chemotherapy was contraindicated. Most patients were pretreated: 19/24 (79%) had previous (radio)chemotherapy, 11 pa-

Table 13.1. Characteristics of 24 patients with peritoneal carcinomatosis from gastric origin undergoing pressurized intraperitoneal aerosol chemotherapy (PIPAC).

Variable	*Value*
Number of patients	24
Sex (M : F)	12 : 12
Age, years (± SD)	56 (± 13)
Histology (Lauren classification)	
Diffuse/ signet ring	18
Mixed	1
Intestinal	5
Extraperitoneal metastasis	4 (17%)
Pleura	3
Liver	1
Peritoneal Carcinomatosis Index (mean ±SD)	16 (± 10)
Karnofsky Index before first PIPAC (mean ±SD)	78 (± 22%)
Previous organ surgery	16/24 (67%)
Previous (radio-) chemotherapy	19 (79%)
≥ 3 lines	4
2 lines	7
1 line	8
contraindication for chemotherapy	3
patient refusal	2
Simultaneous chemotherapy	8 (33%)

tients (46%) were in the third line or fourth line situation. Fourteen patients (58%) had previous gastrectomy or cytoreductive surgery, a further patient had previous intestinal bypass surgery. Eight patients (33%) received PIPAC in combination with systemic chemotherapy.

A total of 60 successful PIPAC procedures were performed, 17 patients (71%) had repeated PIPAC (two patients: five PIPAC; five patients: four PIPAC; three patients: three PIPAC; seven patients: two PIPAC). In three patients, a further PIPAC could not be performed due to bowel adhesions ($n = 3/17$; 18% secondary nonaccess). Mean operating time was 91 ± 34 min. Three intraoperative complications were noted (3/60, 5%): two access lesions (gallbladder puncture necessitating cholecystectomy and small bowel lesion necessitating segment resection) were immediately repaired (CTCAE 2); one severe allergic reaction with acute hypotension was easily controlled with corticoids and volume therapy.

Hospital mortality was 2/24 patients (8%) or 2/60 PIPAC procedures (3%). One patient (ASA IV, Karnofsky 30%, ascites three liters, preoperative GFR 20 ml/min, serum albumin 2.1 g/l) developed postoperative pulmonary edema, refused ICU admission and deceased on POD 3. The second patient, (ASA IV, Karnofsky 40%, ascites 7,000 ml) developed small bowel obstruction after second PIPAC so that symptomatic therapy

Table 13.2. Characteristics of 24 patients with peritoneal carcinomatosis from gastric origin undergoing PIPAC. PIPAC: Pressurized IntraPeritoneal Aerosol Chemotherapy; CRS: CytoReductive Surgery; CTCAE: Common Terminology Criteria for Adverse Events Version 4.0; CR: Complete remission; PR: Partial remission; SD: Stable disease; PD: Progressive disease; CRP: C-reactive Protein; AP: Abdominal pain; R: Renal toxicity; N/V: Nausea-vomiting; SBO: small bowel obstruction.

Patient	Operation	Response	CTCAE grading	Adverse event
1	2× PIPAC, small bowel resection	CR	1	Abdominal pain
2	1× PIPAC	N/A	1	CRP
3	4× PIPAC	CR	1	CRP
4	1× PIPAC, ileostomy	N/A	3	CRP, Cholangitis
5	4× PIPAC	PR	3	Hepatotoxicity, Abdominal pain
6	2× PIPAC	SD	1	CRP
7	4× PIPAC	PD	1	CRP
8	1× PIPAC	N/A	1	Abdominal pain
9	5× PIPAC	CR	1	Abdominal pain, CRP
10	5× PIPAC, adhesiolysis, incisional hernia repair	CR	1	Hepatotoxicity, CRP
11	4× PIPAC	PR	4	Allergy, myolysis
12	3× PIPAC, small bowel resection	PR	3	Hepatotoxicity, Abdominal pain
13	3× PIPAC	CR	1	Abdominal pain, CRP
14	1× PIPAC	N/A	1	CRP
15	2× PIPAC	PR	1	CRP
16	2× PIPAC	PR	1	N/V, CRP
17	3× PIPAC	SD	1	Renal toxicity, CRP
18	2× PIPAC, gastrectomy	CR	1	CRP
19	2× PIPAC	PR	5	CRP, Hepatotoxicity, SBO, death
20	1× PIPAC	N/A	3	CRP, Hepatotoxicity
21	2× PIPAC	PD	3	Hepatotoxicity
22	1× PIPAC	N/A	5	Lung edema, death
23	5× PIPAC	SD	3	Hepatotoxicity, CRP, 2× Access lesion
24	1× PIPAC	N/A	1	Access site extravasation

was decided and patient died on POD 8. Further adverse events are summarized in Table 13.2.

In general, PIPAC was very well tolerated. Elevated postoperative serum C-reactive protein was observed in most patients (16/24, 67%) as a sign of the chemical peritonitis induced by PIPAC (Figure 13.1).

Abdominal pain CTCAE 1 or 2 was noted in 6/24 patients (25%). A patient with preexisting biliary stent developed postoperative cholangitis; another patient developed local erythema at an abdominal port site and transient fever. In one case, an upper gastrointestinal bleeding was suspected but could not be confirmed endoscopically.

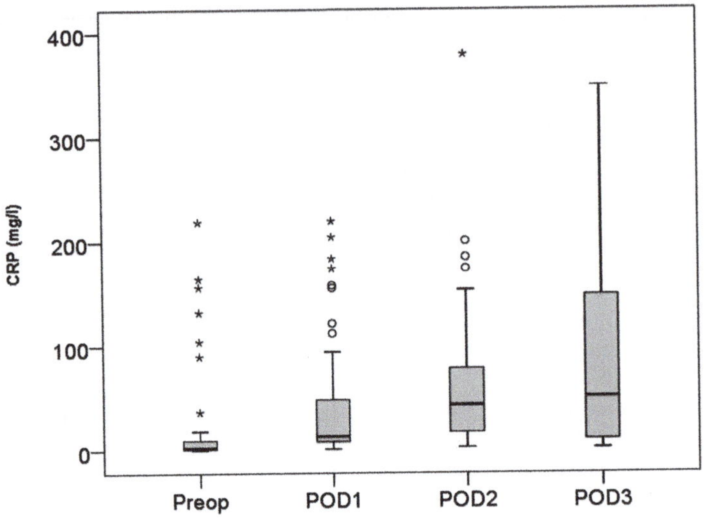

Fig. 13.1. PIPAC is well tolerated. Although the dose applied is only 10% of a usual systemic dose, patients develop a postoperative inflammatory syndrome with elevated C-reactive protein, probably explained by a chemical peritonitis. However, acute and cumulative local toxicities of PIPAC are well controlled and no bowel perforation and no gastrointestinal side effects above CTCAE grade 2 were observed.

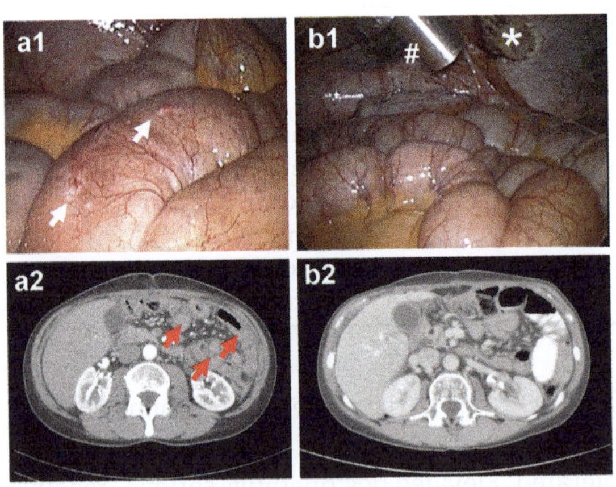

Fig. 13.2. Fifty-one-year-old female patient after R1 gastrectomy, postoperative chemotherapy (FLOT) and radiochemotherapy (5-FU) for gastric cancer, intestinal type, pT3 pN2 pM1 (per). Video-laparoscopy (a1) and CT scan (a2) at first PIPAC showing multiple small bowel involvement (white arrows) and radiological diffuse small bowel thickening (red arrows). At fourth PIPAC, videolaparoscopy shows a complete macroscopic response (b1) and CT a complete radiological response according to RECIST criteria (b2). #: micropump placed into the abdomen during laparoscopy. *: local peritonectomy scar. Multiple biopsies confirm major remission with extensive fibrosis and isolated vital tumor cells. Patient was alive 148 days after first PIPAC with a KI of 90%.

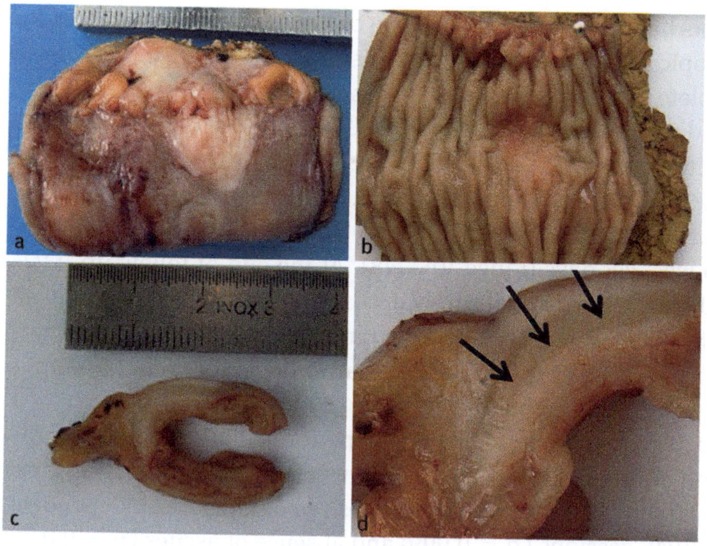

Fig. 13.3. Forty-two-year-old male patient with progressive peritoneal carcinomatosis from signet-ring cell gastric cancer after two lines systemic chemotherapy (ECF and FLOT). Partial pathologic response (PR) after three PIPAC and 4.5 months follow up. Secondary limited small bowel resection was performed in order to remove remaining macroscopic disease. Macroscopy of the surgical specimen: (a) overview of the scarred centimetric peritoneal carcinomatosis node (1.8 × 1.3 × 0.4 cm); (b) mucosal ulceration, histology showed no tumor within the mucosa; (c) perpendicular section through the bowel wall, showing transmural tumor scarring over several milimetres; (d) narrow view, arrows show the direction of penetration of aerosolized chemotherapy. Histology revealed transmural fibrosis with 30% vital tumor cells (major response) down to the submucosa, and the ulceration was healed suggesting penetration of chemotherapy throughout the bowel wall. Patient was alive 386 days after first PIPAC. GC: gastric cancer. PC: peritoneal carcinomatosis. PCI: Peritoneal Cancer Index.

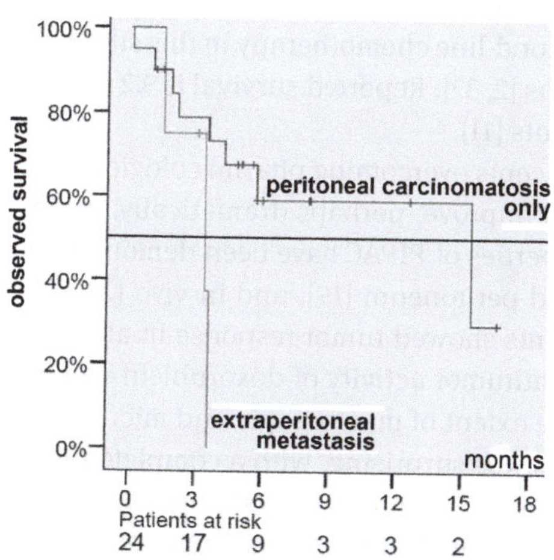

Fig. 13.4. Kaplan–Meier survival curve of 24 consecutive patients after PIPAC salvage therapy with cisplatin and doxorubicin. *x*-axis: survival in months; *y*-axis: cumulative survival. Green line: patients with peritoneal carcinomatosis (PC) plus other metastases. Blue line: patients with peritoneal carcinomatosis without other metastases.

A total of 17 patients having received at least two cycles of PIPAC were eligible for assessment of microscopic tumor response. In six patients (6/17; 35.2%) no vital tumor cells were found (complete histological remission), in six further patients (6/17; 35.2%) partial regression was documented (PR) and in three (3/17, 17.6%) stable disease (SD). In total, clinical benefit rate was 88.2% (15/17 patients with repeated PIPAC) or 60% (intention to treat, 15/ 25 patients scheduled for PIPAC). Examples of tumor regressions are given in Figures 13.2 and 13.3.

Median follow up was 248 days (range 105–748). At the end of follow up, 13/24 patients are alive. Median survival overall survival is 15.4 months. Overall survival after one year is 52%. Three out of 11 deaths occurred in patients with extraperitoneal metastatic disease. In this subgroup of patients, median survival was only 3.5 months (Figure 13.4)

A multivariable logistic regression analysis was performed with survival as the dependent variable and number of PIPAC sessions, Karnofksy Index, presence of extraperitoneal metastasis (yes versus no) and ascites (yes versus no) as the independent variables. Number of PIPAC sessions ($p = 0.009$) and absence of ascites ($p = 0.017$) independently predicted survival in this patient population.

13.3 Discussion

Peritoneal carcinomatosis from gastric cancer is considered an untreatable condition with short life expectancy. Thus, routine gastrectomy has been largely abandoned and platinum-based palliative systemic combination chemotherapy is the first-line therapy of choice in this situation [2]. Recent population-based statistics report a median survival of 4.8 months from timepoint of diagnosis in patients having received palliative chemotherapy [5]. When gastric cancer is progressing after first-line chemotherapy, expected median survival with best supportive care is only 2.5 months [2, 32]. Thus, German guidelines recommend second-line chemotherapy in this situation, with a reported median survival of 4–5 months [2, 32]. Reported survival is 9.2 months after CRS and HIPEC in highly selected patients [11].

It has been predicted that innovative concepts overcoming pharmacologic limitations of intraperitoneal chemotherapy could improve, perhaps dramatically, its efficacy [15]. The superior pharmacological properties of PIPAC have been demonstrated in the animal model [21], ex vivo in diseased peritoneum [19], and in vivo [22]. The first PIPAC application in three human patients showed tumor response in all cases, as a consequence of the well-documented antitumor activity of doxorubicin and cisplatin and the superior local disposition. The extent of macroscopic and microscopic response in these multidrug-resistant tumors was surprising, with a complete remission of peritoneal carcinomatosis in two patients, which was indeed unexpected [22]. In a preliminary series of 18 women with recurrent, platinum resistant ovarian cancer, PIPAC achieved an objective tumor response in 6/8 cases with repeated PIPAC [24].

Now, in gastric cancer, we are documenting objective tumor response in 15/17 (88%) patients after repeated PIPAC, including complete histological regression in six patients (35%). Thus, PIPAC (combined or not with systemic chemotherapy) can induce objective tumor regression in platinum-resistant peritoneal carcinomatosis of gastric cancer.

We observed a median survival of 15.4 months after PIPAC in these patients with advanced-stage disease. Interestingly, in four patients with peritoneal carcinomatosis and further distant metastasis, median survival after PIPAC was only 3.5 months – which is comparable with literature figures. This negative finding indirectly supports PIPAC efficacy since only patients with locoregional disease profited from locoregional therapy. A further argument for PIPAC efficacy is that the number of PIPAC sessions independently predicted survival in our patient cohort. Survival numbers after repeated PIPAC in the salvage therapy situation appear exceptional when compared with a median survival of 4.8 (3.5–5.7) months from timepoint of diagnosis of peritoneal carcinomatosis in population-based statistics for gastric cancer [5]. These encouraging numbers can be explained by patient selection, by outstanding PIPAC efficacy or by a combination of both factors. In contrast, this excellent survival after PIPAC cannot be explained by simultaneous systemic chemotherapy in eight patients, since the historical controls were obtained with patients receiving palliative systemic chemotherapy [5] and concern a recent period (2007–2011).

Most patients were heavily pretreated, indicating that PIPAC may be able to overcome platinum resistance, at least in some patients. The same observation has been made after PIPAC therapy in ovarian cancer [24]. The following factors might contribute to this favourable effect: (a) the intraperitoneal administration route resulting in a better therapeutic index than systemic delivery [12, 19]; (b) a homogeneous drug repartition within the closed abdomen due to the gas carrier [19, 21, 22]; (c) a superior drug penetration into the tumor nodules due to the artificial pressure gradient [18–22], and; (d) repeated application of up to five PIPAC cycles.

In spite of the high local drug concentration and of repeated administration, local PIPAC toxicity appears to be well controlled. In particular, acute and cumulative bowel toxicities appear to be low at the dosage given. No patient developed bowel perforation, and no gastrointestinal symptoms CTCAE > 2 were registered. In the majority of patients, PIPAC did not create peritoneal adhesions. However, abdominal access was not possible after repeated PIPAC in 3/17 patients (17.6%), or in 3/63 procedures (4.7%) so that secondary nonaccess might become a limitation of the PIPAC procedure in the future.

Hospital mortality was limited to two patients in poor general condition (ECOG 3, resp. 4, ASA 4). Cessation of life was caused by disease progression and causal relationship with PIPAC could not be established. In one case, death was due to decompensated ascites with preexisting renal failure; in the other patient it was due to progressive small bowel obstruction after second PIPAC. With a more conservative patient selection, procedure-related mortality does not seem to be a relevant issue after

PIPAC: we did not register any mortality in the last 362 consecutive PIPAC procedures in our institution (data on file).

In accordance with previous observations [23, 24], no significant renal toxicity was documented after PIPAC application in this group of patients. This appears reasonable bearing in mind the 90% dose reduction as compared to conventional systemic chemotherapy. However, PIPAC induced transient liver toxicity in a significant number of patients, confirming drug passage into the portal-venous system and a first-pass liver effect of intraperitoneal chemotherapy. Elevated serum levels of glutamic pyruvic transaminase (ALT, GPT) and/or oxaloacetic transaminase (AST, GOT) > 5× ULN were observed in 6/24 patients (25%).

In a single patient, a significant CK increase (CTCAE grade 3) was recorded without definite aetiology; CK-MB and troponin remained within normal limits. Finally, one patient developed anaphylactic shock during PIPAC, postoperative allergy testing showing metamizol but no platinum reactivity. The systemic inflammatory response to the chemical peritonitis following intraperitoneal chemotherapy caused few general symptoms such as fever or fatigue.

We did not observe typical chemotherapy-related side effects such as alopecia, neurotoxicity, cardiac toxicity and myelosuppression. This suggests that PIPAC might be indicated as a salvage therapy for patients who experienced severe side effects from previous systemic chemotherapy.

These results obtained in gastric cancer are preliminary and must be interpreted conservatively. Due to the framework conditions (off-label use program), most patients were heavily pretreated andsome of them were in critical condition. Eight patients received combined systemic chemotherapy. Thus, the results presented here cannot be extrapolated to all patients with peritoneal carcinomatosis from gastric cancer. Efficacy and safety of PIPAC is currently being investigated in a prospective clinical trial (NCT01854255) at our institution.

In summary, PIPAC was effective in treating this group of patients with recurrent, platinum-resistant peritoneal carcinomatosis from gastric cancer, with a favourable side effects profile. The time window for PIPAC salvage therapy appears to open when peritoneal carcinomatosis becomes resistant to platinum-based SC and to close when therapy-resistant ascites or bowel obstruction develops. Patients with extraperitoneal metastasis do not seem to experience the benefit PIPAC therapy. These data are consistent with our previous experience with PIPAC in patients with peritoneal carcinomatosis of ovarian [23] and appendiceal [22] origin. Together, these data suggest that clinical benefit might be achieved with PIPAC therapy in selected patients with recurrent cancer of various origins having spread to the peritoneum. These preliminary, retrospective results have now to be confirmed within the framework of a prospective study.

Bibliography

[1] Ferlay J, Shin HR, Bray F et al. Estimates of worldwide burden of cancer in 2008: GLOBOCAN 2008. Int J Cancer. 127 (2010) 2893–2917.

[2] Wagner AD, Unverzagt S, Grothe W et al. Chemotherapy for advanced gastric cancer. Cochrane Database Syst Rev. 17 (2010) CD004064. Review.

[3] Yonemura Y, Endou Y, Sasaki T et al. Surgical treatment for peritoneal carcinomatosis from gastric cancer. Eur J Surg Oncol. 36 (2010) 1131–1138.

[4] Sadeghi B, Arvieux C, Glehen O et al. Peritoneal carcinomatosis from non-gynecologic malignancies: results of the EVOCAPE 1 multicentric prospective study. Cancer. 88 (2000) 358–363.

[5] Thomassen I, van Gestel YR, van Ramshorst B et al. Peritoneal carcinomatosis of gastric origin: a population-based study on incidence, survival and risk factors. Int J Cancer. 134, 3 (Feb 1 2014) 622–628.

[6] Sarela AI, Miner TJ, Karpeh MS et al. Clinical outcomes with laparoscopic stage M1, unresected gastric adenocarcinoma. Ann Surg. 243 (2006) 189–195.

[7] Ceelen WP, Flessner MF. Intraperitoneal therapy for peritoneal tumors: biophysics and clinical evidence. Nat Rev Clin Oncol. 7 (2010) 108–115.

[8] Yamaguchi H, Kitayama J, Ishigami H et al. A phase 2 trial of intravenous and intraperitoneal paclitaxel combined with S-1 for treatment of gastric cancer with macroscopic peritoneal metastasis. Cancer. 119 (2013) 3354–3358.

[9] Matharu G, Tucker O, Alderson D. Systematic review of intraperitoneal chemotherapy for gastric cancer. Br J Surg. 98 (2011) 1225–1235.

[10] Macrì A, Fortugno A, Saladino E. Rationale and techniques of cytoreductive surgery and peritoneal chemohyperthermia. World J Gastrointest Oncol. 3 (2011) 169–174.

[11] Glehen O, Gilly FN, Arvieux C et al. Peritoneal carcinomatosis from gastric cancer: a multi-institutional study of 159 patients treated by cytoreductive surgery combined with perioperative intraperitoneal chemotherapy. Ann Surg Oncol. 17 (2010) 2370–2377.

[12] Coccolini F, Cotte E, Glehen O et al. Intraperitoneal chemotherapy in advanced gastric cancer. Meta-analysis of randomized trials. Eur J Surg Oncol. 40, 1 (2014) 12–26.

[13] Mi DH, Li Z, Yang KH et al. Surgery combined with intraoperative hyperthermic intraperitoneal chemotherapy (IHIC) for gastric cancer: a systematic review and meta-analysis of randomised controlled trials. Int J Hyperthermia. 29 (2013) 156–167.

[14] Gill RS, Al-Adra DP, Nagendran J et al. Treatment of gastric cancer with peritoneal carcinomatosis by cytoreductive surgery and HIPEC: a systematic review of survival, mortality, and morbidity. J Surg Oncol. 104 (2011) 692–698.

[15] Dedrick RL, Flessner MF. Pharmacokinetic Problems in Peritoneal Drug Administration: Tissue Penetration and Surface Exposure. J Natl Cancer Inst 89 (1997) 480–487.

[16] Hirose K, Katayama K, Iida A et al. Efficacy of continuous hyperthermic peritoneal perfusion for the prophylaxis and treatment of peritoneal metastasis of advanced gastric cancer: evaluation by multivariate regression analysis. Oncology. 57 (1999) 106–114.

[17] Ung L, Chua TC, Morris DL. Cure for peritoneal metastases? An evidence-based review. ANZ J Surg. 83, 11 (2013) 821–826.

[18] Minchinton AI, Tannock IF. Drug penetration in solid tumors. Nat Rev Cancer. 6 (2006) 583–592. Review.

[19] Solass W, Herbette A, Schwarz T et al. Therapeutic approach of human peritoneal carcinomatosis with Dbait in combination with capnoperitoneum: proof of concept. Surg Endosc. 26 (2012) 847–852.

[20] Facy O, Al Samman S, Magnin G et al. High pressure enhances the effect of hyperthermia in intraperitoneal chemotherapy with oxaliplatin: an experimental study. Ann Surg. 256 (2012) 1084–1088.

[21] Solass W, Hetzel A, Nadiradze G et al. Description of a novel approach for intraperitoneal drug delivery and the related device. Surg Endosc. 26 (2012) 1849–1855.
[22] Solass W, Kerb R, Mürdter T et al. Intraperitoneal Chemotherapy of Peritoneal Carcinomatosis Using Pressurized Aerosol as an Alternative to Liquid Solution: First Evidence for Efficacy. Ann Surg Oncol. 21, 2 (2014) 3504–3511.
[23] Blanco A, Giger-Pabst U, Solass W et al. Renal and hepatic toxicities after pressurized intraperitoneal aerosol chemotherapy (PIPAC). Ann Surg Oncol. 20 (2013) 2311–2316.
[24] Tempfer CB, Celik I, Solass W et al. Activity of Pressurized Intraperitoneal Aerosol Chemotherapy (PIPAC) with cisplatin and doxorubicin in women with recurrent, platinum-resistant ovarian cancer: Preliminary clinical experience. Gynecol Oncol. 132, 2 (2014) 307–311.
[25] Guideline on compassionate use of medicinal products, pursuant to Article 83 of regulation (EC) No 726/2004. London, EMEA/27170/2006.
[26] Vierzehntes Gesetz zur Änderung des Arzneimittelgesetzes vom 29. August 2005 /BGBl. I, p. 2570.
[27] Elias D, Souadka A, Fayard F et al. Variation in the peritoneal cancer index scores between surgeons and according to when they are determined (before or after cytoreductive surgery). Eur J Surg Oncol. 38 (2012) 503–508.
[28] Solass W, Giger-Pabst U, Borgstedt R et al. Pressurized IntraPeritoneal Aerosol Chemotherapy (PIPAC): occupational health and safety aspects. Ann Surg Oncol. 20 (2013) 3504–3511
[29] Oyais A, Solass W, Zieren J, Reymond MA, Giger-Pabst U. Arbeitssicherheits-aspekte der Intraperitonealen Druck-Aerosolchemotherapie (PIPAC): Bestätigung der Unbedenklichkeit. Zbl Chir 2014 Feb 14 (Epub ahead of print).
[30] Rubbia-Brandt L, Giostra E, Brezault C et al. Importance of histological tumor response assessment in predicting the outcome in patients with colorectal liver metastases treated with neo-adjuvant chemotherapy followed by liver surgery. Ann Oncol. 18 (2007) 299–304.
[31] Common Terminology Criteria for Adverse Events (CTCAE) version 4.0; published: May 28, 2009 v4.03. U.S. Department of Health and Human Services, National Institutes of Health, National Cancer Institute; June 14 2010.
[32] Kim HS, Kim HJ, Kim SY et al. Second-line chemotherapy versus supportive cancer treatment in advanced gastric cancer: a meta-analysis. Ann Oncol. 24, 11 (2013) 2850–2854.

13.4 PIPAC-GA1: a Phase-2 trial in the third-line palliative situation

Based on the preliminary observations described above, a Phase-2 trial aiming to assess efficacy and safety of PIPAC in gastric cancer was opened in February 2014 (www.clinicaltrials.gov, NCT01854255). Study title is "Feasibility, efficacy and safety of pressurized intraperitoneal aerosol chemotherapy (PIPAC) with cisplatin and doxorubicin in patients with gastric cancer and peritoneal carcinomatosis: an open-label, single-arm, phase 2 clinical trial".

13.4.1 Objectives

To evaluate the safety and efficacy in terms of the clinical benefit rate (CBR) of PIPAC in peritoneal carcinomatosis (PC) from gastric cancer (GC).

Table 13.3. PIPAC-GA1 study: eligibility criteria.

Ages Eligible for Study	18 Years to 80 Years
Genders Eligible for Study	Male or Females
Accepts Healthy Volunteers	No
Inclusion criteria	At least one line previous chemotherapy
	Recurrent gastric cancer
	Mobile patient
	Informed consent
Exclusion criteria	Ileus
	Necessity of parenteral nutrition
	Extraperitoneal metastases

13.4.2 Study design

Single center, open-label, non-randomized, single-arm, repeated single dose study to explore the efficacy, safety, and CBR of doxorubicin and cisplatin when given as a pressurized intraperitoneal aerosol chemotherapy (PIPAC) to patients (men and women) with advanced gastric cancer and peritoneal carcinomatosis.

13.4.3 Target subject population

Patients with gastric cancer and peritoneal carcinonatosis with disease progression after at least one line of previous IV chemotherapy (Table 13.3).

13.4.4 Investigational product, dosage and mode of administration

Doxorubicin 1.5 mg/m^2 body surface in 50 ml NaCl 0.9% and Cisplatinum 7.5 mg/m^2 in 50 ml NaCl 0.9% q 4–6 weeks, applied intraperitoneally as PIPAC.

13.4.5 Duration of treatment

Three single doses in six-week intervals, duration of treatment is 18 weeks.

13.4.6 Study endpoints

Primary outcome variable

Clinical Benefit Rate (CBR) according to RECIST criteria after three cycles of PIPAC with cisplatin and doxorubicin.

Secondary outcome variables

- The observed survival (OS).
- The median time to progression (TTP) according to RECIST criteria after three cycles of PIPAC with cisplatin and doxorubicin.

- The Peritoneal Carcinomatosis Index (PCI) before and after therapy.
- The degree of histological regression assessed by pathological review.
- Apoptosis as assessed by TUNEL analysis.
- The difference in ascites volume before and after the first, second, and third PIPAC application.

Patient reported outcomes (PROs)

European Organization for Research and Treatment of Cancer (EORTC) quality of life questionnaire (QLQ-C30, German version [1]).

Safety

Safety and tolerability will be assessed by collection of adverse events, according to the Common Terminology Criteria for Adverse Events (CTCAE) [2] including physical examination results, laboratory assessments (chemistry and hematology).

Biological monitoring

Basic research investigating the expression of genes associated with drug resistance.

Statistical methods

The sample size of 50 patients was calculated on the basis of a proportion of patients with a CBR of 40% or more as proof of efficacy of PIPAC in this patient population and of less than 10% as insufficient to continue the assessment. We assumed a risk of $\alpha = 0.05$ (type I error) and $\beta = 0.10$ (type II error), and a dropout rate of 10%. Analysis will be performed using nonparametric tests since we do not assume a normal distribution of data. Safety data will be summarized at each scheduled time point by treatment using descriptive statistics.

13.4.7 Current stage

Twelve patients have been recruited in the study (July 2014).

Bibliography

[1] Quality of Life Questionnaire – C30, http://www.eortc.org, consulted on Aug 14th, 2012.
[2] U.S. Department of Health and Human services, National Institutes of Health, National Cancer Institute. Common Terminology Criteria for Adverse Events (CTCAE) Version 4.0, Published: May 28, 2009 (v4.03: June 14, 2010).

U. Giger-Pabst, W. Solass, C. Demtröder, D. Strumberg, J. Zieren, and M. A. Reymond

14 PIPAC in colorectal cancer

Systemic therapy for metastatic colorectal cancer has undergone significant development in the last 20 years. Therapy regimens consisting of combinations of cytotoxic chemotherapeutic agents have demonstrated greater efficacy and contributed to a significant survival improvement. Oxaliplatin, irinotecan and 5-fluorouracil in combination with or without targeted therapies are recommended first- and second-line therapies of metastatic colorectal cancer [1]. In the third-line setting, data on the beneficial effect on systemic therapy are scarce, evidence being based on retrospective studies and phase II studies (reviewed in [2]). In the third- or fourth-line palliative situation, conventional chemotherapeutic agents such as capecitabine, mitomycin C, and gemcitabine have limited or no activity. Regorafinib, retreatment with oxaliplatin, or rechallenge with EGFR-directed therapy might be options in selected patients. Angiogenesis-inhibitors may prolong survival. Very few randomized clinical trials are available in third- or later lines of treatment in metastatic colorectal cancer so that there is a place for studies comparing investigational therapies with best supportive care (reviewed in [2]).

A particular challenge is the therapy of colorectal cancer patients with peritoneal involvement. Fifteen to 20% of patients with metastatic colorectal cancer show isolated peritoneal carcinomatosis with significant clinical relevance. Their prognosis is poor, with a reported mean survival of less than one year. Moreover, there is a lack of knowledge regarding treatment optimally tailored to individual patients (reviewed in [3]). Only a few studies are available regarding the efficacy of systemic chemotherapy against peritoneal carcinomatosis in colorectal cancer. In these studies, median survival of isolated peritoneal carcinomatosis treated with historical, 5-FU based chemotherapy was between 5.2 and 12.6 months [4–6]. There are only two published studies investigating the efficacy of modern drugs such as oxaliplatin or irinotecan in patients with colorectal peritoneal carcinomatosis. The first study reported a median survival of 12 months (95% CI, 4–20 months) for patients treated with oxaliplatin/irinotecan-based chemotherapy, versus 11 months (95% CI, 6–9 months) for patients treated with 5-FU/LV, and five months (95% CI, 3–7 months) for patients with best supportive care [7]. The second study with systemic administration of a combination of oxaliplatin and 5-FU/LV leucovorin in 40 patients reported a median survival of 22 months (95% CI, 17 to 26 months) [8].

Selected patients with peritoneal carcinomatosis from colorectal cancer can benefit from multimodal therapy combining surgical cytoreduction (CRS) with intraoperative hyperthermic intraperitoneal chemotherapy (HIPEC). Proper patient selection is indeed critical to the success of this combined treatment concept. Selection criteria are the presence of a limited peritoneal carcinomatosis without extraperitoneal metastases with a Peritoneal Cancer Index (PCI) less than 20 as well as the lack of diffuse small bowel involvement, so that a complete macroscopic surgical cytoreduction is possible [3]. This concept has gained in acceptance over the last years, in particular following the publication of a prospective randomized phase III trial analyzing CRS and HIPEC with mitomycin C plus adjuvant chemotherapy with 5-FU/folinic acid compared to systemic chemotherapy with 5-FU/folinic acid and palliative surgery. After a median follow up of 21.6 months, the experimental treatment arm showed a median overall survival of 22.3 months compared to 12.6 months in the standard arm. In the subgroup of patients with complete macroscopic cytoreduction (CC-0/1) median survival was 42.9 months [9, 10].

A frequent criticism of the above study is that old-fashioned drugs were used. In the meantime, new data using intraperitoneal oxaliplatin [11] have confirmed significant efficacy of CRS and HIPEC with a median survival after complete cytoreduction of 63 months versus 24 months in the systemic chemotherapy group, so that the current German S3-guideline recommends CRS and HIPEC in selected patients [1]. Recently, a prospective, multicenter, open-label, single-arm, single-stage Phase-2 study (COMBATAC study) has started, evaluating CRS and HIPEC in peritoneal carcinomatosis of colorectal origin. The primary objective of the COMBATAC study in patients with peritoneal carcinomatosis arising from wildtype KRAS colorectal and appendiceal cancer is to estimate the progression-free survival (PFS). Based on this estimation, it will be determined whether the multimodality treatment with pre- and postoperative systemic chemotherapy plus cetuximab, cytoreductive surgery (CRS) and bidirectional hyperthermic intraoperative chemotherapy (HIPEC) shows sufficient evidence of efficacy for further investigation [12].

A significant challenge remains, namely treating patients with isolated, platinum-resistant colorectal carcinomatosis who do not fulfil the criteria for combined CRS and HIPEC, in particular patients with diffuse small bowel involvement. It is in this particular situation where we applied Pressurized IntraPeritoneal Aerosol Chemotherapy (PIPAC) as an off-label use with oxaliplatin. In this retrospective analysis, we are now reporting the first results obtained with PIPAC and oxaliplatin in the human patient.

14.1 Patients and methods

In fall 2011, we opened an off-label use program for treating patients diagnosed with advanced, therapy-resistant peritoneal carcinomatosis from colorectal cancer with PIPAC. This program was approved by the Ethics Committees of the Ruhr University Bochum, Germany. Access to this off-label use program was limited to patients who had a life-threatening disease with no satisfactory alternative therapies or could not enter a clinical trial. Therefore, only patients left without treatment options or patients whose disease did not respond or relapsed to available treatments, or for whom the treatments were contraindicated or inadequate were included.

Prior to therapy, each patient was evaluated on an individual basis by the multidisciplinary tumor board at the Marien Hospital Herne, Comprehensive Cancer Centre, Ruhr University Bochum, Germany. Specific inclusion and exclusion criteria were not defined a priori. This retrospective review concerns only patients with histologically documented peritoneal carcinomatosis of colorectal origin, who had no option for complete cytoreductive surgery (CRS) and hyperthermic intraperitoneal chemotherapy (HIPEC). Most patients received prior palliative chemotherapy or were medically unfit for systemic palliative chemotherapy or had experienced severe side effects under systemic palliative chemotherapy or had refused to receive systemic chemotherapy. Patients with extraperitoneal metastatic disease were not treated because no effect of a locoregional therapy was expected. Patients with contraindication for general anesthesia and acute infection or sepsis were not treated. Patients with reduced general condition (Karnofsky ≤ 60%), therapy-resistant ascites necessitating iterative drainage and partial small bowel obstruction were not excluded from therapy. All procedures were performed according to the principles of the Helsinki declaration. All patients were extensively informed and signed a consent form.

All interventions were performed under general anesthesia with a single-shot of ceftriaxone 1.5 g IV administered 30 minutes prior to surgery. A venous thromboembolism prophylaxis was given the night before surgery using certoparin 3000 IE 1× s.c. After insufflation of a 12 mm Hg CO_2 pneumoperitoneum with open access or with Veres needle, two balloon safety trocars (5 and 12 mm, Applied Medical, Düsseldorf, Germany) were inserted into the abdominal wall. Ascites were removed and the amount documented. Extent of peritoneal carcinomatosis was determined according to Sugarbaker [13] based on lesion size and distribution. Peritoneal biopsies were taken in all four quadrants for histological examination, and a local partial peritonectomy of several square centimeters was performed routinely to improve accuracy of negative findings. Then, a nebulizer (MIP®, Reger Medizintechnik, Rottweil, Germany) was connected to an intravenous high-pressure injector (Injektron 82M, MedTron, Saarbrücken, Germany) and inserted into the abdomen. The following safety measures were taken to exclude any exposure of the operating team [14, 15]. First, tightness of the abdomen was documented via a zero-flow of CO_2. Second, the procedure was performed in an operating room equipped with laminar air flow. Third, chemotherapy injection was remote-controlled and nobody remained in the operating room during the application. A pressurized aerosol containing oxaliplatin at a dose of 92 mg/m^2 body surface in a 150 ml dextrose solution was applied via nebulizer and injector. Flow rate was 30 ml/min and maximal upstream pressure was 200 psi. The therapeutic capnoperitoneum was maintained for 30 minutes at 37 °C. Then, the chemotherapy aerosol was exsufflated via a closed line over two sequential microparticle filters into the airwaste system of the hospital. Finally, trocars were retracted and laparoscopy ended. No drainage of the abdomen was applied. The PIPAC procedure was repeated after six weeks. Three PIPAC cycles were scheduled for each patient. All interventions were performed by three surgeons (M. A. R., U. G. P. and J. Z.). Survival follow up data were regularly updated by telephone calls. Patients were followed-up until Feb 22nd, 2014 or until death. Clinical, laboratory and anatomopathology data were documented according to GCP rules, including electronic microfilm archiving and digital video recording of the surgical procedures. Anatomopathological response was assessed by independent pathologists considering fibrosis overgrowth and proportion of vital tumor cells, as described elsewhere [16]. Adverse events were graded according to the Common Terminology Criteria for Adverse Events (CTCAE) version 4.0 [17]. Survival was modelled in a Kaplan–Meier survival curve. We used the software SPSS for Windows (SPSS 20.0, SPSS Inc., Chicago, IL, USA) for statistical analysis.

14.2 Results

Between October 2012 and February 2014, a total of 17 consecutive patients with platinum-resistant colorectal peritoneal carcinomatosis were scheduled for PIPAC. Access to the abdominal cavity was possible in all cases. Preoperative patients' characteristics and previous therapy are summarized in Table 14.1.

In all cases, peritoneal carcinomatosis was documented by histology. In most cases peritoneal carcinomatosis was advanced (mean PCI of 16 ± 10). No patients had clinical extraperitoneal disease; in one patient three liver metastases had been previously removed by radiofrequency ablation, without radiological evidence for recurrence.

Table 14.1. Characteristics of 17 patients having received Pressurized IntraPeritoneal Aerosol Chemotherapy with oxaliplatin 92 mg/m^2 body surface for colorectal cancer.

Characteristics	Value
Number of patients	17
Sex (M : F)	10 : 7
Age, years (mean ± SD)	59 ± 12
Karnofsky-Index, % (mean ± SD)	85 ± 13
Mean PCI (± SD)	16 (± 10)
Ascites (> 250 ml)	3/17 (18%)
Extraperitoneal metastasis	0/17
S/P colorectal resection	17/17 (100%)
S/P chemotherapy (platinum-based)	16/17 (94%)
Previous chemotherapy	
none (combined PIPAC & systemic chemo)	1
1 line	5
2 lines	10
3 lines	1
Combined chemotherapy (PIPAC + systemic)	11

Table 14.2. Surgical procedures.

Number of procedures	48
Number of PIPAC	42
Secondary non-access	6
Operating time, min (mean ± SD)	91 ± 34
Intraoperative complication	0

One patient was in reduced general condition (Karnofsky index ≤ 60%, ECOG ≥ 2). All patients were pretreated: 17/18 had previous chemotherapy, 11 patients (65%) were in the third- or fourth-line situation. All patients had previous colorectal surgery. Eleven patients (65%) received systemic chemotherapy in combination with PIPAC.

A total of 42 successful PIPAC procedures were performed (mean number of PIPAC procedures/patient = 2.5). Thirteen patients (76%) had repeated PIPAC (four patients: four PIPAC; four patients: three PIPAC; five patients: two PIPAC). In six patients, a further PIPAC could not be performed due to bowel adhesions at a later stage ($n = 6/17$; 35% secondary non access). Mean operating time was 91 ± 34 minutes. No intraoperative complications were noted (Table 14.2).

Hospital mortality was zero. The following postoperative side effects were recorded: CTCAE 1 = 13 (88%), CTCAE 2 = 0, CTCAE 3 = 4 (12%), CTCAE 4 = 0, CTCAE 5 = 0. Side effects are detailed in Table 14.3.

Symptoms CTCAE 3 were observed only in 4/17 patients (23%), no side effect CTCAE 4 being documented. The most frequent symptom was postoperative pain which was reported in 11 cases. All patients developed a postoperative inflammatory syndrome (with significant CRP increase) but fever was observed in only four cases. Seven patients reported nausea (41%) and a single patient diarrhea (6%). Liver and renal toxicities were minimal (CTCAE 1 in six patients).

A total of 13 patients having received at least two cycles of PIPAC were eligible for assessment of microscopic tumor response. In six patients (6/13; 46%), major pathological tumor response was documented (no tumor cells or isolated tumor cells within fibrosis). In a further five patients (5/13, 38%), a partial pathological response was observed, and in two patients (16%) there was no response to therapy. In total, the clinical benefit rate was 84.6% (11/13 patients with repeated PIPAC) or 64.7% (intention to treat, 11/ 17 patients scheduled for PIPAC). Examples of tumor regressions are given in Figure 14.1.

One patient experienced such a regression that a secondary cytoreductive surgery and HIPEC was possible. Vital tumor cells were found in 3/9 peritoneal and omental biopsies, at macroscopically suspect locations. Four millimetric tumor nodules were removed from the small bowel surface, and no tumor cells were found in these nodules anymore (Figure 14.2).

Table 14.3. Side effects observed in 17 patients after pressurized intraperitoneal aerosol chemotherapy (PIPAC) with oxaliplatin 92 mg/m^2 body surface.

Patient	PIPAC (*n*)	Response	CTCAE	Adverse event
1	4	major	1	CRP, LT
2	4	major	3	CRP, Pain, N/V
3	2	partial	3	CRP, Pain, N/V, Diarrhea
4	3	major	1	CRP, RT, Pain, Fever
5	1	N/A	1	CRP, Pain, N/V
6	1	N/A	1	CRP, Pain
7	4	partial	1	CRP, RT, LT, Pain, Fever
8	1	N/A	1	CRP, CK
9	1	N/A	3	CRP, Pain
10	3	partial	1	CRP, Fever, Pain
11	3	partial	1	CRP, N/V, LT
12	2	no response	1	CRP, RT
13	3	no response	3	CRP, Pain, N/V
14	2	major	1	CRP, Pain, N/V
15	4	major	1	CRP, N/V
16	2	major	1	CRP
17	2	partial	1	CRP, RT, LT, Pain, Fever

PIPAC: Pressurized IntraPeritoneal Aerosol Chemotherapy (PIPAC); CTCAE: Common Terminology Criteria for Adverse Events Version 4.0; CRP: C-reactive Protein; AP: Abdominal pain; RT: Renal toxicity; LT: Liver toxicity.

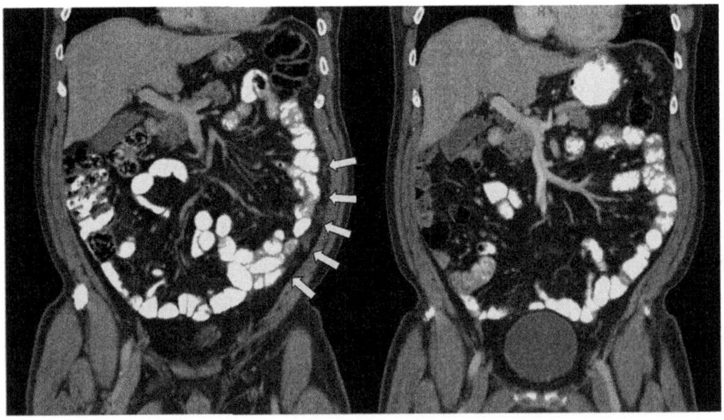

Fig. 14.1. Fifty-eight-year-old patient with metachronous peritoneal carcinomatosis of colorectal cancer 27 months after diagnosis and after systemic chemotherapy (XELOX, then capecitabin alone due to side effects). (a) Abdominal CT scan before PIPAC therapy with extensive peritoneal carcinomatosis (arrows). (b) Complete radiological response according to RECIST criteria after three cycles of Pressurized IntraPeritoneal Aerosol Chemotherapy (PIPAC) q6w with oxaliplatin 92 mg/m^2 at a pressure of 12 mm Hg and a temperature of 37 °C for 30 minutes, combined with systemic chemotherapy (FOLFIRI). Patient is alive one year after first PIPAC with excellent quality of life.

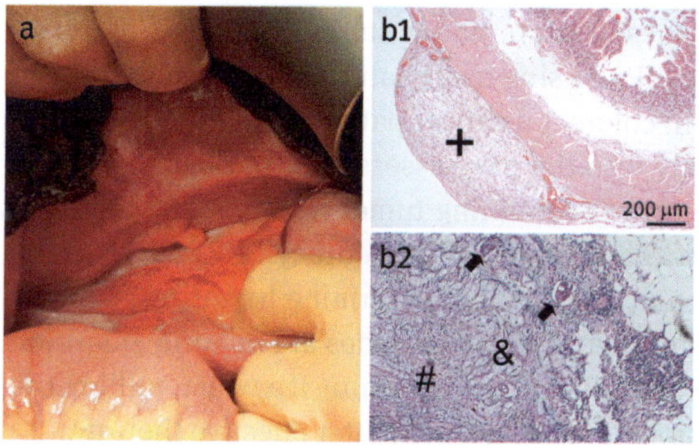

Fig. 14.2. The same patient underwent complete cytoreductive surgery (CC-0) and Hyperthermic IntraPeritoneal Chemotherapy (HIPEC) seven months after first PIPAC. (a) Macroscopy of the left upper abdomen showing limited peritoneal carcinomatosis (Peritoneal Carcinomatosis Index = 3) with diffuse scarring. (b1) Four suspect millimetric nodes on the surface of the small bowel were resected, all of them were tumor-free (+). (b2) Vital tumor cells (arrows) were found in 3/9 peritoneal biopsies and in the omentum, together with extensive fibrosis (#) and large mucous areas (&) as a sign of tumor regression.

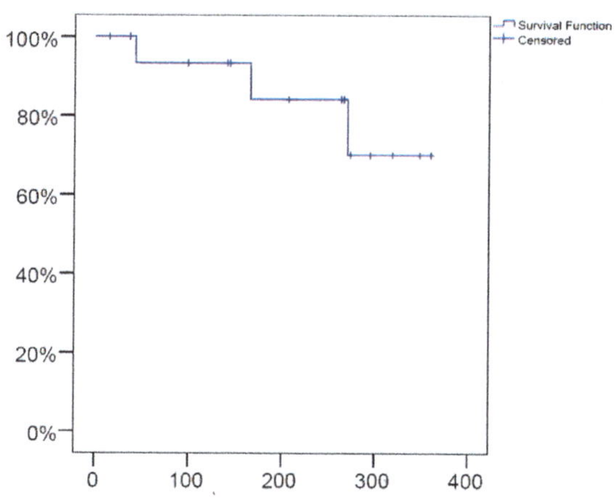

Fig. 14.3. Observed actuarial survival of 17 consecutive patients with peritoneal carcinomatosis of colorectal cancer (mean Peritoneal Carcinomatosis Index = 16) after PIPAC salvage therapy with oxaliplatin. Patients had previously received two lines (median value) of palliative systemic chemotherapy. One-year survival is 70%, 14/17 patients are alive after a mean follow up of 237 days. Median survival has not been reached yet (dotted line). *X*-axis: survival in days. *Y*-axis: cumulated survival.

Mean follow up was 237 days. At the end of follow up, 14/17 patients are alive. Median overall survival has not been reached, one-year overall survival is 70%. (Figure 14.3)

14.3 Discussion

The first in-human data on the application of Pressurized IntraPeritoneal Aerosol Chemotherapy (PIPAC) with doxorubicin and cisplatin have delivered encouraging results in ovarian cancer and gastric cancer. Phase-2 trials [18] are currently ongoing to investigate the reproducibility of these results under study conditions. Here we present the first results obtained with PIPAC using oxaliplatin as a salvage therapy in advanced peritoneal carcinomatosis in colorectal cancer patients.

An important finding of this study was the easy assessment of objective tumor response already six weeks after therapy. Determining tumor response in peritoneal carcinomatosis is difficult because of the relatively low accuracy of RECIST criteria in this situation (see page 68). We found it difficult to determine tumor response by repeated PCI determination, since changes in the tumor nodes are not only quantitative, but also qualitative. For example, it is difficult to determine if a white, millimetric peritoneal node is still an active tumor node or only a scar after effective therapy.

These preliminary data in a small group of (self-)selected patients shows a superior objective tumor response (pathological response rate of 65%) in the salvage situation in platinum-resistant tumors. PIPAC with oxaliplatin can obviously induce tumor response in advanced peritoneal carcinomatosis of colorectal origin. This finding might first appear puzzling since these tumors were resistant to platinum-based systemic chemotherapy. Further pharmacological data have indeed to be gathered in the large animal model, and thereafter in a Phase-1 dose-escalation study in the human patient, in order to document the pharmacological rationale for the observed effect. However, this effect exists and it appears reasonable to attribute the high response rate observed to the relatively high dose of oxaliplatin applied within the peritoneal cavity (92 mg/m^2 body surface), but also to the improvement of the therapeutic index by the local administration of intraperitoneal chemotherapy [19]. Taking advantage of physical properties such as the application of the drug as an aerosol, or applying an artificial intraperitoneal hydrostatic pressure, further improve the pharmacological properties [20]. Finally, repeating PIPAC allows delivery of chemotherapy cycles analogous to systemic chemotherapy.

Acute local toxicity appears to be well controlled, since only 4/17 patients reported abdominal pain CTCAE > 2, and since no bowel perforation was observed in 42 applications. In this small group of patients, we cannot exclude the possibility that repeated PIPAC with oxaliplatin induces a cumulative bowel toxicity but this toxicity appears clinically acceptable.

In colorectal cancer liver metastasis, overall survival correlates with pathological tumor response after systemic chemotherapy [16]. We observe a similar correlation in peritoneal metastases of colorectal origin, the overall one-year survival of 70% being in accordance with the superior pathological tumor response. Importantly, this survival is calculated from the time point of first PIPAC application and not from the time point of diagnosis of peritoneal carcinomatosis.

Eleven patients received salvage systemic chemotherapy in parallel to PIPAC. This appears logical since metastatic colorectal cancer is a systemic disease and PIPAC is only a locoregional therapy. In analogy, the principle of bidirectional chemotherapy is also increasingly accepted for cytoreductive surgery and HIPEC in colorectal cancer [11]. Of course, combined use of systemic palliative chemotherapy together with

PIPAC is a methodological limitation for assessment of PIPAC efficacy. However, one should remember the low response rate of systemic chemotherapy in the salvage situation [2] to evaluate the possible influence of systemic therapy on platinum-resistant peritoneal carcinomatosis. At the same time, this report provides first evidence of the possibility to combine systemic chemotherapy with PIPAC in multimodal therapy cycles. For this purpose and in a first step, we chose the following schedule: PIPAC on week one, day two; then systemic chemotherapy from week two, day one until week four, day five; then two weeks recovery time; then second PIPAC on week six, day two. This schedule was repeated at least three times.

It was possible to perform complete cytoreductive surgery in one patient after four combined cycles of systemic chemotherapy and PIPAC. We are aware of three further patients with appendiceal cancer having received PIPAC who had secondary cytoreductive surgery.

Safety data are favourable in this small group of patients. No hospital mortality was observed, and the procedures were remarkably well tolerated. The main problem was postoperative abdominal pain, which was severe (CTCAE 3) in four patients. This is obviously explained by the chemical peritonitis induced by PIPAC. This side effects appears clinically more important after PIPAC with oxaliplatin with a dose of $92\,mg/m^2$ than in our experience after PIPAC with a combination of cisplatin ($1.5\,mg/m^2$) and doxorubicin ($7.5\,mg/m^2$).

Of course, these preliminary results should be interpreted with caution. They might be helpful for optimizing patient selection criteria but should now be confirmed in prospective controlled studies. They should not be interpretated as proof of PIPAC's superiority over salvage systemic chemotherapies in this desperate situation.

In summary, the results of this retrospective analysis in a small cohort of patients support the rationale for further studies on palliative treatment with PIPAC for colorectal cancer patients with platinum-resistant peritoneal carcinomatosis who do not meet the inclusion criteria for CRS and HIPEC.

Bibliography

[1] Pox C, Aretz S, Bischoff SC et al. [S3-guideline colorectal cancer version 1.0]. Z Gastroenterol. 51, 8 (Aug 2013) 753–854.

[2] Nielsen DL, Palshof JA, Larsen FO, Jensen BV, Pfeiffer P. A systematic review of salvage therapy to patients with metastatic colorectal cancer previously treated with fluorouracil, oxaliplatin and irinotecan +/- targeted therapy. Cancer Treat Rev. 2014 Feb 28. pii: S0305–7372(14)00026–00027. doi: 10.1016/j.ctrv.2014.02.006. [Epub ahead of print] Review.

[3] Piso P, Arnold D. Multimodal treatment approaches for peritoneal carcinosis in colorectal cancer. Dtsch Arztebl Int. 108, 47 (Nov 2011) 802–808.

[4] Chu DZ, Lang NP, Thompson C, Osteen PK, Westbrook KC. Peritoneal carcinomatosis in nongynecologic malignancy. A prospective study of prognostic factors. Cancer. 63 (1989) 364–367.

[5] Sadeghi B, Arvieux C, Glehen O, Beaujard AC, Rivoire M, Baulieux J et al. Peritoneal carcinomatosis from non-gynecologic malignancies: results of the EVOCAPE 1 multicentric prospective study. Cancer. 88 (2000) 358–363.
[6] Jayne DG, Fook S, Loi C, Seow-Choen F. Peritoneal carcinomatosis from colorectal cancer. Br J Surg. 89 (2002) 1545–1550.
[7] Pelz JO, Chua TC, Esquivel J, Stojadinovic A, Doerfer J, Morris DL et al. Evaluation of best supportive care and systemic chemotherapy as treatment stratified according to the retrospective peritoneal surface disease severity score (PSDSS) for peritoneal carcinomatosis of colorectal origin. BMC Cancer. 10 (2010) 689.
[8] Lee DH, Oh SY, Lee YR, Huh SJ, Yoon HH, Kim SH, Lee S, Lee JH, Kim Y, Kim HJ, Kwon HC. A Phase II Study of Modified FOLFOX4 for Colorectal Cancer Patients with Peritoneal Carcinomatosis. Cancer Res Treat. 43, 4 (Dec 2011) 225–230.
[9] Verwaal VJ, van Ruth S, de Bree E, van Sloothen GW, van Tinteren H, Boot H, Zoetmulder FA: Randomized trial of cytoreduction and hyperthermic intraperitoneal chemotherapy versus systemic chemotherapy and palliative surgery in patients with peritoneal carcinomatosis of colorectal cancer. J Clin Oncol 21, 20 (2003) 3737–3743.
[10] Verwaal VJ, Bruin S, Boot H, van Slooten G, van Tinteren H: 8-year follow up of randomized trial: cytoreduction and hyperthermic intraperitoneal chemotherapy versus systemic chemotherapy in patients with peritoneal carcinomatosis of colorectal cancer. Ann Surg Oncol 15, 9 (2008) 2426–2432.
[11] Elias D, Lefevre JH, Chevalier J, Brouquet A, Marchal F, Classe JM et al. Complete cytoreductive surgery plus intraperitoneal chemohyperthermia with oxaliplatin for peritoneal carcinomatosis of colorectal origin. J Clin Oncol – Off J Am Soc Clin Oncol 27 (2009) 681–685.
[12] Glockzin G, Rochon J, Arnold D, Lang SA, Klebl F, Zeman F, Koller M, Schlitt HJ, Piso P. A prospective multicenter phase II study evaluating multimodality treatment of patients with peritoneal carcinomatosis arising from appendiceal and colorectal cancer: the COMBATAC trial. BMC Cancer. 13 (Feb 7 2013) 67. doi: 10.1186/1471–2407-13–67.
[13] Jacquet P, Sugarbaker PH. Clinical research methodologies in diagnosis and staging of patients with peritoneal carcinomatosis. In: Sugarbaker PH (ed). Peritoneal carcinomatosis: principles of management. Boston: Kluwer Academic publishers; 1996. pp. 359–374.
[14] Solass W, Giger-Pabst U, Borgstedt R et al. Pressurized IntraPeritoneal Aerosol Chemotherapy (PIPAC): occupational health and safety aspects. Ann Surg Oncol. 20 (2013) 3504–3511.
[15] Oyais A, Solass W, Zieren J, Reymond MA, Giger-Pabst U. Arbeitssicherheits-aspekte der Intraperitonealen Druck-Aerosolchemotherapie (PIPAC): Bestätigung der Unbedenklichkeit. Zbl Chir 2014 Feb 4 [Epub ahead of print].
[16] Rubbia-Brandt L, Giostra E, Brezault C et al. Importance of histological tumor response assessment in predicting the outcome in patients with colorectal liver metastases treated with neo-adjuvant chemotherapy followed by liver surgery. Ann Oncol. 18 (2007) 299–304.
[17] Common Terminology Criteria for Adverse Events (CTCAE) version 4.0; published: May 28, 2009 v4.03. U.S. Department of Health and Human Services, National Institutes of Health, National Cancer Institute; June 14 2010.
[18] http://www.clinicaltrials.gov. Ovarian cancer: NCT01809379, gastric cancer: NCT NCT01854255.
[19] Ceelen WP, Flessner MF. Intraperitoneal therapy for peritoneal tumors: biophysics and clinical evidence. Nat Rev Clin Oncol. 7, 2 (Feb 2010) 108–115.
[20] Solass W, Kerb R, Mürdter T, Giger-Pabst U, Strumberg D, Tempfer C, Zieren J, Schwab M, Reymond MA. Intraperitoneal chemotherapy of peritoneal carcinomatosis using pressurized aerosol as an alternative to liquid solution: first evidence for efficacy. Ann Surg Oncol. 21, 2 (Feb 2014) 553–559.

W. Solass, U. Giger-Pabst, C. Demtröder, D. Strumberg, J. Zieren, and M. A. Reymond

15 PIPAC in mesothelioma

Malignant peritoneal mesothelioma is a rare disease. Patients typically present with abdominal pain (33%), increasing abdominal girth (31%), new onset hernia (12%), pain (5%), or a variety of other clinical symptoms such as anorexia, dyspnea, fever and abdominal mass [1, 2]. Due to unspecificity of symptoms, peritoneal mesothelioma is often diagnosed at an advanced stage. At this stage, patients may experience small bowel obstruction, perforation or severe ascites, which require emergency surgery. Peritoneal mesothelioma might also be diagnosed incidentally during laparoscopy for another reason. Peritoneal malignant mesothelioma is often reported in men and women with no known asbestos exposure. Peritoneal mesothelioma is divided into three major histological types: epitheloid, sarcomatoid or mixed type mesothelioma [3].

Despite the combined systemic palliative therapy with cisplatin and pemetrexed, the median survival of patients with peritoneal mesothelioma remains poor (between 8–14 months) [1]. Cytoreductive surgery with hyperthermic intraperitoneal chemotherapy (HIPEC) is indicated only in patients in good general condition and with limited disease and is associated with long-term survival in selected cases. The Pressurized IntraPeritoneal Aerosol Chemotherapy (PIPAC) has superior pharmacological properties [4] and has shown encouraging results in peritoneal carcinomatosis from ovary, stomach and colon cancers. We now report the first results of PIPAC in patients with peritoneal mesothelioma.

15.1 Patients and methods

Between 26 June 2012 and 17 March 2014, 23 PIPAC applications were carried out in ten patients with peritoneal mesothelioma within the framework of off-label use applications. Analysis was retrospective. No specific inclusion or exclusion criteria were defined, and indication was decided on an individual, case-by-case basis in our interdisciplinary tumor board. In eight patients peritoneal mesothelioma was progressive after platinum-based, systemic combination chemotherapy. No patient had an indication for CRS and HIPEC. Median age was 59 ± 13 years. Karnofsky index was 83 ± 20%. Mean PCI was 18 ± 12. During the procedure, 7.5 mg/m^2 cisplatin and doxorubicin 1.5 mg/m^2 were administered at 12 mm Hg and 37 °C for 30 minutes. The follow up was carried out until 27 March 2014 or until death. Target variables were overall survival and histological tumor response.

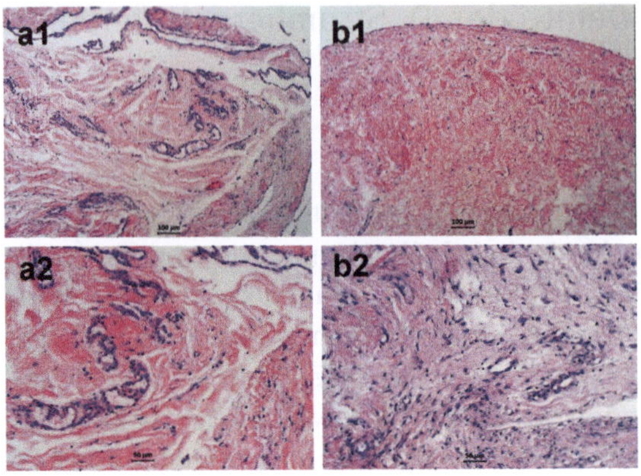

Fig. 15.1. Forty-two-year-old female patient with malignant peritoneal mesothelioma. Peritoneal biopsies before (a1, a2) and after (b1, b2) PIPAC with cisplatin 7.5 mg/m^2 and doxorubicin 1.5 mg/m^2 body surface. (a1) and (a2): infiltration of a malignant mesothelioma; (b1) and (b2): peritoneum with a linear fibrosis below the mesotheliom and discrete chronic inflammation. No vital tumor tissue. Secondary CC-0 cytoreductive surgery was performed after third PIPAC, and the patient is alive eight months after first PIPAC with objective major pathological response at forth PIPAC.

15.2 Results

In all cases, the surgical approach was possible. None of the 23 interventions led to an intraoperative complication. Mean operative time (PIPAC alone) was 87 minutes. PIPAC has been repeated in eight patients (4×: $n = 1$; 3×: $n = 3$; 2×: $n = 4$). One patient had combined PIPAC and PITAC (intrapleural) treatment; another a combined pleurectomy and PIPAC. One patient in poor general condition (Karnofsky 40%) died in the hospital because of disease progression after second PIPAC. The same patient developed postoperative tumor lysis syndrome. Otherwise, no side effect CTCAE > 2 was documented. Of the eight patients with repeated PIPAC, six showed an objective response in histology (Figure 15.1).

Mean follow up was 7.9 months. At the end of follow up, eight patients were alive. Actuarial survival after 317 days was 78%, median survival has not been reached (Figure 15.2). Importantly, this survival is not calculated from diagnosis of peritoneal mesothelioma, but from the time point of first PIPAC. Eight out of ten patient had previously received guideline-based therapy with systemic cisplatin and pemetrexed.

15.3 Conclusions

These preliminary findings in a small retrospective cohort of patients are promising. PIPAC with doxorubicin and cisplatin (about 10% of a systemic dose) can induce a

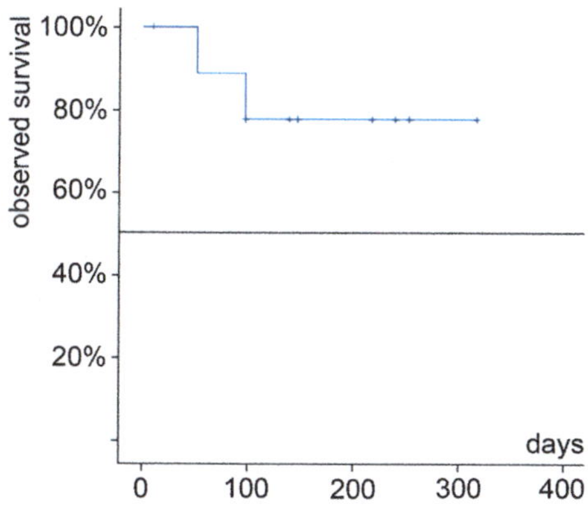

Fig. 15.2. Observed actuarial survival of ten consecutive patients with peritoneal mesothelioma after PIPAC salvage therapy with cisplatin and doxorubicin. Eight patients had previously received palliative systemic chemotherapy with cisplatin and permetrexed. Eight out of the ten patients are alive after a mean follow up of 236 days. Median survival has not been reached yet after 317 days (dotted line). *X*-axis: survival in days. *Y*-axis: cumulated survival.

tumor regression in pretreated, progressive peritoneal mesothelioma. Overall survival in this (self-) selected patients group is encouraging high.

Beside of the superior pharmacological properties of PIPAC, these encouraging survival results might be also explained by repeated PIPAC application. Longer survival times were documented in patients with malignant mesothelioma after repeat HIPEC application. Patients who underwent repeat HIPEC had a significantly improved median survival (80 months) versus single HIPEC (27.2 months). A lower peritoneal carcinoma index and complete cytoreduction were also associated positively with survival [2].

PIPAC is well tolerated, and combination with intrathoracic surgery is possible. Efficacy and safety of PIPAC in peritoneal mesothelioma should now be evaluated under study conditions.

Bibliography

[1] Chua TC, Yan TD, Morris DL. Surgical biology for the clinician: peritoneal mesothelioma: current understanding and management. Can J Surg. 52, 1 (Feb 2009) 59–64. Review.

[2] Wong J, Koch AL, Deneve JL, Fulp W, Tanvetyanon T, Dessureault S. Repeat cytoreductive surgery and heated intraperitoneal chemotherapy may offer survival benefit for intraperitoneal mesothelioma: a single institution experience. Ann Surg Oncol. 21, 5 (May 2014) 1480–1486.

[3] Tannapfel A (ed). Malignant Mesothelioma. Springer, Berlin Heidelberg, 2011.

[4] Solass W, Kerb R, Mürdter T, Giger-Pabst U, Strumberg D, Tempfer C, Zieren J, Schwab M, Reymond MA. Intraperitoneal chemotherapy of peritoneal carcinomatosis using pressurized aerosol as an alternative to liquid solution: first evidence for efficacy. Ann Surg Oncol. 21, 2 (Feb 2014) 553–559.

K. Odendahl, W. Solass, C. Demtröder, U. Giger-Pabst, C. Tempfer, D. Strumberg, A. Münker, and M. A. Reymond

16 Quality of Life after PIPAC

Patient symptoms resulting from cancer progression and tolerability of treatment-related toxicities are of critical importance when considering whether a new treatment produces a clinically meaningful outcome for patients. Recently, a working group of the ASCO agreed that if a therapy is less toxic than prevailing treatments, a smaller improvement in efficacy is acceptable. Conversely, a highly toxic therapy should be accompanied by an expectation of substantially greater benefit to provide a clinically meaningful outcome to patients [1].

Intraperitoneal pressure aerosol chemotherapy (Pressurized IntraPeritoneal Aerosol Chemotherapy, PIPAC) is an innovative, palliative therapy of Peritoneal Carcinomatosis (PC). Preliminary results from small retrospective series concerning tumor response and survival are encouraging. However, according to the ASCO recommendation above, information on the quality of life (QOL) of patients with peritoneal carcinomatosis treated with PIPAC is critical.

This is a single-center retrospective study on a cohort of 48 consecutive patients treated with PIPAC as off-label salvage therapy for peritoneal carcinomatosis. Consecutive patients were selected on a retrospective basis, with the condition that they received at least two PIPAC applications, in order to be able to determine an evolution.

The selected 48 patients (M : F = 23 : 25, age 58 ± 10 years) were treated with 158 PIPAC procedures in six-week intervals. The primary tumor was stomach (18), colon (9), ovary (7) and others (14). The patients had previously treated, platinum-resistant peritoneal carcinomatosis. As a rule, peritoneal carcinomatosis was advanced (PCI = 15 ± 9).

Assessment of quality of life was performed with a validated instrument, the QLQ30 questionnaire of the EORTC. Questionnaires were filled out by the patients alone. The document was handed to the patient by a study nurse the day before PIPAC therapy.

Questionnaire compliance was 100% at baseline and after six weeks, then declined to 71% after 12 weeks and 35% after 18 weeks.

The global quality of life score, physical and health condition at the beginning of treatment was significantly reduced (65 ± 20%) as compared to normal controls. Six weeks after the first PIPAC the global quality of life score deteriorated slightly further (63 ± 19%). Later in the evolution, this global score improved after second PIPAC (after three months, 70 ± 18%) and third PIPAC (after 4.5 months, 70 ± 16%, Figure 16.1).

Gastrointestinal symptoms (nausea or vomiting, constipation, diarrhea, anorexia scores) remained stable under PIPAC therapy (Figure 16.2).

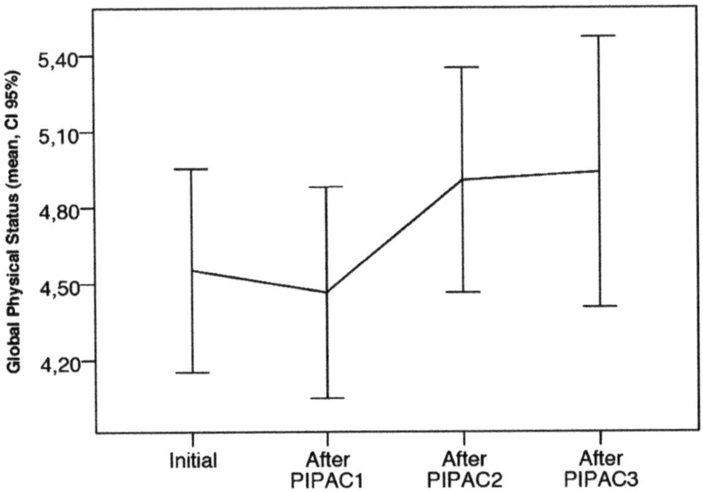

Fig. 16.1. QLQ-30 Global physical status score. The score deteriorates in the first six weeks, increases then slightly until 4.5 months after first PIPAC. Worst possible value = 1, best possible value = 7.

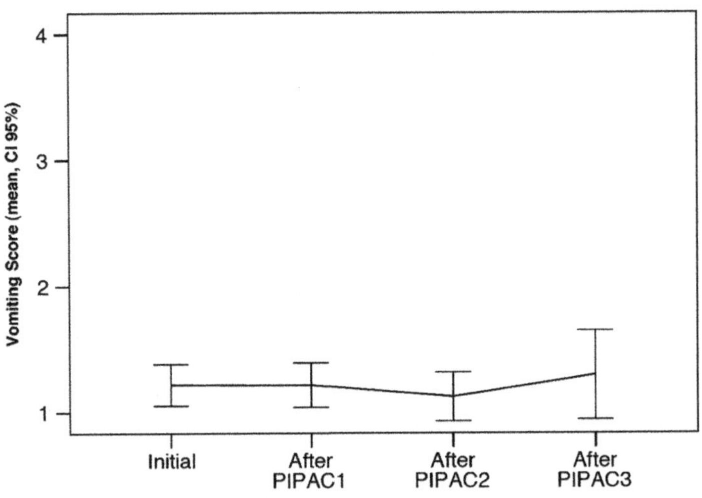

Fig. 16.2. Gastrointestinal smyptoms: vomiting. Symptoms remain stable during therapy. Best possible value = 1, worst possible value = 4.

The pain score increased slightly during PIPAC therapy, in particular in patients with colorectal peritoneal carcinomatosis treated with oxaliplatin 92 mg/m^2 body surface (Figure 16.3).

These preliminary data obtained in (self-) selected patients with advanced peritoneal carcinomatosis suggest that global quality of life is conserved under PIPAC therapy. In fact, all three global scores (quality of life, physical performance and global health status) slightly improve under therapy.

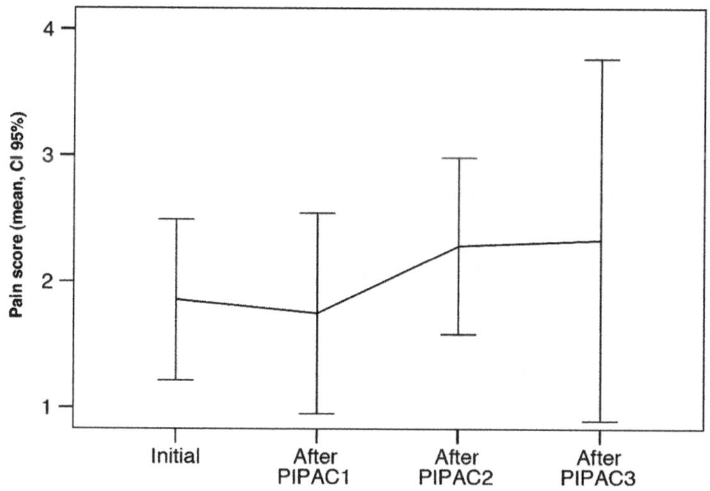

Fig. 16.3. QLQ-30 pain score. Pain diminishes during the first six weeks, then increases slightly over the initial value. Best possible value = 1, worst possible value = 4.

Disease-related gastrointestinal symptoms such as nausea and vomiting, constipation, diarrhea and anorexia can be stabilized for at least 4.5 months under repeated PIPAC application at six-week intervals. PIPAC barely induces therapy-related symptoms (in particular few gastrointestinal side effects), with the exception of moderate, transient increase of pain.

As expected, the global physical score of patients with advanced peritoneal carcinomatosis is reduced, and is comparable with the score reported in a large population of patients with advanced colorectal cancer [2]. To interpretate our data, it is important to notice that disease progression in advanced cancer induces a rapid and continuous deterioration of global health status and physical performance. For example, in patients with advanced colorectal cancer under symptomatic therapy, the mean QLQ-30 physical performance deteriorated by 8.6 points at eight weeks and by 12.5 points at 16 weeks. Similarly, the global health score deteriorated by 7.1 points at eight weeks and by 15.2 points at 16 weeks [2]. Progressive deterioration of quality of life with advanced colorectal cancer was confirmed in another, independent study [3].

Thus, the observed stabilization of quality of life, physical performance and global health status under PIPAC can be interpreted as an encouraging finding, even though the improvement does not reach statistical significance in this small cohort of patients.

Quality of life is difficult to measure and interpret, even when using validated instruments. In particular, defining a clinically meaningful change score in global quality of life measures is challenging. Moreover, limitations in some studies relate to a "response" bias – patients who feel better may be more inclined to respond. In recent years, interest has therefore shifted to focus on a patient's specific symptom burden and engaging the patient in reporting directly on his or her symptoms. Recently, an ASCO working group expressed the view that serial assessment of specific cancer-related symptoms, using validated instruments and shorter, more cancer-specific surveys, can define a clinically meaningful outcome for patients [1]. In the present group of patients, we observed no clinically significant deterioration of gastrointestinal symptoms, using comparisons between pre- and post-treatment. This appears favorable for two reasons: first, peritoneal carcinomatosis usually induces severe gastrointestinal symptoms with rapid degradation; second, it does not seem that PIPAC induces significant gastrointestinal symptoms, an important observation for a locoregional, intraperitoneal therapy with cytotoxic drugs.

However, these results are preliminary, retrospective and obtained in a relatively small cohort of patient. Therefore, they must be interpreted with caution and should be confirmed within the framework of larger prospective studies.

Bibliography

[1] Ellis LM, Bernstein DS, Voest EE et al. American society of clinical oncology perspective: raising the bar for clinical trials by defining clinically meaningful outcomes. J Clin Oncol. 32, 12 (Apr 20 2014) 1277–1280.

[2] Au HJ, Karapetis CS, O'Callaghan CJ et al. Health-related quality of life in patients with advanced colorectal cancer treated with cetuximab: overall and KRAS-specific results of the NCIC CTG and AGITG CO.17 Trial. J Clin Oncol. 27, 11 (Apr 10 2009) 1822–1828.

[3] Wong CK, Lam CL, Poon JT, Kwong DL. Clinical correlates of health preference and generic health-related quality of life in patients with colorectal neoplasms. PLoS One. 8, 3 (2013) e58341. doi: 10.1371/journal.pone.0058341. Epub 2013 Mar 13.

M. A. Reymond

17 PIPAC and HIPEC

An important and frequently asked question is a possible concurrence between HIPEC and PIPAC therapy concepts. This discussion is not only raised by medical issues, but also by the process of innovation.

John B. McKinlay has defined seven stages in the career of a medical innovation [1]:

1. Promise: first optimistic reports appear in the press.
2. Adoption: the procedure is used by more clinicians.
3. Acceptance: the procedure is widely accepted and endorsed.
4. The New Standard: the procedures becomes a standard of care. The first critical reports are published.
5. Evaluation: randomized controlled trials are performed.
6. Defense: opponents try to discredit negative study results.
7. Erosion: the innovation's career is terminated.

HIPEC has reached stage 4, perhaps 5, whereas PIPAC's development is lagging well behind, at stage 2. This explains why reactions from the regulatory, medical and scientific communities are so different for both procedure.

At the present stage of development, we do not see any concurrence between PIPAC and HIPEC, and this for two reasons:

1. PIPAC cannot be combined with cytoreductive surgery, and;
2. HIPEC is evidence-based in selected cases, PIPAC is not.

Thus, both procedures are complementary, at least at the present stage of development and under the condition that indication for HIPEC is decided according to evidence and current guidelines. For example, in colorectal cancer we do not indicate PIPAC therapy when the PCI is fewer than 20, in the absence of diffuse small bowel involvement.

Contraindications for combined cytoreductive surgery and HIPEC are numerous. In many patients where HIPEC is not indicated, PIPAC can be evaluated as an alternative. The criteria are detailed in Table 17.1.

Of course, the postoperative morbidity increases with the number of patients' comorbidities, independently of the surgical procedure. This is also true after PIPAC application. On the one hand, in individual patients with Karnofsky Index < 50%, we observed an impressive clinical improvement and some longer survival periods (up to two years). On the other hand, all cases of hospital mortality belonged to this group of patients. The risk of indicating PIPAC in patients who are already in the process of dying should not be underestimated, and this has to be seriously discussed with

Table 17.1. Contraindications for HIPEC and PIPAC. Many patients who have contraindications for HIPEC therapy can be treated with PIPAC.

Contraindication	HIPEC	PIPAC
Karnofsky Index	> 70%	> 50%
Nonresectable intraabdominal metastases	yes	no
Extraabdominal metastases	yes	yes
Diffuse small-bowel involvement	yes	no
Infiltration of the retroperitoneum or pancreas	yes	no
Infiltration of the mesentery root	yes	no
Infiltration of the hepatoduodenal ligament	yes	?
Short bowel syndrome	yes	yes
Small bowel obstruction (> 3 stenoses)	yes	yes
Cardiac contraindications	yes	no
Renal function impairment	yes	no
Hepatic function impairment	yes	no
Active infection	yes	yes

the patient and this family. Since we do not indicate PIPAC anymore in patients with Karnofsky < 50%, hospital mortality (after 362 consecutive procedures) is zero.

Without any doubt, evidence-based data for PIPAC are lagging behind those for HIPEC, a procedure where results of prospective randomized trials are already available. However, the HIPEC community is experiencing difficulties in setting up and recruiting patients for such trials. It is difficult to convince patients to enter the study and to stratify the patients, the procedure, the drugs and the methods of application. Moreover, determination of time to progression is extraordinarily difficult in small-volume peritoneal carcinomatosis. The situation is more advantageous for PIPAC, where objective tumor response assessment is possible after six weeks, where surgery and drug administration are fully standardized, and where operative trauma is minimal. Moreover, expected survival time is shorter after PIPAC than after HIPEC, since PIPAC has a palliative intent and is applied so far only in the salvage situation in advanced peritoneal carcinomatosis. Therefore, it is reasonable to expect that the degree of evidence for PIPAC will catch up relatively rapidly. Experience collected in the first prospective trials in ovarian and gastric cancers shows that patient recruitment for PIPAC is relatively easy: the first single-center study was closed 12 months after opening, after having recruited all 50 patients. The study protocol for the first randomized trial with PIPAC in ovarian cancer is already under redaction, and the trial is expected to start recruiting in 2015.

An important limitation of cytoreductive surgery and HIPEC is the aggressive character of the procedure, with the related morbidity and mortality. The benefit of therapy is limited to selected patients, and patients have to wait several months until preoperative quality of life is restored. This is of course an important point of criticism against this combined procedure. In our experience, many patients have difficulties going for a combined cytoreductive surgery and HIPEC, and are seeking a more gentle alternative. Of course, these patients should be motivated to accept CRS and HIPEC if the indication is given. However, should they refuse this therapy, PIPAC therapy could be offered to them.

17.1 PIPAC as a neoadjuvant therapy before HIPEC

So far, PIPAC has only been indicated in the salvage situation, when evidence-based therapy was exhausted. In particular, patients should have received at least two lines of palliative chemotherapy in ovarian cancer, and one line in gastric cancer. Moreover, indication for cytoreductive surgery and HIPEC was excluded in all patients.

In our retrospective registry, we noticed several patients who received secondary cytoreductive surgery and HIPEC, so that PIPAC was obviously useful as "neoadjuvant therapy" in individual cases (Table 17.2).

These individual observations have to be confirmed in prospective cohorts, and secondary complete cytoreduction might be chosen as a secondary endpoint in future studies.

So far, cytoreductive surgery combined with HIPEC has been reserved to selected patients with limited peritoneal carcinomatosis, with a curative intent after complete cytoreduction (CC0). Recently, it has been claimed that HIPEC might be indicated as postoperative adjuvant therapy in high-risk patients for developing metachronous peritoneal carcinomatosis [2, 3]. Although the rationale for adjuvant, prophylactic intraperitoneal chemotherapy in these patients is given, both the risks and benefits of such procedures should be carefully evaluated. The possibility of achieving the same therapeutic effects with a minimally-invasive procedure such as PIPAC is realistic and should also be considered.

Taken together, at the present point in time, we see complementarities between HIPEC and PIPAC approaches. Combined cytoreductive surgery and HIPEC is a curative therapeutic approach that can be offered to a limited number of selected patients.

Table 17.2. PIPAC as a neoadjuvant therapy before HIPEC.

Origin of peritoneal carcinomatosis	Number of patients
Gastric cancer	2
Appendiceal cancer	3
Colorectal cancer	2
Malignant mesothelioma	1
Pseudomyxoma peritonei	1
Carcinoma unknown origin (CUP)	1
Total	10 patients

PIPAC is a palliative procedure that can be offered to a large number of patients. Further indications (nedoadjuvant, adjuvant) of both procedures should be determined by adequate studies.

Bibliography

[1] Mc Kinley JB. From "promising report" to "standard procedure": seven stages in the career of a medicasl innovation. Milbank Mem Fund 59 (1981) 371–411.

[2] Baratti D, Kusamura S, Deraco M. Prevention and early treatment of peritoneal metastases from colorectal cancer: second-look laparotomy or prophylactic HIPEC? J Surg Oncol. 109, 3 (Mar 2014) 225–226.

[3] Saladino E, Fleres F, Mazzeo C, Pruiti V, Scollica M, Rossitto M, Cucinotta E, Macrì A. The role of prophylactic hyperthermic intraperitoneal chemotherapy in the management of serosal involved gastric cancer. Anticancer Res. 34, 4 (Apr 2014) 2019–2022.

N. Jonscher, M. Hummels, U. Giger-Pabst, E. Karljalainen, J. Zieren, N. Büchner, M. A. Reymond, and M. Beshay

18 Pressurized IntraThoracic Aerosol Chemotherapy (PITAC)

The feasibility of Pressurized Intraperitoneal Aerosol Chemotherapy (PIPAC) has been now demonstrated in the human patient. The first applications in ovarian, gastric and colorectal peritoneal carcinomatosis have delivered promising results, including superior pharmacological properties with high local concentration of doxorubicin in tumor nodes, objective pathological tumor response in about two thirds of patients in the salvage situation, median survival time over one year and good ascites control. Moreover, significant regressions have been observed in peritoneal mesothelioma (see Chapter 15).

Malignant pleural effusion is defined by the presence of malignant cells in the pleural fluid or pleural tissue. Many cancers can metastasize to the pleura at an advanced stage. The incidence of malignant pleural effusion is estimated at approximately 400,000 patients per year in Europe, about 56,000 of them in Germany. The most common cause of malignant pleural effusions are lung cancer (40%), breast cancer (25%), lymphoma (10%), ovarian cancer (5%) and gastrointestinal cancers (5%). Standard therapy is drainage of the pleural effusion and pleurodesis, in order to prevent a recurrence of the effusion. Further treatment options include pleurectomy, thoracentesis, temporary or permanent pleural catheter insertion, and thoracoscopic pleurodesis. There is so far no clear evidence for efficacy of cytoreductive surgery combined with intraoperative hyperthermic thoracic chemotherapy (HITOC) in this indication. Prognosis of patients with pleural carcinomatosis is dismal, with a mean survival of four months and a one-year survival rate of 18% (reviewed in [1]).

Mesothelioma is an insidious mesothelial neoplasm originating in the pleura, pericardium, peritoneum, or tunica vaginalis, with approximately 80% of cases involving the thorax. The predominant cause of malignant mesothelioma is exposure to asbestos. The incidence of mesothelioma in the United States is estimated to be approximately 2,000–3,000 cases per year, with an increasing incidence worldwide, secondary to the proliferation and poor regulation of industrial and household utilization of asbestos. A nihilistic attitude regarding mesothelioma has persisted among many physicians because of significant associated morbidity and mortality, as well as poor response to standard therapeutic interventions. Novel treatment paradigms, however, offer hope for enhanced palliation, improved tumor responses, and prolonged survival. These options include standard therapeutic interventions for malignant pleural mesothelioma (MPM) such as surgery, chemotherapy, and radiation therapy, as well as experimental approaches such as targeted therapy, immunotherapy, and gene-based therapies (reviewed in [2]).

Novel approaches to manage mesothelioma and malignant pleural effusions are desperately needed and the pleural space provides a unique platform as an easily accessible body cavity for developing and assessing these treatments and their responses. In this setting, novel intrapleural chemotherapeutic approaches such as immunotherapeutic and genetic treatments have been investigated, as well as those under current clinical development. While responses have been demonstrated to variable degrees with all these approaches, it is expected that only an integrated multimodality approach incorporating these methods with other antineoplastic interventions will ultimately ensure the best responses and patient outcomes (reviewed in [3]).

Against this background, there is a rationale for testing the applicability of pressurized aerosol chemotherapy within the pleural cavity, with the aim of improving delivery of various therapeutic agents into the pleural space. We now report the first in-human applications of therapeutic pressurized chemotherapy aerosol (PITAC) within the pleural cavity.

18.1 Patients

This is a retrospective analysis of preliminary data obtained within the framework of an off-label use program in the salvage therapy situation. No inclusion or exclusion criteria were defined a priori, and indications were selected on a case-by-case, individual basis in the interdisciplinary tumor board. Patients were extensively informed about the procedure and signed an informed consent. The Institutional Review Board was informed about the procedures and did not express any objections.

18.2 Technique

A double-lumen tube is inserted and the ipsilateral lung excluded. A two-trocar technique is used and remote-controlled aerosol nebulisation is performed in analogy to the PIPAC standard operating procedures. Cisplatinum 7.5 mg/m^2 and doxorubicin 1.5 mg/m^2 body surface are applied at a pressure of 12 mm Hg for 30 minutes at a temperature of 37 °C (Figure 18.1).

18.2.1 First in-human use

A 74-year-old female patient suffering peritoneal and pleural cacinomatosis of ovarian origin was admitted with symptomatic ascitis and bilateral pleural effusion. We first performed combined PIPAC application in the abdomen and PITAC in the right thorax. It was possible to apply the same intrathoracal CO_2 pressure as during PIPAC (12 mm Hg) without significant intraoperative problems. During the procedure, the pa-

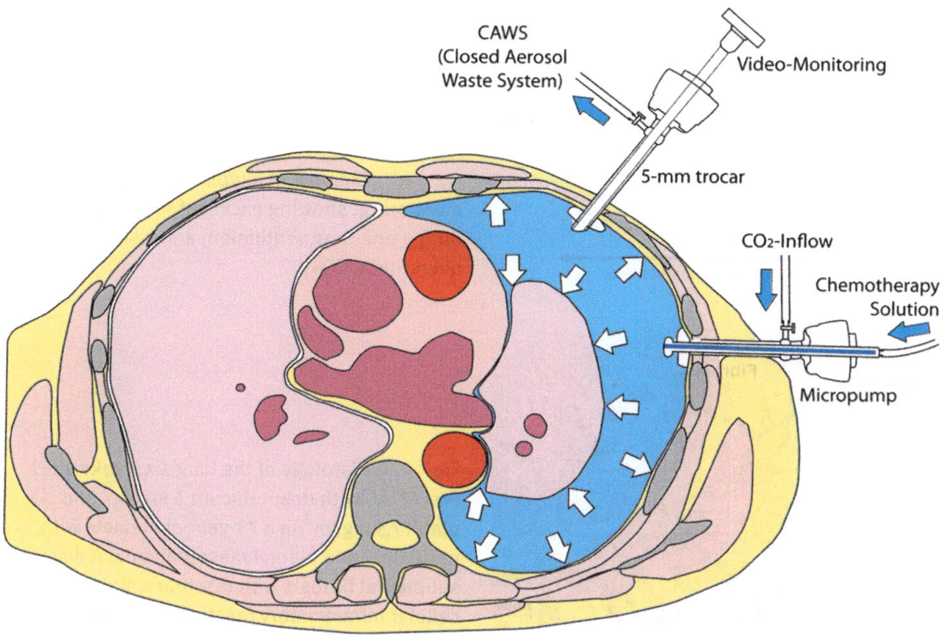

Fig. 18.1. Technique of Pressurized IntraThoracic Aerosol Chemotherapy (PITAC). A capnothorax of 12 mm Hg is established. A chemotherapy aerosol is generated at the tip of a mechanical micropump introduced through a balloon trocar, and maintained for 30 minutes at 37 °C. Then, the toxic aerosol is exsufflated over a secure system (CAWS: Closed Aerosol Waste System) into the outside environment.

tient needed low-dose catecholamines. FiO_2 was 50%, peak ventilation pressure was 18 mbar with a PEEP of 5 mm Hg. Some hypercarbia developed with an end-tidal CO_2 of 37 mm Hg at the end of the procedure. After four weeks, PITAC was performed on the left side. After two months follow up, no significant pleural effusion was detected anymore.

18.3 Results

Between April 2012 and April 2014, we applied 10 PITAC in six patients for malignant pleural effusion of gastric origin ($n = 4$), ovarian origin ($n = 1$) or malignant mesothelioma. In four instances, PIPAC was combined with one-sided PITAC. The patient with malignant peritoneal and pleural mesothelioma had three PITAC, one on the left side, two in the right side, as well as four PIPAC, combined in four procedures in six-week intervals over six months.

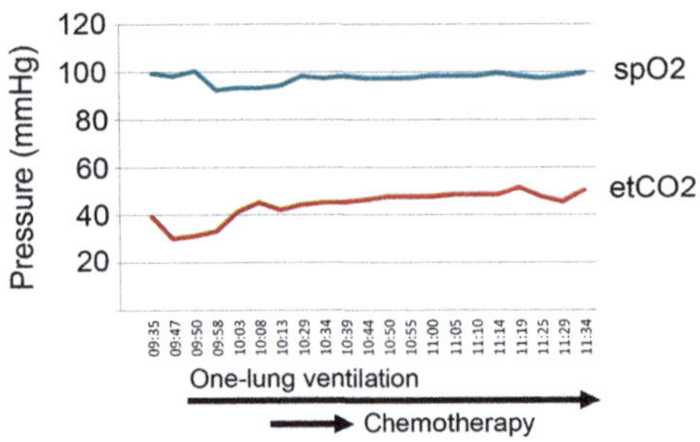

Fig. 18.2. Example of a typical intraoperative monitoring, showing excellent oxygenation during one-lung ventilation, and a slow increase of end-tidal CO_2.

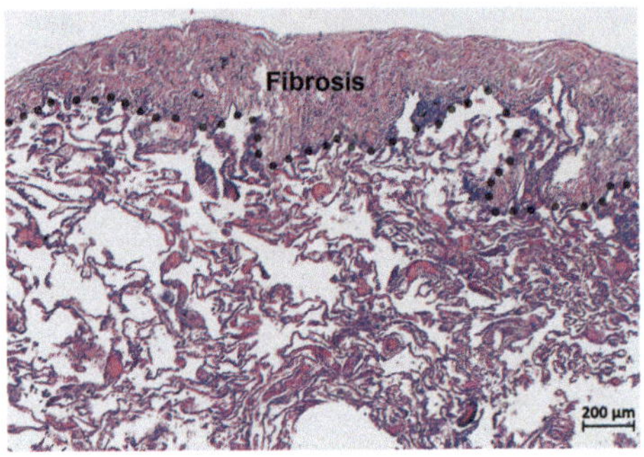

Fig. 18.3. Histology of the lung six weeks after first PITAC with doxorubicin 1.5 mg/m^3 and cisplatin 7.5 mg/m^2 in a 73-year-old female with peritoneal and pleural mesothelioma. A discrete subpleural fibrosis with discrete lymphoplasmocellular inflammatory reaction is observed.

The operating time for PITAC alone was 100 ± 25 min, and the operating time for combined PITAC and PIPAC procedures was 189 ± 29 min. No intraoperative complications were noted, and the procedure was well tolerated in all patients (Figure 18.2).

Hospital mortality was zero. No postoperative complications CTCAE > 2 were noted. Control of the pleural effusion was achieved in all cases.

The numbers are too small to make any statement on tumor response. Moreover, only a single patient had a repeated PITAC in the same side: Out of multiple pleural biopsies, one showed major pathological response of the mesothelioma, the other biopsies were tumor-free. In the histology, only a superficial subpleural fibrosis was observed (Figure 18.3).

PITAC is feasible in the human patient. No cardiovascular collapse nor any signs of tension pneumothorax were observed. PITAC can induce regression of pleural effusion. Further studies with pleural effusion of ovarian origin and pleura mesothelioma are needed.

Bibliography

[1] Ried M, Hofmann HS. The treatment of pleural carcinosis with malignant pleural effusion. Dtsch Arztebl Int 110, 18 (2013) 313–318.

[2] Haas AR, Sterman DH. Malignant pleural mesothelioma: update on treatment options with a focus on novel therapies. Clin Chest Med. 34, 1 (Mar 2013) 99–111.

[3] Haas AR, Sterman DH. Intracavitary therapeutics for pleural malignancies. Clin Chest Med. 34, 3 (Sep 2013) 501–513.

N. Khalili-Harbi, A. Herbette, W. Solass, U. Giger-Pabst, E. Engin, A. Giese, M. Dutreix, and M. A. Reymond

19 Future applications of therapeutic capnoperitoneum

Technically, a pressurized therapeutic aerosol can be applied not only within body cavities such as the peritoneal or the pleural space, but also within hollow organs such as the esophagus, the stomach, the intestine, the bladder or the bronchial system.

From the theoretical point of view, the application of a therapeutic substance as an aerosol under pressure should achieve similar results. To prove this hypothesis we performed the first feasibility experiments in the large animal model.

19.1 Study design

This is an experimental, in-vivo study in the large animal model, investigating the feasibility of a therapeutic capnoperitoneum in the urinary bladder and in the esophagus.

19.2 Regulatory background and animals

This study was authorized by the Animal Committee of the State of Thüringen, Germany. Under the supervision of a veterinarian we operated on three female German pigs (approximately 70 kg) under anesthesia, following regular protocols.

19.2.1 Staining

For each animal 1.29 mg of Cy5-labelled Dbait (1 : 1 dilution with nonfluorescent Dbait) were diluted in 10 ml of NaCol 0.9%. The solution was stained with a single droplet of methylene blue.

19.2.2 Macroscopy

Macroscopic analysis was performed immediately after autopsy, at the end of the procedure. Organs (esophagus with proximal stomach; urinary bladder) were surgically removed, opened and pictures taken. Mucosa was screened for possible injuries, lesions or rupture, as was the muscular wall.

19.2.3 Microscopic analysis

For analysis, formalin-fixed specimens were stained with H&E according to usual protocols. For microscopic fluorescence analysis, sampled were fixed with PFA 4% for 20 minutes at room temperature (RT), followed by exposure to Triton 0.5% for 10 minutes at RT. Then, samples were washed out in SVF diluted in PBS solution for one hour at RT. After washing, samples were incubated with secondary anti-mouse FITC (Sigma-Aldrich Chimie Sarl., Lyon, France) diluted 1/100 for 45 minutes at RT. Nuclei were counterstained with Dapi 0.5 lg/ml for five minutes at room temperature. Analysis was performed with an inverted microscope.

19.3 Pressurized IntraVesical Aerosol Chemotherapy (PIVAC)

High risk nonmuscle invasive bladder cancer (NMIBC) includes both papillary disease and carcinoma in situ (CIS). Patients with fully resected papillary NMIBC have no evidence of disease, but might develop intravesical tumor recurrence later. In contrast, patients with carcinoma in situ (CIS) have active disease and therapy should induce complete tumor response for the longest period of time. Many patients with high risk papillary disease have concomitant carcinoma in situ that may not be recognized [1]. Transurethral resection of the bladder tumor (TURBT) is the standard initial treatment for NMIBC. For optimal visualisation of tumors, fluorescence techniques should be used with low threshold, especially in the case of suspicion of carcinoma in situ (CIS). Increased completeness of the resection will lead to less persisting disease and less need for adjuvant treatment. A re-TURBT should be done when in doubt of radical resection (judged by the pathologist or the surgeon). However, even after a radical resection, recurrence (30–80%) and progression (1–45%) are commonly seen. Intravesical chemotherapy provides direct contact of the agent with the bladder mucosa and clearly has improved the outcome, especially in high-risk disease. A single postoperative instillation (SPI) with chemotherapy is only indicated in low-risk disease. BCG (Bacille Calmette-Guérin) is the treatment of choice for high-grade disease. BCG should be given as maintenance. An awareness of deterioration of the prognosis after progression is of great importance. In BCG failures, cystectomy is strongly advised. Chemotherapy in combination with hyperthermia seems to be a new promising treatment (reviewed in [2]).

Against this background, in analogy to peritoneal and pleural surface malignancies, the outstanding pharmacological properties of pressurized aerorosol chemotherapy might be of great help. In order to further investigate this question, we designed and built a prototype allowing creation of a therapeutic pressurized aerosol within the urinary bladder and performed the first feasibility study in the large animal model (Figure 19.1).

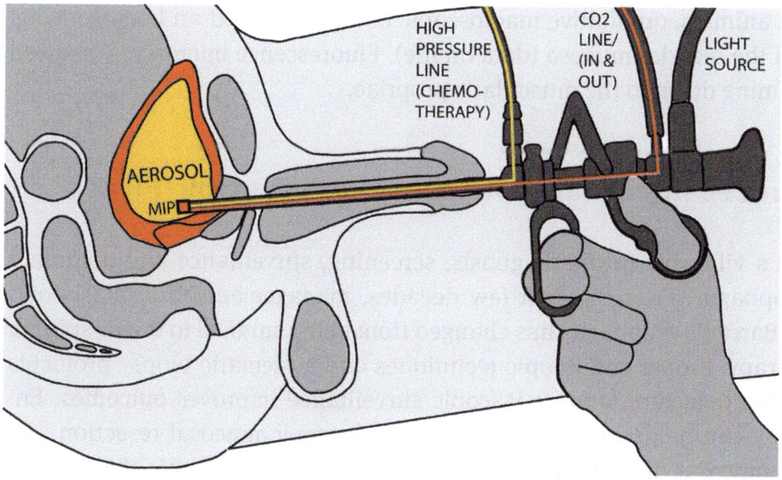

Fig. 19.1. Principle of Pressurized IntraVesical Aerosol Chemotherapy (PIVAC). First, a specifically designed cytoscope is introduced into the bladder. Second, a pressurized CO_2 environment is created, creating a maximal exposure of the mucosal surface. Third, a therapeutic aerosol is produced at the tip of the instrument.

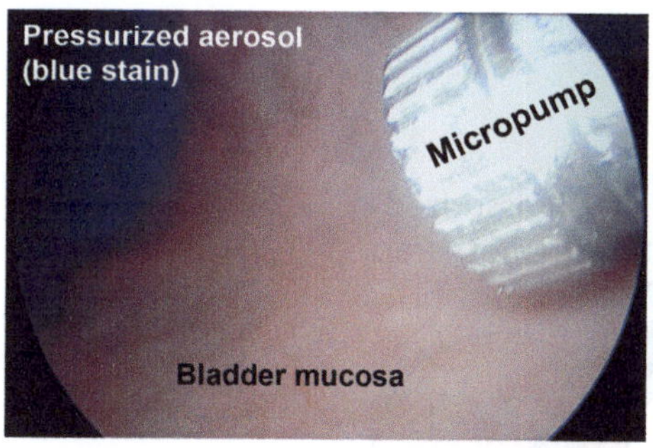

Fig. 19.2. Intraoperative picture of PIVAC in the large animal model (pig), during aerosolization of a diluted methylene blue solution into the urinary bladder. The pattern observed is similar to intraoperative views during intraperitoneal administration.

After obliterating the urethra with a balloon, a working space was created within the urinary bladder with CO_2 at a pressure of of 12 mm Hg. Then, the micropump (MIP®, Reger Medizintechnik, Rottweil, Germany) was introduced into the baldder. In order to allow video monitoring of the procedure, a balloon trocar (Applied Medical, Düsseldorf, Germany) was introduced into the bladder through the abdominal wall, under laparoscopic control. Intravesical application of the pressurized therapeutic aerosol was possible without technical difficulties. An homogeneous blue staining was observed macroscopically (Figure 19.2).

The pressurized aerosol was maintained for 30 minutes. After exsufflation, the animals were euthanized, a laparotomy performed and the bladder removed for further analysis.

In all three animals, qualitative macroscopic analysis showed an homogeneous blue staining of the bladder mucosa (data on file). Fluorescence microscopy showed Cy5 nuclear staining down to the muscularis propriae.

19.4 Pressurized IntraLuminal Aerosol Chemotherapy (PILAC)

Endoscopy has a vital role in the diagnosis, screening, surveillance and treatment of Barrett's esophagus. Over the past few decades, management of dysplasia and early cancer in Barrett's esophagus has changed from being surgical to organ-sparing endoscopic therapy. Proper endoscopic techniques and systematic biopsy protocols improve dysplasia detection, and endoscopic surveillance improves outcomes. Endoscopic therapy can be tissue acquiring (as in endoscopic mucosal resection and endoscopic submucosal dissection) or ablative (as with photodynamic therapy, radiofrequency ablation and cryotherapy). Treatment is usually multimodal, combining endoscopic resection of visible lesions with one or more mucosal ablation techniques, followed by long-term surveillance. Such treatment is safe and effective. Development

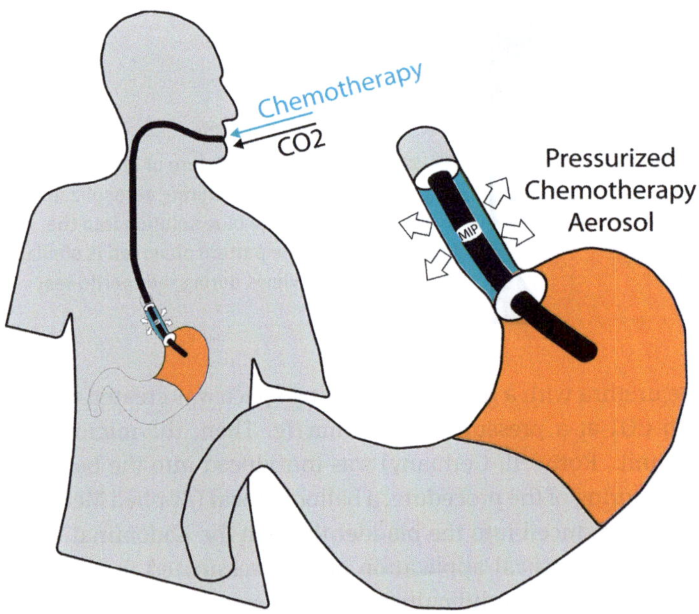

Fig. 19.3. Pressurized IntraLuminal Aerosol Chemotherapy (PILAC). A double balloon catheter is introduced into the stomach, the distal balloon inflated and the device retracted until the esogastric junction is blocked. Then, the proximal balloon is inflated, and a pressurized CO_2 environment is created in the distal esophagus, between both balloons. Finally, the therapeutic aerosol is created over a mircopump (analogous to PIPAC) and maintained for a given period of time.

of safer wide-field resection techniques, which would effectively remove all Barrett's esophagus and obviate the need for long-term surveillance, is needed (reviewed in [3]).

Against this framework, in analogy to other application fields, pressurized aerosol therapy might be an interesting option that should be the object of further research. To investigate the feasibility of application of a therapeutic pressurized aerosol in the distal esophagus, we designed and built a prototype for experiments in the large animal model. The prototype consists of three elements: (a) a flexible tube, equipped with two inflatable balloons (one proximal, one distal), similar to a Sengstaken–Blakemore tube; (b) a CO_2 line to create the capnoperitoneum (connected to a standard insufflator for laparoscopic surgery), and; (c) the MIP® (Reger Medizintechnik, Rottweil, Germany) to generate the therapeutic aerosol. For monitoring purpose, a gastroscopy was first performed, and a 10–12 mm Hg laparoscopy balloon trocar (Applied Medical, Düsseldorf, Germany) inserted into the stomach and tightly fixed. The prototype was then placed under laparo-endoscopic control (Figures 19.4 and 19.5).

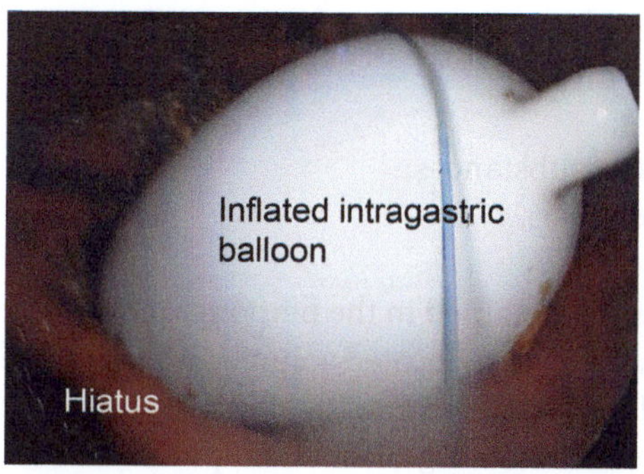

Fig. 19.4. Intraoperative intracavitary view of the stomach (over an intragastric trocar placed by laparoscopy) showing the distal balloon inflated at the esogastric junction, tightening the distal esophagus.

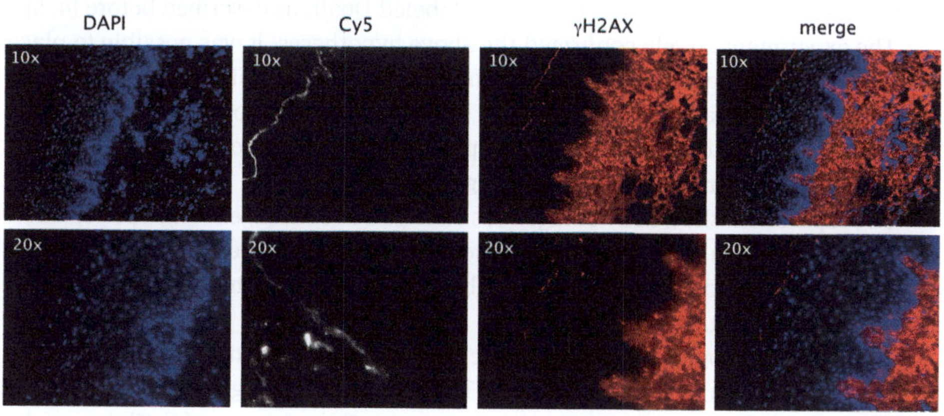

Fig. 19.5. Diffusion of therapeutic substance into the esophageal wall. Cryosection of pig esophagus, red: Dbait-Cy5 staining, blue: Dapi (nucleus). After nebulization of Dbait, staining reveals homogeneous mucosal and submucosal fluorescence down to the muscularis mucosae.

Microscopic analysis showed homogenous distribution of Dbait within the esophagus mucosa. The proximal esophagus showed a Dbait presence up to 400–600 µm depth (Figure 19.5). Similar findings were documented in the distal segment of the esophagus (data not shown).

19.5 Discussion

This experiment was designed to investigate the feasibility of application of a pressurized aerosol therapy within the distal esophagus in a large animal model, simulating the anatomical conditions to be expected in the human patient. An important prerequisite was to be able to use the same physical conditions as planned in clinical practice, in particular the same pressure of the capnoperitoneum, the same dilution volume of the staining substance, the same surgical devices, and so on. Moreover, the target organs had about the same structure and dimension, in particular concerning the anatomy of the esophagus and of the bladder wall.

Specifically, we were interested in determining:

1. the technical feasibility of the procedure;
2. the homogeneity of distribution of the test substances;
3. the depth of penetration of the test substances.

The hypotheses were that, by analogy to results obtained in the peritoneal cavity [4], the stain would distribute homogeneously within the allocated volume and penetrate the esophageal wall beyond the mucosal layer. In order to allow both macroscopic and microscopic assessment, we used a double staining of the therapeutic aerosol with methylene blue and with fluorescence-labeled Dbait, as described before [4, 5].

The experiment largely confirmed the above hypotheses. It was possible to place the device correctly and to nebulize the therapeutic agent within the distal esophagus. Moreover, the balloons did not harm the esophageal mucosa, and the artificial hydrostatic pressure of 12 mm Hg of the capnoperitoneum did not cause any mucosal lesion nor muscular rupture of the esophageal wall.

The experiment showed a homogenous distribution of the agent and a penetration into the tissue down to 600 µm, which means that the cells were staining down to the muscularis propria. Thus, it was possible to distribute the therapeutic substance within the expected target volume.

Beside morphological findings, a bioactivity of Dbait within the parietal cells (mucosa and submucosa) was demonstrated. The phosphorylated gamma-H2AX reveals nuclear activation of DNA-PK, and thus a genotoxic effect of therapy [6]. These results are encouraging since they show an activation of the DNA repair system, which in theory could induce beneficial therapeutic effects.

Another potential advantage of this innovative approach is that PILAC or PIVAC application can be repeated, for example during follow up endoscopies in patients with high-risk dysplasia or carcinoma in situ.

In the next experimental step, we now intend to treat human tissue ex vivo with PILAC. For this purpose, we will apply a therapeutic Dbait aerosol into a surgical specimen of the distal esophagus immediately after resection in patients with Barret adenocarcinoma.

Bibliography

[1] http://www.fda.gov/downloads/Drugs/NewsEvents/UCM348395.pdf, consulted on 30.4.2014.

[2] van Lingen AV, Witjes JA. Current intravesical therapy for non-muscle invasive bladder cancer. Expert Opin Biol Ther. 13, 10 (Oct 2013) 1371–1385.

[3] Repaka A, Chak A. Endoscopic management of Barrett esophagus. Nat Rev Gastroenterol Hepatol. 8, 10 (Sep 6 2011) 582–591.

[4] Solass W, Hetzel A, Nadiradze G, Sagynaliev E, Reymond MA. Description of a novel approach for intraperitoneal drug delivery and the related device. Surg Endosc. 26, 7 (Jul 2012) 1849–1855.

[5] Solass W, Herbette A, Schwarz T, Hetzel A, Sun JS, Dutreix M, Reymond MA. Therapeutic approach of human peritoneal carcinomatosis with Dbait in combination with capnoperitoneum: proof of concept. Surg Endosc. 26, 3 (Mar 2012) 847–852.

[6] Quanz M, Chassoux D, Berthault N, Agrario C, Sun JS, Dutreix M. Hyperactivation of DNA-PK by double-strand break mimicking molecules disorganizes DNA damage response. PLoS One. 4, 7 (Jul 21 2009) e6298.

W. Solass, U. Giger-Pabst, J. Zieren, and M. A. Reymond

20 Occupational health and safety aspects

Local drug administration has been used as a therapeutic modality for many years and for a broad spectrum of indications. In particular, intraperitoneal chemotherapy is increasingly used in clinical practice. The goal of intraperitoneal chemotherapy is to increase drug exposure of cancer cells within the peritoneal cavity while minimizing systemic toxicity [1].

Treating peritoneal diseases with aerosolized drugs has a number of advantages. First, aerosolized chemotherapy provides a direct, minimally invasive means for targeted delivery to different regions of the peritoneum. Second, this route of administration delivers a high dose to the target site. Third, aerosolized intraperitoneal chemotherapy causes fewer adverse effects than intravenous administration. Thus, PIPAC opens new avenues in the therapy of peritoneal carcinomatosis, an unmet medical need [2].

However, delivering chemotherapy as an aerosol might cause an increased risk of exposure to health care workers as compared with other administration routes. This is due to the difficulty of controlling the spread of aerosols during PIPAC which in turn contributes to the risk of leakage and unwanted exposition. To prevent any harm to health care workers, we have identified and evaluated potential hazards concerning occupational exposures during PIPAC performance. In a second set of experiments, we have simulated PIPAC in the laboratory and in the operating room. In addition, we have applied PIPAC in the human patient using chemotherapeutic drugs and measured contamination levels under real clinical conditions.

20.1 Methods

20.1.1 Ethical, legal and regulatory background

The study protocol was submitted to the Institutional Review Board (IRB, Common Ethics Committee of the Westfalian Wilhelms-University Münster and of the Westfalian Medical Chamber). The IRB recommended performing the first PIPAC therapy with volunteers, which were extensively informed and trained in the PIPAC procedure.

20.1.2 Methodology

The following steps were defined: identification of hazardous substances and dose; identification of possible exposure ways; simulation of the PIPAC procedure with non-toxic aerosols and smoke; redaction of a Standard Operating Procedures (SOP); second simulation according to the SOP; informing and training of the health care workers; performance of the first two PIPAC procedures with chemotherapeutic substances, and; workplace measurements under real conditions.

20.1.3 Nebulizer

The micropump (MIP®, Reger Medizintechnik, Rottweil, Germany) has been described elsewhere (5). In brief, it consists of several components, including an injector, a tube and a nozzle. The nozzle has a diameter of 0.2 mm. A pressure of up to 20 bar is delivered upstream of the nozzle, using an industry-standard contrast medium injector (Injektron 82M, MedTron, Saarbrücken, Germany, including a remote control device MT1130/1).

20.1.4 Operating room characteristics

The PIPAC procedure was performed within an operating room (OR) equipped with laminar air flow. The volume of the OR was approximately 168 m^3. Air flow was 1.8 × 106 L/h. Room temperature was 22.3–22.6 °C. Relative humidity was 36–37%. Atmospheric pressure was 994 hPa. Vacuum was generated with a pressure of −0.85 bar (Dräger, Lübeck, Germany) (Table 20.1).

Table 20.1. Assumptions for determination of exposure.

Parameter	***Value***
Room temperature	22 °C
Inhalation rate	1.5 m^3/hour
Body weight	70 kg
Body surface	1.7 m^2
Duration of therapy	30 to 60 min./application; one therapy/day
Total amount of applied CO_2	3 to max. 6 liter
Duration of exposure (presence of OR-Team)	No routine presence; if intervention required, max. 20 minutes/procedure
Technical details of application	
Pressurizing in injector:	< 20 bar
Pressure at the nozzle:	0.16 bar
Duration of nebulizing:	ca. 5 min
Total applied volume:	150 ml per chemotherapeutic cycle
Diameter of nozzle:	0.2 mm

20.1.5 Chemotherapy

We have focused on the application of two chemotherapeutic agents: cisplatin and doxorubicin. Chemotherapy was applied as follows: nebulization over 3–6 minutes of 7.5 mg cisplatin/m^2 body surface followed immediately by the aerosolization of 1.5 mg doxorubicin/m^2 body surface into the abdominal cavity filled with CO_2 at a pressure of 16 to 20 mbar (12 to 15 mm Hg) at a temperature of 37 °C followed by 30 minutes steady-state before exsufflation.

20.1.6 Experimental protocol

Two PIPAC procedures were performed in two consecutive patients within the same operating room. Between the procedures, the room was cleaned according to the hospital's standard hygiene and surface cleaning protocols.

Each procedure was structured into four consecutive phases.

- Phase 1: CO_2 Insufflation over an industry-standard trocar (Kii Access System, Applied Medical, Darmstadt, Germany), with a target pressure of 16 mbar (12 mm Hg). The access system was secured with an intraabdominal balloon and an extraabdominal obturator, ensuring tightness of the abdomen and steadiness of the pressure. Two 5 mm working trocars were inserted.
- Phase 2: Introduction of a micropump (MIP®, Reger Medizintechnik, Rottweil, Germany) through the access trocar and aerosol formation of the chemotherapy solution into the abdominal cavity using the high-pressure injector.
- Phase 3: The system was kept in steady-state for 30 minutes at a constant pressure and temperature. The abdomen is hermetically sealed and the total gas flow is minimal (< 0.1 to 0.2 L7min due to body resorption of CO_2).
- Phase 4: At the end of the procedure, the gas from the abdomen was released directly into the hospital's waste air system over one of the trocars a closed line and an aerosol/smoke filter (pores 0.027 µm, model 03110-10, mtp, Neuhausenob Eck, Germany).

Toxicology analysis

The probe sampling system used was a Gravikon VC25 device combined with a dust detector (Ströhlein, Kaarst, Germany). Air was collected on a cellulose nitrate filter with a diameter of 50 mm, with a flow of 22.5 m^3/h. Toxicological research analysis of cisplatin levels was performed according to a standard protocol (NIOSH 7300). The detection limit was 0.3 µg/sample. Sampling and analysis were performed by engineers of the Division for Hazardous Substances at the Laboratory for Environmental and Product Analysis of DEKRA Industrial GmbH in Stuttgart (Germany), an independent certification organization.

20.2 Results

20.2.1 Identification of hazardous substances and dose

In short, cisplatin is highly poisonous. It can provoke anaphylactic reactions, irritates eyes and skin, and has no transdermal absorption. Furthermore, it irritates airways, and has a cumulative toxic effect on kidney, bone marrow and the inner ear. It is probably carcinogenic to humans (Table 20.2).

Doxorubicin is hazardous to human health by provoking mucosal inflammation, leucopenia as well as dilative cardiomyopathy. Additionally, it induces DNA mutation and is carcinogenic to humans (Table 20.3). The total dose applied during PIPAC (see

Table 20.2. Toxicological characteristics of cisplatin.

Parameter	*Value*
CAS-/EG Number	15663–27-1/239–733-8
Formula	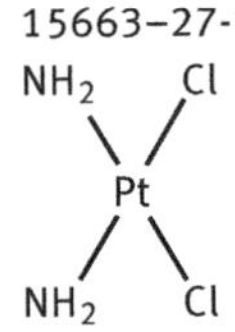
Molecular weight	300.06 g/mol
Melting point	270 °C; dark yellow powder at room temperature
Boiling point	Not applicable
Steam pressure	Not applicable
Water solubility	2.530 g/L [25 °C]
LD50 oral	20 mg/kg (rat) 32 mg/kg (mouse)
NOAEL[1]	No data
Important toxicological details	– Acute toxicity: very toxic – Skin and eye irritation – No evidence for transdermal absorption – Cumulative damage of kidney, bone marrow and inner ear – No evidence for carcinogenity in human – Evidence for carcinogenity and teratogenity in mouse and rat – Level of carcinogenity: 2A – Anaphylactic reactions reported – Sensibilisation of skin and airways
Total amount of applied cisplatin	15 mg in 150 ml NaCl 0.9%
Concentration of applied solution	0.1 mg/ml = 0.1 g/L = 0.01%
Total applied amount of cisplatin	150 ml
Workplace exposure limits	Germany: not available Netherlands: 0.00005 mg/m^3

above) is approximately 10% of a usual systemic chemotherapy dose. There is no legal exposure limit for either of these two substances in Germany. However, in the Netherlands, the maximally allowed air concentration for cisplatin is < 0.00005 mg/m^3.

Table 20.3. Toxicological characteristics of doxorubicin.

Parameter	***Value***
CAS-/EG Number	23214-92-8/245-495-6 25316-40-9/246-818-3 (Hydrochloride)
Formula	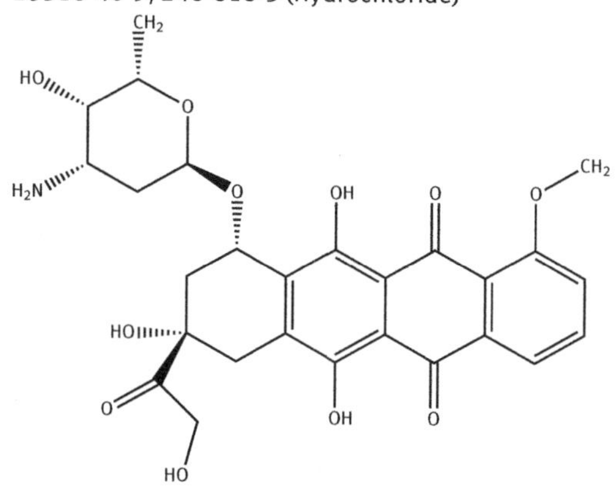
Molecular weight	543.52 g/mol
Melting point	205 °C (Degradation); crystalline red powder at room temperature
Boiling point	Not applicable
Steam pressure	Not applicable
Water solubility	0.0928 g/L [25 °C]
LD50 oral	570 mg/kg (mouse)
NOAEL1	No data
Important toxicological details	– Acute toxicity: harmful – Dilatative cardiomyopathy – Inflammation of mucosa – Leucopenia – Evidence for carcinogenicity in animals – Evidence for mutagenicity in animals – Level of carcinogenicity 2A
Total amount of applied doxorubicin	3 mg in 50 ml NaCL 0.9% solution
Concentration of applied solution	0.06 mg/ml = 0.06 g/L = 0.006%
Total applied amount of doxorubicin	50 ml
Legal upper limit for working place	Germany: no upper legal limit

20.2.2 Identification of possible exposure ways

The preparation of the chemotherapeutic agents in the hospital pharmacy and their transport in adequate containers to the operating room is scheduled according to the German recommendations (12). Both agents are provided in a closed delivery system (special injection syringes filled with NaCl 0.9% solution). Identified exposure ways are ocular, dermal and inhalative exposition. Other possibilities were reasonably excluded.

20.2.3 First PIPAC simulation with NaCl 0.9% solution

Before performing the first clinical PIPAC application, the procedure was simulated in the operating room using a laparoscopy training phantom and NaCl 0.9% aerosol.

Working steps were written down and risk analysis performed within an interdisciplinary team including physicians (surgeons and anesthesiologists), scrub nurses, hospital technicians, nebulizer engineers and occupational health experts. Possible mechanical failures related to the injector, the infusion tube, the nebulizer itself, the laminar flow system and the tightness of the abdomen were identified. In case of any failure of the procedure, appropriate security measures were taken and defined. On this basis, a standard operating protocol was established that served as a basis for the second simulation.

20.2.4 Second PIPAC simulation with smoke and an artificial leak

The second simulation was performed in the operating room under strict implementation of the standard operating procedures simulating the abdomen with a sealed plastic container of similar dimensions. An aerosol of CO_2 and smoke with the same pressure as during laparoscopy (using identical, industry-standard technical instruments [access trocars, video camera, grasping forceps]) was applied. We were able to perform the complete procedure without any incident; in particular, the system remained tight. Then, a maximal leakage (an access trocar was fully opened) was simulated. The smoke escaping from the leak was flowing downward to the floor and into the lateral outflow windows of the hospital air waste system (Figure 20.1).

20.2.5 Information and training of the team of volunteers

On the basis of the successful simulations, it was decided to schedule two patients for the first PIPAC procedures. Information meetings allowing open, interactive discussion were organized since the planned procedures had raised emotional concerns, in particular among scrubbing nurses and cleaning workers. On the basis of these dis-

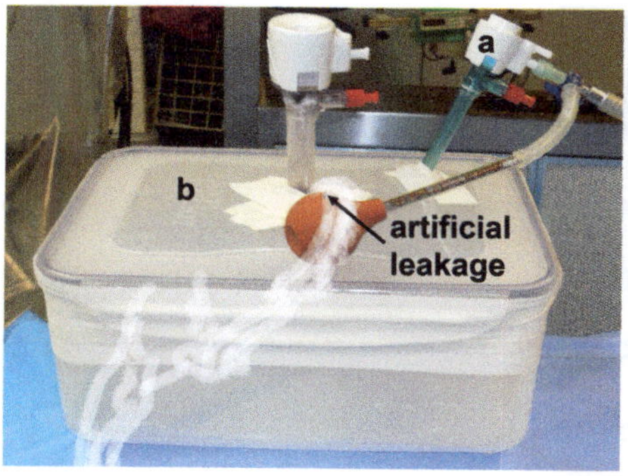

Fig. 20.1. PIPAC simulation with smoke and artificial leakage: sealing access trocars (a) were introduced into a sealed plastic box (b) with the same volume dimensions as the human abdominal cavity. The box was pressurized with CO_2 and steam. Via an artificial leakage (open access trocar), the steam (white bold) was observed to be directed to the floor and not randomly distributed within the operating room. This is caused by the laminar air flowing downwards from the ceiling to the floor.

cussions, we decided to restrict the first procedure to volunteers within the framework of a special shift under exclusion of other simultaneous surgical procedures. Before the first procedure, the team of volunteers received interdisciplinary training according to the standard operating procedures.

20.2.6 Performance of the first PIPAC procedures with chemotherapy

The first PIPAC procedure worldwide was performed on 5 November 2011 under the supervision of a safety officer and included workplace air measurements. The standard operating protocols were strictly implemented; in particular, nobody remained within the operating room during the PIPAC procedure, which was remote-controlled. The nebulizer functioned as expected and the system remained airtight. At the end of the procedure, the chemotherapy aerosol was exhausted into the air waste system of the hospital and released into the environment (Figure 20.2).

Air contamination of the operating room with platinum was measured. Air was sampled during two consecutive PIPAC procedures (Figure 20.3).

The results are summarized in Table 20.4. Air analysis showed no traces of cisplatin, neither at the position of the surgeon nor at the position of the anesthesiologist.

20.3 Conclusions

Chemotherapy is an essential component of modern, multimodal cancer therapy. However, many drugs used to fight cancer are mutagenic, teratogenic and carcinogenic in experimental systems.

Of course, development of PIPAC has raised concerns about the risk of occupational inhalation linked to the application of toxic aerosols. To assess this problem, it was not possible to rely on existing safety standards, since PIPAC had not been performed before. However, we could compare – to some extent – intraperitoneal

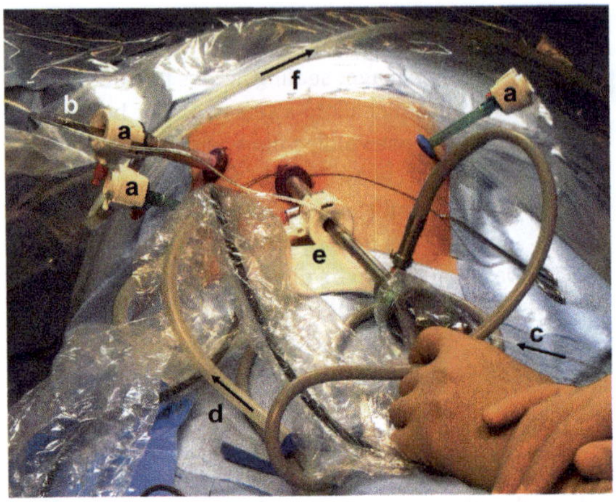

Fig. 20.2. First PIPAC under real conditions. Access trocars (a) with the nebulizer (b) in situ. The chemotherapeutic agents were transported from the injector to the nebulizer via a high-pressure infusion line (c). CO_2 was injected into the abdominal cavity via a standard gas line (d) and the trocar (e); (camera trocar). At the end of the procedure, the chemotherapeutic capnoperitoneum was desufflated via line (f) over an aerosol filter into the air waste system of the hospital. Dark arrows indicate the flow direction of the gas and chemotherapeutics, respectively.

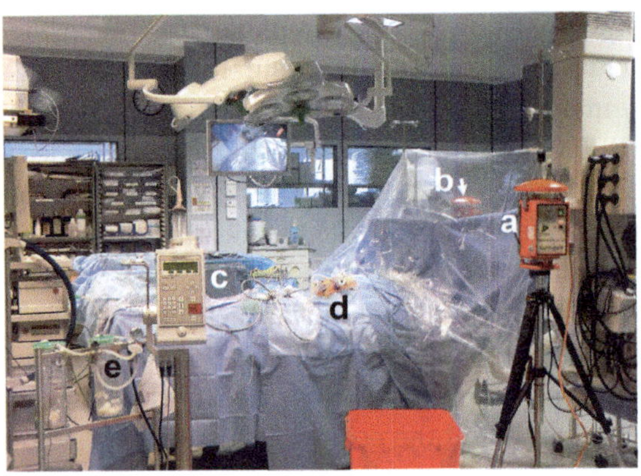

Fig. 20.3. Operating room (OR) set up for first PIPAC and safety measurement. The OR is equipped with laminar airflow. The abdomen is tight. The procedure is remote-controlled. Environmental air sampling was undertaken at the surgeon's (a) and anesthesiologist's (b) working positions. The pressure injector (c), sealing trocars and nebulizer in situ (d) and also the exsufflation line (e) are shown. To minimize any possible chemotherapeutic exposure of the anesthesiology crew, a vertical transparent curtain dividing the laminar air flow was hanged between the patient's head and the site of chemotherapy application.

aerosol chemotherapy to aerosolized chemotherapy in lung cancer. In this latter setting, aerosolized chemotherapy has been delivered in a well-ventilated room with an air filtering system [3]. Alternatively, a mobile filter air cleaning system combined with

Table 20.4. Measurement of platinum concentration in the operating room. Notes: To allow a precise analysis of the limit of determination (LoD), probe sampling was performed during two operations but only when chemotherapeutic drugs were applied. In the meantime, sampling was paused. Measurement locations: 1 Anesthesiologist's position – patient head; 2 Surgeon's position – patient abdomen.

Measurement points	*1*	*2*
Probe N°	0511-01	0511-02
Date	05.11.2011	05.11.2011
Start [hh:mm]	12:15	12:15
End [hh:mm]	16:38	16:38
Duration [h]	2.4	2.4
Air pressure [hPa]	994	994
Temperature [°C]	22.5	22.5
Volume stream $[m^3/h]$	22.5	22.5
Partial gas volume $[m^3]$	54.2	54.0
Platinum in inhalable dust [mg/Pr.]	0.3	0.3
Limit of Determination (LoD) [mg/Pr.]	0.3	0.3
Relative LoD $[mg/m^3]$	0.000006	0.000006
Analysis [mg/Pr.]	< 0.3	< 0.3
Concentration $[mg/m^3]$	< 0.000006	< 0.000006
Platinum calculated as cisplatin Concentration $[mg/m^3]$	< 0.000009	< 0.000009

a collecting tent was also effective in preventing propagation of aerosol during inhalation of nebulized liposomal cisplatin [4]. Chemotherapy levels in the air were below workplace exposure limits. Other recent phase I studies have demonstrated the feasibility and safety of aerosol delivery of doxorubicin [5] and gemcitabin [6] in lung cancer patients.

In occupational settings, environmental monitoring of exposure to toxic aerosols seems to be superior to biological monitoring. It offers the possibility of simultaneous determination of components of mixtures, is simple to interpret, and evaluates short-term exposure to environmental irritants [7]. Thus, estimation of exposure under real conditions was an important step to provide a safe working environment during PIPAC. The total chemotherapy dose was a tenth of a systemic dose delivered intravenously. The aerosol was applied within the closed abdomen, and no leakage occurred. No cisplatin contamination in the air was detected.

Since PIPAC is applied within a closed system, the risk of skin contamination with chemotherapy is minimal (e.g. following a manipulation error with the contrast medium injector, or use of inadequate, low-pressure infusion tubing, etc.). This risk can be reduced by providing one-block systems (nebulizer and infusion tubing), and by training and drilling in order to minimize human errors. In the case of leakage, skin contamination with chemotherapy solutions would be adequately met by wearing special chemotherapy gloves and protection glasses. A special set to remove spilled chemotherapy solution is available in the OR. The operating room has to be cleaned afterwards, as is routinely the case because of biological risks such as blood contamination, and so on. Tissues, tubes, lines and other devices such as operation drapes and sponges have to be disposed of into special sealed and labelled containers.

In summary, this study shows that the risk of occupational exposure to chemotherapy during PIPAC has been reduced to a minimum so that the procedure complies with German occupational safety regulations. This is an important precondition for beginning Phase 2 and Phase 3 clinical studies in order to define the possibilities and limits of PIPAC in the therapy of peritoneal carcinomatosis. Strict application of the standard operating procedures, repeated measurement of exposure levels and continuous education of physicians and nurses will be necessary with the increasing use of this new therapeutic strategy, in order to avoid any harm.

Following the implementation of all equipment, organizational aspects and procedures as described above, any other team starting with PIPAC should perform a toxicological work-place analysis. This analysis has to be scheduled prior to the routine application of PIPAC in order to ensure that it can be performed in accordance to local regulations.

20.4 Second assessement

As soon as PIPAC procedures were initiated in a second hospital (St. Mary's Hospital in Herne, Westfalia, Germany), environmental measurements were repeated. A specialized, independent institution (Dräger Analytical) was commissioned to assess a possible release of hazardous substances during PIPAC therapy. Platinum concentration was used as a tracer for possible contamination of the circulating air.

The probe sampling system used was a Gravikon PM 4-2device combined with a dust detector (Ströhlein, Kaarst, Germany). Air was collected on a cellulose nitrate filter with a diameter of 50 mm, with a flow of 4 m^3/h. The absolute detection limit for platinum was 0.0005 mg, corresponding to 0.00013 mg/m^3 for 4 m^3 air. Blind analysis of the test and control samples was performed by Kiwa Control GmbH, Rostock, Germany, by flameless atomic absorption spectrometry (AAS), executed with inductive coupled plasma (ICP-OES). All probes remained negative. Thus, this second assessment confirmed the harmlessness of PIPAC therapy from the occupational health perspective, in an independent institution [8].

20.5 Biological monitoring

Biomonitoring is in the context of occupational health a secondary prevention measure for the identification of individual load after exposure to hazardous substances. For many hazardous materials, including many chemotherapeutic drugs, the individually recorded load is quantifiable by biomonitoring and thus assessable. The aim of biomonitoring is to take appropriate measures (improvement of technical, organizational and personal prevention) to reduce the burden and the health hazard (reviewed in [9]).

In particular, biomonitoring should be taken into consideration in activities

- where direct skin contact with hazardous substances is possible;
- for which exposure to hazardous substances with long biological half-life is present;
- when there is exposure to carcinogenic or mutagenic substances;
- where the hazardous substances are difficult to measure in the air;
- in case of accidental exposition to hazardous substances.

These conditions (a nonexhaustive list) are clearly given for health workers administering PIPAC to patients. Therefore, after 500 PIPAC procedures, blood was sampled from the five surgeons and gynecologists having performed all PIPAC in our institution. Samples were taken by the company physician. Serum concentrations of doxorubicin and cisplatin were determined by an independent laboratory. All samples remained negative, meaning that no traces of cisplatin or doxorubicin could be detected (data on file).

Bibliography

[1] Markman M. Intraperitoneal antineoplastic drug delivery: rationale and results. Lancet Oncol. 4, 5 (May 2003) 277–283. Review.

[2] Canis M, Matsuzaki S, Bourdel N et al. Peritoneum and laparoscopic environment. Bull Cancer 94 (2007) (12): 1043–1051.

[3] Zytostatika im Gesundheitsdienst. Informatiuon zur sicheren Handhabung von Zytostatika. GUV-I 8533. Deutsche Gesetzliche Unfallversicherung, Berlin 2008.

[4] Wittgen BP, Kunst PW, Perkins WR et al. Assessing a system to capture stray aerosol during inhalation of nebulized liposomal cisplatin. J Aerosol Med. 19, 3 (Fall 2006) 385–391.

[5] Otterson GA, Villalona-Calero MA, Sharma S et al. Phase I study of inhaled Doxorubicin for patients with metastatic tumors to the lungs. Clin Cancer Res. 13, 4 (Feb 15 2007) 1246–1252.

[6] Lemarie E, Vecellio L, Hureaux J et al. Aerosolized gemcitabine in patients with carcinoma of the lung: feasibility and safety study. J Aerosol Med Pulm Drug Deliv. 24, 6 (Dec 2011) 261–270.

[7] Jakubowski M. Biological monitoring versus air monitoring strategies in assessing environmental-occupational exposure. J Environ Monit. 14, 2 (Feb 2012) 348–352.

[8] Oyais A, Solass W, Zieren J, Reymond MA, Giger-Pabst U. [Occupational Health Aspects of Pressurised Intraperitoneal Aerosol Chemotherapy (PIPAC): Confirmation of Harmlessness.]. Zentralbl Chir. 2014 Feb 4. [Epub ahead of print] German.

[9] Arbeitsmedizinische Leitlinie „Biomonitoring". S1-Leitlinie der Deutschen Gesellschaft für Arbeitsmedizin und Umweltmedizin. http://www.dgaum.de/fileadmin/PDF/Leitlinien/002--027l_S1_Biomonitoring_2013-03.pdf, consulted on 28.4.2014.

U. Giger-Pabst and M. A. Reymond

21 PIPAC: Risks and dangers

PIPAC and PITAC are in our expertise safe procedures that can be performed with a low morbidity. Overall hospital mortality in all consecutive procedures since first PIPAC (n = 576) is 1.5%. All hospital death occurred in patients with advanced peritoneal carcinomatosis and poor general condition and were attributed to disease progression. In a single case, a causal relationship was determined between PIPAC application and postoperative death in a patient with massive ascites necessitating repeated punctions. The patient developed postoperative bacterial peritonitis that was shown to be a iatrogenic bowel perforation at relaparotomy. Thanks to a more stringent patient selection, we have recorded no hospital mortality during the last 362 consecutive PIPAC or PITAC procedures anymore (including primary and secondary non-access cases, data on file). Thus, PIPAC was safe in this retrospective series with 576 procedures, and posttherapeutic mortality in nonselectioned patients is comparable with numbers reported after systemic chemotherapy [1]. However, as with any surgical procedure, PIPAC and PITAC have specific risks that have to be addressed in detail in order to prevent danger for the patient.

21.1 Bowel access lesions

Primary and secondary non-access cases represent 11.9% of the procedures. Thus, a significant number of patients could not benefit from PIPAC therapy, and this is a limitation of the procedure.

However, access was possible in 88.1% of the intended procedures so that this limitation should not be over-interpreted. Although we were trained to perform open-access laparoscopy, we found it more convenient to install capnoperitoneum with a Veres-needle in the left upper quadrant. This was followed by the blind introduction of a 5 mm blunt trocar (Applied Medical) under camera control. Using this technique, we recorded eight bowel lesions; seven of them were recognized and immediately repaired. For repair, a mini-laparotomy is performed at the trocar site and the bowel loop is sutured with 4-0 monofilament stitches. All sutures healed properly. In this situation, we recommend postponing PIPAC application (see below).

21.2 Simultaneous PIPAC and cytoreductive surgery

We started PIPAC application in analogy to cytoreductive surgery (CRS) and HIPEC, by associating organ surgery with PIPAC application during a single procedure. Unfortunately, we observed in several patients the occurrence of unusual postoperative

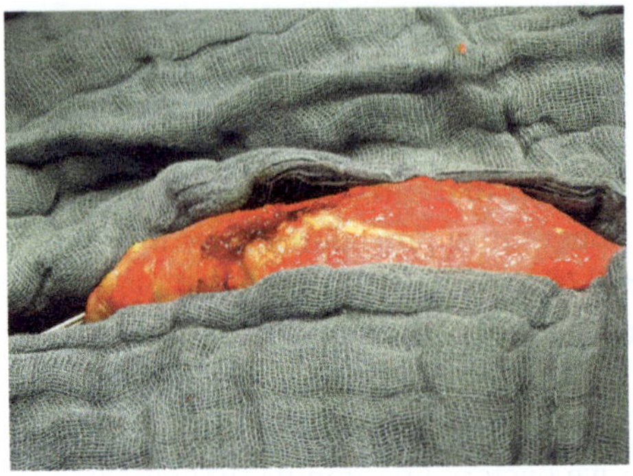

Fig. 21.1. Example of a small bowel fistula after combined, simultaneous cytoreductive surgery and PIPAC. Macroscopy shows a third grade burning of the small bowel wall, probably caused by the local effect of chemotherapy (here: cisplatin 7.5 mg/m^2 and doxorubicin 1.5 mg/m^2 body surface).

anastomotic leakages after bowel resection. We also noted bowel perforations after superficial resection of peritoneal nodules from the bowel surface, followed by serosal sutures (Figure 21.1). These complications are reported in detail in Chapters 12 (PIPAC and ovarian cancer) and 13 (PIPAC and gastric cancer).

All patients recovered after adequate complication management, including prolonged intensive care therapy. No hospital mortality was recorded in these patients. These complications were analyzed, and a causality with PIPAC was considered to be possible. The hypothesis is that the high tissue concentration of cytotoxic drugs is impairing wound healing. Therefore, we stopped combining cytoreductive surgery with PIPAC.

In a second step, we scheduled PIPAC 5–7 days after cytoreductive surgery, in order to prevent such complications and to keep the advantage of combined intraoperative chemotherapy. However, the abdominal access was impaired by significant postoperative adhesions already at this early timepoint. Moreover, a further patient developed a bowel perforation. Therefore, we stopped combining cytoreductive surgery and PIPAC and we strongly discourage other surgeons from doing so.

We observed a single small bowel perforation after PIPAC alone, in 500 consecutive procedures (incidence of two per thousand). In this lady with a large amount of therapy-resistant ascites, a double perforation of the anterior and posterior walls of the same small bowel loop was documented at relaparotomy, in the immediate vicinity of the access port. We assume that the bowel was injured by the surgeon during the access maneuver (insufflation of capnoperitoneum with the Veres needle), and that the double perforation was not chemotherapy-induced.

21.3 Port-site metastases

We are aware of the development of three port-site metastases in the first 500 consecutive PIPAC applications in 256 patients, which gives an incidence of 0.6% of procedures or 1.1% of patients. This number is low and comparable with the incidence of port-site metastases reported in modern laparoscopic cancer surgery [2] (Figure 21.2).

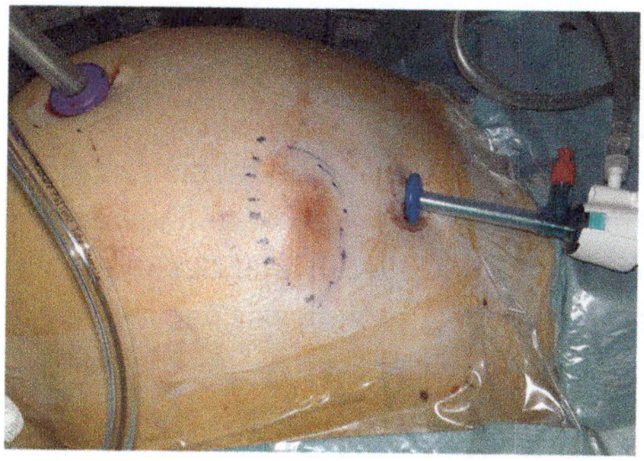

Fig. 21.2. Example of a port-site metastasis in a 53-year-old. male patient with peritoneal carcinomatosis from gallbladder cancer and therapy-resistant ascites.

21.4 Tumor invasion of the laparotomy scar

In a single patient, we observed a tumoral invasion of the former median laparotomy wound four weeks after PIPAC with doxorubicin and cisplatin. This laparotomy wound was not used for laparoscopic access so it is unclear if there is a causal relationship between PIPAC and this abdominal wall invasion (Figure 21.3).

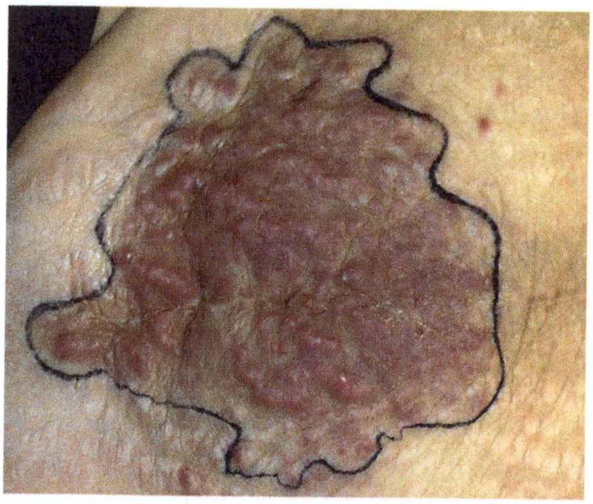

Fig. 21.3. Tumor invasion of the laparotomy scar in a 61-year-old. woman with advanced peritoneal carcinomatosis (PCI= 39) of ovarian origin. It is unclear if there is a relationship with PIPAC. Abdominal wall invasion is a relatively common event in advanced ovarian cancer.

In another female patient with advanced peritoneal carcinomatosis of ovarian origin, abdominal wall recurrence developed in the mini-laparotomy wound after secondary repair of an incisional hernia. Together, the incidence of laparotomy wound recurrence is 2/500 (0.4%) procedures or 0.8% consecutive patients in this retrospective analysis.

21.5 Subcutaneous toxic emphysema

In the case of gas leakage along the trocar into the subcutaneous tissue, the toxic aerosol can create a subcutaneous emphysema. This implies that the skin is hermetically closed. This risk has to be evaluated specifically and carefully during and after PIPAC since doxorubicin is applied: severe subcutaneous necrosis have been reported after paravenous infusion of anthracyclines.

Seven patients have reported the delayed development of an erythema around a trocar site (incidence of 1.4% procedures). These complications appeared about two weeks postoperatively, and disappeared spontaneously one week later. A single case of necrosis was observed, and no specific therapy but local cooling was necessary. All patients recovered spontaneously.

21.6 Therapy-resistant ascites

PIPAC can induce a regression of ascites in peritoneal carcinomatosis patients. However, there might be an important limitation to PIPAC application in massive, therapy-resistant ascites necessitating repeated drainage. In patients with low albuminemia (under 2 g/dl), repeated ascites drainage provides short-term symptomatic improvement, but pejorates the hydrostatic and osmotic balance in the debilitated patient. PIPAC requires complete ascites evacuation before application. After removal of several liters of ascites, the risk of a cardiovascular decompensation is real. Application of toxic intraperitoneal chemotherapy might even pejorate the situation. There might be a need for intensive care therapy in order to support circulation and diuresis, and this might become a difficult experience for both the patient, his family, the nurses and the medical team.

21.7 Small bowel obstruction

In peritoneal carcinomatosis as well as in other cancers, tumor growth increases energy consumption. Cancer cells are programmed to rely on aerobic glycolysis to support their proliferation and anabolic growth [3]. Increased tumor metabolism is harming healthy organs by stealing their energy resources. This process, commonly described as cachexia, results in modified body metabolism with loss of fatty tissue and of muscle mass [4]. Moreover, peritoneal carcinomatosis causes progressive intestinal dysfunction by infiltration of the bowel wall. Patients report ill-defined abdominal pain, nausea and anorexia which in turn impair an adequate oral nutritional intake [5]. Vomiting is observed when malignant bowel obstruction develops and finally patients have to receive parenteral nutrition [6]. Systemic chemotherapy also induces gastrointestinal symptoms [7]. Chemotherapy acts on all rapidly dividing cells including tumor cells but also normal cells lining the GI tract, susceptible to damage and growth inhibition. This can result in patients experiencing clusters of gastrointestinal symptoms such as anorexia, nausea, vomiting, diarrhea, and so on [8]. In peritoneal carcinomatosis, all these three pathways together contribute to the development of the cachexia-anorexia syndrome and finally to death.

Although many patients are referred for PIPAC therapy in the situation of small bowel (sub)obstruction, we believe that PIPAC is not able to relieve such bowel occlusion. The therapeutic window is already closed and the time necessary for inducing tumor response is not available anymore. Applying a toxic substance directly on the dilated bowel might even cause severe side effects. Therefore, we are not treating patients with small bowel obstruction, patients with a nasogastric tube or a percutaneous gastrostomy, and we are cautious with the indication for PIPAC therapy when patients need a parenteral nutrition over a central intravenous catheter.

21.8 Secondary CRS and HIPEC

The peritoneum is now being accepted as an organ from which cancer can be resected for cure, in particular for colorectal cancer when the extent of peritoneal carcinomatosis is limited and the patient in good general condition. In many patients treated with PIPAC so far, the indication for cytoreductive surgery (CRS) and and Hyperthermic IntraPEritoneal Chemotherapy (HIPEC) had been excluded by laparoscopy performed by experienced peritoneal surgeons. In a handful of patients, it then became possible to perform secondary CC0 or CC1 cytoredutive surgery after (repeated) PIPAC application. These secondary procedures were not only performed at our own institution, but also in other expert German centers for peritoneal diseases (Figure 21.4).

On the one hand, this new possibility is more potential progress on the way toward a better multidisciplinary therapy of peritoneal carcinomatosis. PIPAC might become a neoadjuvant therapy for patients who are primarily not candidates for CRS and HIPEC, allowing secondary cytoreduction.

On the other hand, performing cytoreductive surgery in the presence of aggressive tumor biologies (e.g. signet-ring cells) might also have drawbacks: in two patients with appendiceal signet ring cancer and major histological response after PIPAC ther-

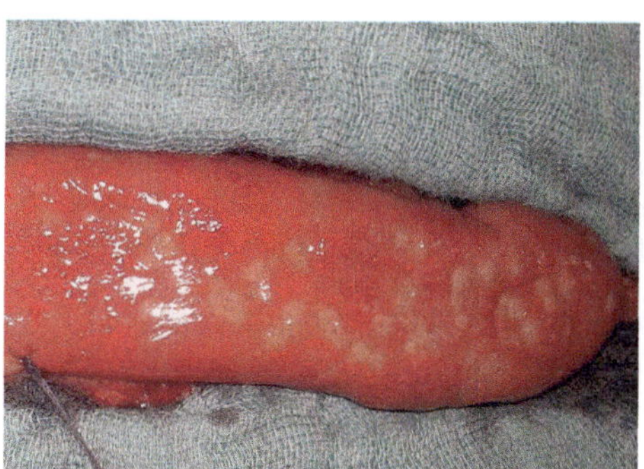

Fig. 21.4. Example of a macroscopic regression of diffuse metastatic small bowel involvement in a 44-year-old male patient with signet-ring appendical cancer, after four PIPAC with oxaliplatin 92 mg/m^2 body surface. This patient had secondary CC1 cytoreductive surgery associated with HIPEC with oxaliplatin eight months after first PIPAC.

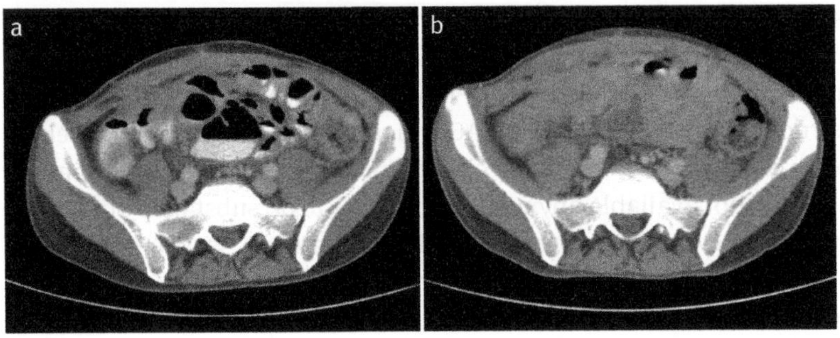

Fig. 21.5. Same patient as above with appendiceal signet-ring adenocarcinoma. (a) Postoperative abdominal CT immediately after cytoreductive surgery showing no radiological evidence for peritoneal carcinomatosis. (b) The same patient was admitted to the hospital five weeks later because of small bowel obstruction. CT is showing massive tumoral involvement.

apy, peritoneal carcinomatosis developed explosively after secondary cytoreductive surgery and HIPEC (Figure 21.5).

The peritoneum presents a first-line of defense to the organism in the implantation of intraperitoneal tumor cells. This protective function might remain important even in the presence of focal peritoneal invasion. Creating surgical wounds in this situation might be deleterious since these wounds are rich in growth factors, angiogenesis factors, and so on, which will stimulate tumor growth. It has to be noted that this risk is not directly related to PIPAC application, but rather to cytoreductive surgery and HIPEC in biologically aggressive tumors. Tumor cell entrapment may explain the rapid progression of peritoneal surface maligancioes in patients with aggressive tumors and incomplete cytoreduction. This might explain the poor results of cytoreductive surgery and HIPEC in peritoneal carcinomatosis of signet ring cancers of gastric and appendiceal origin.

Bibliography

[1] Qi WX, Tang LN, He AN, Yao Y, Shen Z. Incidence and risk of treatment-related mortality in cancer patients treated with EGFR-TKIs: a meta-analysis of 22 phase III randomized controlled trials. Respir Med. 107, 8 (Aug 2013) 1280–1283.

[2] Balli JE, Franklin ME, Almeida JA, Glass JL, Diaz JA, Reymond M. How to prevent port-site metastases in laparoscopic colorectal surgery. Surg Endosc. 14, 11 (Nov 2000) 1034–1036. Review.

[3] Vander Heiden MG, Cantley LC, Thompson CB. Understanding the Warburg effect: the metabolic requirements of cell proliferation. Science. 324, 5930 (2009) 1029–1033.

[4] Suzuki H, Asakawa A, Amitani H, Nakamura N, Inui A. Cancer cachexia–pathophysiology and management. J Gastroenterol. 48, 5 (May 2013) 574–594. doi: 10.1007/s00535-013-0787-0. Epub 2013 Mar 20. Review.

[5] Klein C, Stiel S, Bükki J, Ostgathe C. [Pharmacological treatment of malignant bowel obstruction in severely ill and dying patients: a systematic literature review]. Schmerz. 26, 5 (Sep 2012) 587–599.

[6] O'Connor B, Creedon B. Pharmacological treatment of bowel obstruction in cancer patients. Expert Opin Pharmacother. 12, 14 (Oct 2011) 2205–2214.

[7] Suzuki H, Asakawa A, Amitani H, Nakamura N, Inui A. Cancer cachexia–pathophysiology and management. J Gastroenterol. 48, 5 (May 2013) 574–594. doi: 10.1007/s00535-013-0787-0. Epub 2013 Mar 20. Review.

[8] Cherwin CH. Gastrointestinal symptom representation in cancer symptom clusters: a synthesis of the literature. Oncol Nurs Forum. 39, 2 (Mar 2012) 157–165.

M. A. Reymond

22 Outlook

"Nescire autem quid antequam natus sis acciderit,
id est semper esse puerum".
– Cicero

One century ago, cancer surgery was limited to resection of the primary tumor and most patients developed a recurrence. Fifty years ago, additional removal of lymphatic drainage areas allowed drastic reduction in the recurrence rate. It is unlikely that further improvement of surgical techniques will allow supplementary survival gain. Now the time has come to treat the anatomic body cavity as a whole in order to prevent millions of remaining tumor cells implanting and growing in surgical wounds.

A growing body of evidence is showing the beneficial effects of perioperative systemic chemotherapy on survival, and perioperative systemic chemotherapy should be included in the management of cancer patients. However, the effect of systemic chemotherapy on peritoneal carcinomatosis is obviously limited so that novel therapeutic approaches are needed.

This is the rationale for the development of locoregional chemotherapy procedures including EPIC, NIPS, HIPEC, HITOC and others. The optimal form of intraperitoneal chemotherapy remains to be determined. The question now is how intraperitoneal chemotherapy should be distributed in order to be most effective, and least toxic.

The ideal intraperitoneal chemotherapy procedure should have following qualities and properties:

- a minimally invasive procedure
- the possibility to repeat the procedure
- an excellent distribution within the body cavity
- a deeper penetration into tumor nodes
- a low dosis of chemotherapy to limit local toxicity and side effects
- no need for cytoreductive surgery
- efficacy in the presence of diffuse small bowel invasion
- objective and early assessment of tumor response
- short-term combination with systemic chemotherapy possible
- administration of a large range of active substances.

Ideally, the procedure should be a generic procedure allowing customization for various indications and further developments in the future.

After having read this book, the reader might now recognize that Pressurized IntraPeritoneal Aerosol Chemotherapy (PIPAC) and derived procedures fulfill most of the criteria above. It is legitimate to claim that PIPAC has superior pharmacologic properties versus both intraperitoneal lavage and systemic chemotherapy for treating peritoneal carcinomatosis. It is also legitimate to claim that PIPAC can induce regression of diffuse, platinum-resistant peritoneal carcinomatosis. Of course, it is much too early to claim PIPAC will allow a quantum leap in therapy of surface malignancies.

However, peritoneal carcinomatosis is indeed an unmet medical need and there is an urgent need for novel and better therapies in this fatal situation. Thus, it is realistic to expect that PIPAC and derived technologies will now be tested in numerous cancer types, in different anatomical locations, with many drugs and biologicals, in different indications, under various physico-chemical conditions and in various combinations with other therapeutic modalities. The most exciting property of PIPAC technology is its generic character: PIPAC is versatile and can be used to transport an almost unlimited range of therapeutic substances to the target tumor tissue: drugs, antibodies, nanomolecules or viruses.

22.1 Radio- and Chemosensibilizers

In particular, applying radio- and chemosensibilizers like Dbait as a pressurized aerosol appears an interesting potential approach. Clinical studies are already ongoing on neoadjuvant radiochemotherapy in locally nonresectable pancreatic cancer. Dbait could be applied during initial staging laparoscopy, and followed by conventional radiochemotherapy.

22.2 Nanodrugs

The use of nanodrugs has been claimed to be a highly potent approach to improving the efficacy of intraperitoneal chemotherapy. PIPAC offers unique conditions for such application in a closed environment and under optimal occupational health safety conditions. Application of FDA/EMEA approved nanocarriers is in theory already possible as an off-label use on an individual patient basis.

22.3 Multimodal therapy

Obviously, systemic chemotherapy has a poor biodisponibility in peritoneal nodules. Conversely, PIPAC induces only low systemic chemotherapy AUCs, because of the small dose applied, and of the locoregional administration. Moreover, the surgical trauma caused by PIPAC is minimal and therefore there is no delay before starting with postoperative systemic chemotherapy. These are ideal preconditions for developing combined locoregional and systemic chemotherapy cycles. Bidirectional chemotherapy approaches are already increasing in acceptance today.

22.4 Preventive application in cancer

Clearly, PIPAC is a minimally-invasive approach with a low side effect profile. This property makes this technology attractive for therapy in the palliative situation, where the patients not only want to live but also to live well. By analogy, this minimally-invasive technique with low side effect profile might be suitable for primary or secondary prophylaxis of peritoneal carcinomatosis in high-risk situations such as advanced gastric and ovarian cancer, or perforated colorectal cancer.

22.5 Applications outside cancer therapy

So far, we have had no time and no resources to further investigate PIPAC applications outside the cancer area. However, domains like analgesia (in particular when PIPAC might become an ambulatory procedure) or prevention of postoperative adhesions are interesting topics for further research projects.

At the end of this writing, we would like to insist once more that there is no innovation without evaluation. The pitfall to be avoided is the acceptance of preliminary, nonrandomized data as proof of PIPAC's superiority. Further validation of this stimulating therapeutic approach will require numerous studies, which cannot be performed by a single research group. The funding of this research will also remain a constant challenge, taking into account the resistance of opinion leaders in the oncology community. However, the reality of scientific data has a strong normative effect: if PIPAC is working, it will become a standard, if not, PIPAC will be abandoned. We invite the medical and scientific community to answer this question.

U. Giger-Pabst and M. A. Reymond

23 How to start a PIPAC program at your own institution?

We currently receive numerous demands from various academic institutions and cancer centers to start a clinical PIPAC program. This is one of the reasons why we decided to write the present "Book of PIPAC". We hope to facilitate this process by providing physicians with all necessary information in a compact form.

23.1 Regulatory aspects

An important prerequisite for starting safely with a PIPAC program is to observe strictly all ethical, legal and regulatory requirements. Although some guidelines such as the Declaration of Helsinki are universal, most regulations are national. Therefore, it is not possible to provide here a guide for all interested physicians worldwide.

However, we are in the position to give information on the legal and regulatory situation in Germany and, by extension, some hints for European countries.

23.1.1 Compassionate use program or off-label use?

PIPAC is an innovative, experimental therapy which is not evidence-based. We had doubts about the regulatory conditions under which PIPAC can be performed. In particular, it was not clear to us if PIPAC therapy is, at the present stage of development, considered as a compassionate therapy or an off-label use of approved drugs. Therefore, we asked for regulatory counselling from the German federal Drug Administration [1]. After detailed exchange, we were informed that application of approved drugs with PIPAC is considered as an off-label use, from the regulatory point of view.

This is major information since many, not to say the majority, of cancer drugs are applied off-label in clinical oncology. From the regulatory point of view, it is the freedom of the physician to administrate a drug in indications which are not supported by high-level scientific evidence. In many oncological indications, in particular in rare tumors, therapy is supported by data from retrospective studies, phase-I or phase-II trials. Off-label use allows performance of an unlimited number of therapies on an individual basis, for example following the recommendation of the interdisciplinary tumor board in a certified cancer center.

This being written, physicians should refrain from performing any prospective scientific analysis of the results obtained in patients using off-label therapies. In particular, therapeutic decisions should be always taken on an individual basis and no general inclusion or exclusion criteria should be defined a priori. Should the physician breach these rules and publish the results, the suspicion can be made that he is performing a clinical study without authorization, which can lead to an investigation of the competent authority, and to an administrative fine. Should the physician apply nonapproved medications in more than a handful of patients, and should he analyze and publish these results, so could he become the object of a criminal procedure.

23.1.2 Drug or medical product?

Since the main mechanism of action of PIPAC therapy is pharmacological, application of drugs with PIPAC is primarily regulated by the German Arzneimittelgesetz (German Drug Act). For clinical studies with PIPAC, it is enough to comply with the German Drug Act. To exemplify this, it is possible to compare the micropump with a syringe: the study will investigate the effects of the drug administered, not of the syringe. However, the syringe has to be certified in order to prove its safety and performance. Thus, the German Medizinproduktgesetz (German Medicinal Product Act) also applies to the micropump itself, in particular concerning the need for CE certification or FDA approval.

23.1.3 CE certification

EC Directive 93/42/EEC requires manufacturers of Class I, IIa, IIb and III devices to obtain certification from a Notified Body before using the CE mark and placing the product on the market [2]. In September 2012, the micropump (MIP®, Capnomed, Germany) has received CE certification as a Class IIa device. Class IIa devices are of a medium risk that may require assessed quality systems to the ISO 9000/EN46000 standards. These devices are invasive in their interaction with the human body. PIPAC technology is, at the present point in time (April 2014), not FDA-approved.

It is important to note that the micropump (MIP®) is only certified for application pressures of maximum 20 bar. MIP® are single-use instruments that shall not be resterilized because of the risk of fatigue and rupture of the material. Any repeated use, application of pressure over 20 bar or modifications of the instrument leads to loss of warranty.

23.1.4 Reimbursement

Reimbursement rules and procedures differ widely between countries. In Germany, the G-DRG system is applied for therapies necessitating inpatient stay. According to the G-DRG system, reimbursement depends on a grouping process. The grouper summarizes diagnosis and procedure(s) and allocates a case weight for a particular inpatient stay, depending on various parameters. This case weight determines in turn the amount of money that will be reimbursed to the hospital.

For peritoneal or pleural carcinomatosis patients, the following diagnoses are usually entered into the system:

- peritoneal (or pleural) carcinomatosis
- primary tumor (e.g. gastric cancer)
- when indicated: malignant ascites (or malignant pleural effusion).

Then, therapy is coded as follows:
- diagnostic laparoscopy (or thoracoscopy)
- intraperitoneal (or intrapleural) instillation of chemotherapeutic or immunomodulatory agents (not HIPEC!)
- multiple peritoneal/pleural biopsies
- if performed: local parietal peritonectomy (or pleurectomy).

In most cases, with the current (2014) DRG version, the grouper indicates the DRG G12A.

In Switzerland, the reimbursement procedure is very similar. For patients from other EC countries, the reimbursement varies greatly. If the patient has to go to another EC country in order to receive a special treatment (such as PIPAC or PITAC), he needs the prior approval of the competent institution; in general the health insurance. Provided this approval is gained, costs of PIPAC therapy are then covered. Importantly, should the treatment not be available in time in the country of residence, the health insurance shall grant the authorization for treatment in another EC member state. We have treated patients from several EC member states, and the health insurances have granted the patients with the corresponding authorization (questionnaire E112), with the notable exception of Denmark.

23.2 Technology access

PIPAC technology is not available freely on the market. The reason is not that the inventors want to restrict the use of this technology, but that, at this stage, PIPAC efficacy and safety still has to be assessed in adequate clinical studies. Therefore, users ready to participate to clinical development and validation of PIPAC and derived technologies will be given priority. Minimal prerequisites for getting access to PIPAC technology are participation in a training course with credentials, as well as agreement to enter patient data into an independent registry (see below).

23.3 Occupational health and safety

A special chapter in this book is dedicated to occupational health and safety aspects. We highly recommend strictly implementing all safety measures and recommendations we are giving. In particular, hospitals starting PIPAC programs are urged not to perform PIPAC in operating rooms without laminar flow. Scheduling environmental measurements and biomonitoring of the team will determine objectively if the preventive measures are sufficient to prevent any contamination of the environment, and thus hazards for the medical team.

23.4 In-house Information and training

Early, complete and transparent information about a future peritoneal carcinomatosis therapy program is a precondition for success. Surgeons having implemented HIPEC in their hospital are aware of the psychological dimension of such an endeavour. In our experience, the two main psychological hurdles are the resistance of the team to offer aggressive care to end-stage patients, and fears concerning potential occupational health hazards. We have heard of several examples of HIPEC programs having been stopped, at least temporarily, for various reasons. So far, it has been possible to implement PIPAC successfully in Germany, Switzerland, France and Russia. In all centers, implementation was facilitated by previous experience of the team with HIPEC.

Training of the team is an important part of the implementation process. We found it useful to start with a small team of volunteers. When members of the team recognize the positive therapy effects in the patient, concerns begin to vanish and commitment to therapy improves progressively.

23.5 Research

We intend to create a research network together with physicians interested in PIPAC in order to create synergies and, if possible, to develop common research projects (including common grant applications). For this purpose, a scientific society will be created that will create the framework conditions for organizing research meetings, supporting grant application writings, and so on. This association will also address ethical issues in therapy of peritoneal carcinomatosis, and will try to create contacts with patients' advocate groups, with the aim of better defining patient-driven endpoints for clinical trials. For accompanying research, this society will invite an independent advisory board with national and international experts.

Already now, surgeons, gynaecologists, oncologists and other interested physicians are invited to get in touch with the PIPAC community. Contact information is available from the website http://www.pipac.de.

Bibliography

[1] http://www.bfarm.de/DE/Home/home_node.html, consulted on April 29th, 2014.
[2] http://ec.europa.eu/enterprise/policies/european-standards/harmonised-standards/medical-devices/index_en.htm, consulted on April 29th, 2014.

U. Giger-Pabst and M. A. Reymond

24 Training and Standard Operating Procedures

24.1 Training

Training courses are offered on a regular basis. Schedules and locations are available on the PIPAC website, http://www.pipac.de.

The aim is to prepare each participant to start a PIPAC program at his own institution. Course topics are:
- clinical pharmacology background
- principles of Pressurized IntraPeritoneal Aerosol Chemotherapy
- clinical Results
- safety aspects
- live surgery
- patient interviews
- practical training with phantoms.

At the end of the course, a certificate is delivered to each participant. This certificate is required to order PIPAC technology.

24.2 Safety checklist for PIPAC

We are routinely following a safety checklist in the operating room. This checklist has to be completed by two individuals in dialog (four eyes principle).

---

1. Before starting:
1. Patient name OK?
2. Surgical procedure OK?
3. Chemotherapeutic drugs in the operating room? Check-up labeling with patient name and dose and containers.
4. Safety material available?
5. All team members with glasses, gloves and protective clothing?
6. Waste container available?
7. Protective sheet on the floor under the injector?
8. Laminar air flow in function?

2. Preparing application:

9. Video documentation activated.
10. Abdomen tight with 12 mm Hg CO_2 (max. CO_2 Flow = 0.1 to 0.2 L/min corresponding to body resorption).
11. Place 5 mm trocar: apply red cap to the balloon port.

12. Closed aerosol waste system (CAWS) with filters installed at 5 mm port? Clamps closed? Port valve closed? Microparticle filter placed at the extremity of the CAWS, wall connection plugged in?
13. Video camera in 5 mm trocar?
14. Place 12 mm trocar: apply red cap applied to the balloon port.
15. CO_2 tube adapted to 12 mm trocar (port open)?
16. PCI and ascites volume documented?
17. Diagnostic biopsies taken in all four quadrants?
18. Local peritonectomy performed?
19. Research samples taken; samples identified?
20. Micropump (MIP®) inserted into the 12 mm port, free-floating, no bowel contact?
21. Is the connecting line a high-pressure line?
22. High-pressure line firmly screwed to the micropump? Cover sheet bonded to the micropump [MIP]®?
23. Instruments, clothing, gloves and stitches for closing abdomen prepared?
24. Place first chemotherapy syringe into the high-pressure injector (first agent to be determined).
25. Exsufflate air from the syringe?
26. Connect the high-pressure line to the syringe, bond the cover sheet to the syringe?
27. Set up the injector: syringe volume, pressure maximum 20 bar; flow 30 ml/min.
28. Check-up remote monitoring devices.
29. All team members leave the operating room.

3. Chemotherapy application:

30. Remote-controlled application of first chemotherapy product.
31. A single person enters the operating room.
32. Exchange chemotherapy syringe in the high-pressure injector (second agent to be determined)?
33. Exsufflate air from the syringe?
34. Connect the high-pressure line to the second syringe, bond the cover sheet to the syringe?
35. Set up the injector: syringe volume, pressure maximum 20 bars; flow 30 ml/min.
36. Remote-controlled application of second chemotherapy product.
37. Wait 30 minutes.

4. Completing the procedure:

38. A single person enters into the operating room.
39. Stopping CO_2 insufflator.
40. Activate CAWS system (open port and pinchcock), proceed to closed exsufflation of the toxic aerosol.
41. Do not use standard suction device!
42. The team re-enters the operating room.
43. All disposable material is eliminated into the labeled chemotherapy waste container.
44. Closure of the injection sites (absorbable sutures).
45. Documentation of the procedure as usual.
46. For study patients, completing the Case Report Forms (CRFs).
47. DVD with video documentation is burned, labeled and stored.

24.3 Peritoneal and pleural carcinomatosis index

24.3.1 Extent of Pleural Carcinomatosis (EPC) score

The Extent of Pleural Carcinomatosis (EPC) consists of an incremental scale from 0 to 3 that reflects the morphologic extent of diaphragmatic, costoparietal, and visceral pleural involvement as evidenced during thoracoscopic visualization. For each pleural surface, a score of 0 represents no disease; a score of 1 represents focal disease (thickening or tumor nodules) covering a small, distinct part of the pleural surface; a score of 2 represents extensive disease covering most of the pleural surface; and a score of 3 represents diffuse disease covering most or all of the pleural surface. The sum of individual scores for each of these surfaces provides a maximum EPC score of 9.

24.4 Registry data

Registries have recently drawn a lot of attention to the provision of "real-world" data on medical devices. When data collection is carried out in a complete and valid way, registry studies may in fact offer valuable insights about the safety, application and quality of innovative health care (reviewed in [1]). Historical models of such registries are, for example, the AO database for development of osteosynthesis implants and devices [2]. Current examples of registries are the Peritoneum Registry of the German Society for General and Gastrointestinal Surgery [3] or the NOTES registry of the EURO-NOTES registry [4].

The PIPAC/PITAC Clinical Registry (http://www.pipac.de) was established as a worldwide database to allow the monitoring of the results of Pressurized IntraPeritoneal and IntraThoracic Aerosol Chemotherapy. The questionnaire describes patient data, diagnostics and therapy prior to PIPAC including peritoneal or pleural scores, details of locoregional chemotherapy, intraoperative and postoperative complications, and anatomopathology results including tumor response grading and follow up including survival data. All physicians trained in PIPAC technology are strongly encouraged to contribute to the registry with their own cases. The registry is owned by an independent, nonprofit organization for quality control at the University of Magdeburg. Access to their own cases is possible to registered users, and each user receives yearly the results from the own hospital versus the benchmark. Login data are provided during the training courses.

Recently, it was agreed to coordinate the efforts of the HIPEC registry of the German Society for General and Gastrointestinal Surgery with the PIPAC registry, in order to obtain a compatible database.

Bibliography

[1] Sauerland S, Brockhaus AC, Fujita-Rohwerder N, Saad S. Approaches to assessing the benefits and harms of medical devices for application in surgery. Langenbecks Arch Surg. 399, 3 (Mar 2014) 279–285.
[2] http://www.aofoundation.org, consulted on 29.4.2014.
[3] http://www.dgav.de/studoq/hipec-register.html, consulted on 29.4.2014.
[4] Arezzo A, Zornig C, Mofid H et al. The EURO-NOTES clinical registry for natural orifice transluminal endoscopic surgery: a 2-year activity report. Surg Endosc. 27, 9 (Sep 2013) 3073–3084.

Index

A
abdominal access 155
– bowel lesions 207
– Veres-needle 207
access lesions 150
adhesions 48, 80, 137, 155, 217
– non-access 207
aerosol 73, 83
– droplet size 76, 84, 85
– droplets 83
– gravitational sedimentation 85
– heated 86
– inertial impaction 85
– monodisperse, polydisperse 84
– physical laws 84, 85
– possible exposure 200
– propellant 84
– risk for health workers 195
– time airborne 85
– toxic 201
ageing population 1
alanine aminotransferase 130, 136, 152
albumin 17, 18, 22
alopecia 141, 156
anaphylaxis 156
anastomotic leakage 104, 208
angiogenesis-inhibitors 51, 161
animal models
– large animal 77, 92, 100
– small animals 97
anorexia 6, 175, 210
anthracyclines 135
– Epirubicin 1, *see also* unde doxorubicin
appendiceal cancer 169, 211
Area Under the Curve, AUC 41
– plasma/peritoneal ratio 42
ascites 32, 36, 137, 141, 155, 156, 210
– cirrhotic 22
– malignant 13, 22, 86
– therapy with bevacizumab 51
– therapy with catumaxomab 50
aspartate aminotransferase 136

B
Bevacizumab 51
bidirectional chemotherapy 46, 54, 162, 217
bilirubin 136
bleeding 151
body mass index 27
bowel obstruction 156, 211
bowel perforation 104, 207
bowel toxicity 155
butyrate sodium 80

C
CA 19-9 71
CA-125 141
cachexia 6
capecitabine 1
carboplatin 132
Carcino-Embryonic Antigen (CEA) 71
cardiac toxicity 156
caring 2
caron dioxide
– heated 80
Catumaxomab 50, 135
CE certification 86
chemoresistance 6, 127
– platinum 1, 41
chemosensibilization 112
chemosensibilizers 216, *see also* Dbait
chemotherapy 8
– neo-adjuvant 30
– resistance 21
– side effects 6
– systemic palliative 35, 41, 135, 147, 161, 171
chloroquine 113
cholangitis 151
cisplatin 1, 36, 41, 43, 49, 79, 149, 158, 171, 197, 203
– hazards 198
– in malignant mesothelioma 171
– pharmacology 131
clinical benefit rate 71, 154, 158, 165
clinical studies
– phase-1 7
– phase-2 7
– PIPAC 89
clinical trials 2
collagen 21

colorectal cancer 55, 67, 161
– tumor markers 71
COMBATAC study 162
completeness of cytoreduction 57
completeness of cytoreduction score 53
consensus statement 55
– peritoneal carcinomatosis 5
consumption 38
convection 37, 39, 86
cost effectiveness 57
creatinine 136
CRP 137
CT scan 71
CTCAE 160
CT-scan 27, 28
– accuracy 32
cytokeratins 20
cytology
– peritoneal 32
cytoreductive surgery 5, 6, 31, 32, 35, 53
– combination with HIPEC 53
– extent of the procedure 53
– mortality 58
– patient selection 54, 56, 58
– safety 58

D
data registry 55, 225
Dbait viii, 113
– bioavailability 112
– biological effect 113
– tissue penetration 112
– toxicity 113
death 2, 6, 8, 155
desmosomes 20
diffusion 19, 37–39
DNA double strand breaks 106, 132
DNA-PK 112
docetaxel 147
dose 39
Doxorubicin 41, 42, 79, 123, 133, 149, 158, 197
– combination with Cisplatin 41
– combination with mitomycin C 42
– hazards 198
– pharmacology 132
– plasma concentration after PIPAC 122
– systemic exposure after PIPAC 121
– tissue penetration after PIPAC 121
– tumor concentration after PIPAC 122
drug clearance 40
drug metabolism
– first pass effect 83
drug uptake 37

E
E-cadherin 20
efficacy 158
electrolytes 38
encapsulating peritoneal sclerosis 49
endothelium 18
energy
– kinetic 38
– thermal 38
EpCAM 50
EPIC, Intraperitoneal chemotherapy 35, 46
epirubicin 1
Epithelial-mesenchymal transition 19
experimental
– drugs 2
– therapy 2
extraperitoneal metastatic disease 148

F
FDG-Positron emission tomography (PET) 29, 68, 71
fever 49, 51, 137
fibroblasts 12, 21
fibrosis 19
first-pass hepatic toxicity 127
fluid transport 18
FU (fluorouracil) 1, 36, 75, 147, 161, 162

G
gamma-glutamyltransferase 136
gamma-H2AX 112
gas embolism 73
gastric cancer 56
– tumor markers 70
gastrointestinal symptoms
– after PIPAC 175
gemcitabine 135
glucose 38
glycocalyx 17
glycosaminoglycans 11, 17
greater omentum 14
guideline 32, 58
– CRS and HIPEC 53

H
HeLa cells 92
high-pressure injector 87
– hazards 88
HIPEC 2, 35, 49, 54
– in malignant mesothelioma 171
hope 2, 5, 9
hormonal changes 24
hospital stay
– after PIPAC 121
hyperglycemia 38
hyponatremia 38
hypoxia 41

I
ileus
– postoperative 58
immunoradiotherapy 51
incisional hernia 209
incurability 2
information 2
interdisciplinary tumor board 7
Internet 1
– discussion fora 2
interstitial fluid pressure 40
interstitial fluid/tissue pressure 21, 37
interstitium 18
– retoperitoneal 18
intraabdominal abscess 49, 58
intraoperative analgesia
– bupivacain 80
intraperitoneal chemotherapy 6, 31, 36, 41
– analgesia 83
– ascites 47
– choice of the drug 41
– CHPP 44
– dose/effect erlationship 41
– EIPL 46
– limitations 47
– local toxicity 47, 48, 52
– locoregional toxicity 41
– nanodrugs 53
– NIPS 45
– normothermic 49
– occupational health safety 201
– perioperative 44
– pharmacokinetic properties 42
intraperitoneal cytolytic virotherapy 52
intraperitoneal drug concentration 41
intraperitoneal hydrostatic pressure 18, 168
intraperitoneal immunotherapy 35, 50
– IL-2 80
intraperitoneal pressure 123
– artificial hydrostatic 83
– portal venous flow 132
– renal blood flow 132
– tissue penetration 86
intraperitoneal tumor xenograft 91
intraperitonealchemotherapy
– intraabdominal abscess 46
intrapleural chemotherapy 80
intratumoral fluid pressure 40
irinotecan 1, 147, 161

L
laminar air 196
laparoscopic nebulizers 83
laparoscopy 27
– diagnostic 30
laparotomy 27
laparotomy scan recurrence 209
leakage 209
learning curve 57
lidocaine 83
lipids 39
lipophility 38
liposomes 40
liver toxicity 156
– PIPAC with oxaliplatin 165
lung function testing 27
lymphatic 52
lymphatic drainage 79, 215
lymphatic stomata 12, 13, 15
lymphatic vessels 19
lymphatics 13, 21
lymphocytes 15

M
macromolecules 39, 41
macrophages 14, 15, 21
Magnetic Resonance Imaging (MRI) 28
marketing 2
medical need 6
membrane transport 17
mesothelioma 31, 43
– epitheloid 171
– malignant peritoneal 171

mesothelium
– barrier to invasion 79
– cells 11
meta-analysis 55
– ovarian cancer 56
metastases
– extraperitoneal 7, 19
microenvironment, tumoral 21
micropump 74, 88
milky spots 14, 15
mitomycin C 42, 162
mitoxanthron 75
mortality 137, 165
multimodal therapy 161, 216
myelosuppression 141, 156

N
nanodrugs 52, 216
nausea 165
neuropathy 8
neurotoxicity 141, 156
nonmeasurable disease 68
nozzle 84, 86

O
ocupational health 195
off-label use 2, 219
osmosis 22
ovarian cancer 55, 56
– tumor markers 70
oxaliplatin 1, 36, 38, 132, 161, 168
– effect of hyperthermia 43

P
paclitaxel 49, 52
pain 8, 49, 51, 80, 104, 137, 169, 176, 210
palliative care 6–8
– definition 8
palliative surgery 31
palliative therapy 1
pathological tumor response 165
patients
– expectations 2
pemetrexed 171
peritoneal cancer index (PCI) 30, 164
peritoneal carcinomatosis
– incidence 5
– natural course of disease 50
– Natural history 67
– prophylaxis 217
– survival 67
peritoneal dialysis 13, 49
peritoneal sclerosis 49
peritoneal wounds
– tumor recurrence 96
peritonectomy 40
peritoneum
– inflammation 12
– integrity 12
– ontology 11
– parietal 11, 12, 48, 103
– surface 11
– visceral 11, 13, 48, 103
peritoneum-plasma barrier 17
peritonitis 22
piezoelectric element 74
PILAC 190
PIPAC
– cellular electroporation 113
– cycles 133
– drug dose determination 132
– morbidity 207
– mortality 207
– Safety data in colorectal cancer 169
– systemic toxicity 104
– toxicity 133
PIPAC applications
– colorectal cancer 161
– gastric cancer 147
– mesothelioma 171
– ovarian cancer 135
PIPAC-GA1 158
PIPAC-OV1 study 143
PIPAC-OV2 study 145
PIPAC-OV3 study 146
PITAC 183
PIVAC 188
platinum 86, 135
– resistance 155
pleural effusion 137, 148
pleural fibrosis 50
pore 18, 40
– theory 18
portal venous flow 133
port-site recurrences 79, 208, 210
postoperative ileus 104
pressure
– capillary 21

– gradient 19, 21
– hydrostatic 18, 19
– hydrostatic intraperitoneal 79
– intraabdominal 19
– oncotic 23
– osmotic 18
progress
– technical 2
prospective randomized trials
– ovarian cancer 46
protein 18, 19, 22, 23
– plasma 17
pseudomyxoma peritonei 31, 54
pulmonary embolism 58

Q
QLQ30 questionnaire 175
quality of life 2, 6
– after PIPAC 175

R
radiation therapy 8
radiochemotherapy 35
radiofrequency ablation 164
radiosensibilizers 216, *see also* Dbait
radiotherapy 21
randomized controlled trial 5, 49, 51, 56
– EPIC 46
– ICARuS 47
– ovarian cancer 57
RECIST criteria 67
registry
– PIPAC 89, 225
Regorafinib 161
renal failure 8, 131
– after HIPEC 58
renal toxicity 127, 156
– PIPAC with oxaliplatin 165
retention 38
rhabdomyolyse 156

S
safety 158
safety measures
– biomonitoring 204
– CAWS Closed Aerosol Waste System 116
– gloves and glasses 203
– information and training 200
– laminar air flow 87, 196
– leakage 200
– remote-control 201
– risk analysis 200
– spilled chemotherapy 204
– standard operating protocol 200
– tightness of the abdomen 87, 197
– workplace air measurements 201
sclerosing peritonitis 49
side effects 8, 177
signet ring cancer 149, 212
silicium chips 84
small bowel fistula 208
small bowel obstruction 171, 210
solute 19, 38, 41
standard of care 1, 36
subcutaneous toxic emphysema 209
surface exposition 48, 76, 103
surface tension 84
survival 5, 6, 123
– peritoneal carcinomatosis 5
symptoms 2
systemic chemotherapy 1, 7, 35, 41, 135, 147, 161, 171
– side effects 1, 175

T
taurolidin 76, 79, 84
taxanes 135
– Docetaxel 1, 44
– Paclitaxel 43
therapeutic capnoperitoneum
– definition 73, 77
– intraoperative analgesia 80
therapeutic index 168
therapeutic pneumoperitoneum
– applications 79
therapy
– active 8
– curative 8
therapy-resistant ascites 210
thromboembolism prophylaxis 148
thrombosis 58
tissue compliance 18
tissue penetration 36, 38, 40, 42, 53
– cisplatin 43, 104
– limitations 47
– paclitaxel 43
topotecan 135
toxic effects 104

trabectedin 135
treatment
– active 8
treatment-related toxicities 175
trocar
– balloon 87, 197, 202
tumor cell dissemination 15, 19, 79, 208, 212
tumor response assessment 67
– histological response 69
– laparoscopy 68
– RECIST criteria 67
– tumor markers 70
– tumor regression grading (TRG) 70

U
ultrasound 29

V
vaccinia virus (VACV) 52
vascular endothelial growth factor (VEGF) 22, 47, 51
vessels 21, 52
– capillaries 17
virotherapy 35
viscosity 74, 75
vomiting 51, 175, 210

W
wound healing 79
– influence of PIPAC 208
– tumor recurrence 97

X
Xenograft tumor model
– intraperitoneal 96

Printed and bound by CPI Group (UK) Ltd, Croydon, CR0 4YY
13/09/2026
14960858-0001